HEALTH COMMUNICATION

D0217727

Health Communication provides coverage of the major current areas of interest in the field of health communication, including interpersonal, organizational, and health media. It takes an in-depth approach to health communication research by analyzing and critically evaluating research conducted across multiple paradigmatic perspectives.

This edited textbook includes chapters covering such topics as:

- interpersonal health communication issues, challenges, and complexities in health communication,
- communication aspects of health behaviors and conditions,
- organizational issues in health communication, and
- media and eHealth research.

Chapters have been contributed by noted researchers and educators in health communication and represent the current state of the field. They offer pedagogical features that will prove useful to students and instructors of health communication, such as case studies, summary boxes, suggestions for in-class activities, discussion questions, and lists of additional resources.

A companion website provides online resources for use with this text, including:

For students:

- Test questions
- Downloadable flash cards
- Exam study guides

For instructors:

- PowerPoint slides
- Sample syllabi
- Sample assignments

Developed for use in upper-level health communication courses, this text represents the breadth and depth of health communication theory and research as it exists today.

Nancy Grant Harrington is a Professor in the Department of Communication and Associate Dean for Research in the College of Communication and Information at the University of Kentucky.

HEALTH COMMUNICATION

Theory, Method, and Application

Edited by Nancy Grant Harrington

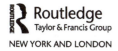

NEW YORK AND LONDON

First published 2015
by Routledge
711 Third Avenue, New York, NY 10017

and by Routledge
2 Park Square, Milton Park, Abingdon, Oxon, OX14 4RN

Routledge is an imprint of the Taylor & Francis Group, an informa business

Library of Congress Cataloging in Publication Data
Health communication (New York, N.Y.)
  Health communication : theory, method, and application
  / edited by Nancy Grant Harrington.
     pages cm
  Includes bibliographical references and index.
  1. Communication in medicine.   2. Health in mass media.   I. Harrington, Nancy Grant, editor of compilation.   II. Title.
  R118.H43254 2014
  362.1—dc23

                                                              2014002628

ISBN: [978–0–415–82455–2] (hbk)
ISBN: [978–0–415–82454–5] (pbk)
ISBN: [978–0–203–36682–0] (ebk)

Typeset in Times New Roman
by RefineCatch Limited, Bungay, Suffolk

Cover artwork: *Mirror Impulses* by Regan Hatfield © 2013. Used with permission of the artist.

I dedicate this book to Lewis Donohew, my mentor, my colleague, and my dear friend. Without his guidance and support, I would not be where I am today.

Contents

Notes on Contributors

Melissa H. Abadi (Ph.D., University of Kentucky) is an Associate Research Scientist at the Pacific Institute for Research and Evaluation—Louisville Center. Her work addresses health behavior promotion and applied behavior change theory, primarily focusing on substance use prevention among youth and young adults.

Katherine Atwood (Sc.D., Harvard School of Public Health) is a Research Scientist at the Pacific Institute for Research and Evaluation—Louisville Center. Her work focuses on the prevention of risky sexual behaviors among adolescents in both international and domestic settings.

Marjorie M. Buckner (M.S., Texas Christian University) is a doctoral candidate in the College of Communication and Information at the University of Kentucky. Her work explores expressions of dissent in organizational and instructional contexts.

Carma L. Bylund (Ph.D., Northwestern University) is Associate Director, Medical Education at Hamad Medical Corporation, Doha, Qatar, and Associate Professor of Communication Studies at Weill Cornell Medical College-Qatar. Dr. Bylund's research and teaching focus on improving healthcare communication.

Elisia L. Cohen (Ph.D., University of Southern California) is Associate Professor and Chair in the Department of Communication at the University of Kentucky and a member of its Markey NCI-Designated Cancer Center. Her work addresses mediated and interpersonal communication strategies to reduce health disparities in medically underserved communities.

Pamela K. Cupp (Ph.D., University of Kentucky) is a Research Associate Professor at the University of Kentucky and a Research Scientist at the Pacific Institute for

Research and Evaluation. Her work for the past three decades has focused on strategies to reduce risky behaviors of adolescents and young adults.

Ashley P. Duggan (Ph.D., University of California, Santa Barbara) is an Associate Professor in the Communication Department at Boston College, and she holds a secondary appointment at Tufts University School of Medicine. Her work addresses the integration of interpersonal communication processes and healthcare contexts, including provider/patient interactions and family conversations about health and illness.

Joy Goldsmith (Ph.D., University of Oklahoma) has been conducting research on communication and illness, specifically in the context of palliative care and hospice, for the last decade. Her numerous publications in clinical as well as communication journals address health clinician curriculum, nurse training in communication, team-based communication in healthcare, and family caregiver communication.

Nancy Grant Harrington (Ph.D., University of Kentucky) is the Douglas A. and Carole A. Boyd Professor of Communication in the Department of Communication and Associate Dean for Research in the College of Communication and Information at the University of Kentucky. Dr. Harrington's research focuses on persuasive message design in a health behavior change context, particularly as it relates to risk behavior prevention/health promotion and interactive health communication using computer technology.

Katharine J. Head (Ph.D., University of Kentucky) is an Assistant Professor in the Department of Communication Studies at Indiana University-Purdue University Indianapolis. Her work addresses health communication strategies in the cancer prevention context, including health message design, community intervention design and evaluation, mHealth and eHealth technologies, and interpersonal influences in health decision making.

Donald W. Helme (Ph.D., University of Kentucky) is an Associate Professor and Director of Undergraduate Studies in the Department of Communication at the University of Kentucky and an Adjunct Research Professor in the Division of Public Health Sciences, Department of Social Science & Health Policy, of the Wake Forest University School of Medicine. Dr. Helme's work concerns media-based community and classroom interventions focusing on risk behavior prevention and health promotion among adolescents and young adults.

Evelyn Y. Ho (Ph.D., University of Iowa) is an Associate Professor of Communication Studies and Asian Pacific American Studies at the University of San Francisco.

Her research intersects health, culture, and communication, especially regarding holistic and alternative medicine use in the United States.

Gretchen Norling Holmes (Ph.D., University of Kentucky) is Director, Research & Academics at the University of Kentucky, College of Medicine, Center of Excellence in Rural Health and a 2014 National Rural Health Association Fellow. Her work addresses provider–patient communication with emphases on rapport, rural health, and health literacy.

Nicholas T. Iannarino (M.A., University of Dayton) is a doctoral candidate in the College of Communication and Information at the University of Kentucky. His work addresses the social experience of severe and chronic illness in close interpersonal relationships, the use of technology in health promotion, and the role of news coverage in crisis events.

Christopher J. Koenig (Ph.D., University of California, Los Angeles) is an Assistant Professor in the Department of Medicine at the University of California, San Francisco and the San Francisco Veterans Affairs Medical Center. His work uses qualitative and mixed methods to study provider–patient communication, patient-centered care, and chronic illness management.

Seth M. Noar (Ph.D., University of Rhode Island) is a Professor in the School of Journalism and Mass Communication at the University of North Carolina, Chapel Hill, and a member of its Lineberger Comprehensive Cancer Center. His work addresses health behavior theories, message design and mass media campaigns, and eHealth applications.

Adam J. Parrish (M.A., University of West Florida) is a doctoral candidate in the College of Communication and Information and a Research Analyst at the University of Kentucky Rural Cancer Prevention Center in the UK College of Public Health, Department of Health Behavior. His research interests include entertainment-education, media misinformation, and message design.

Kevin Real (Ph.D., Texas A&M University) is an Associate Professor in the Department of Communication at the University of Kentucky. His work stands at the intersection of health and organizational communication, including communication in healthcare organizations and occupational safety and health.

Rachael A. Record (M.A., University of Kentucky) is a doctoral candidate in the College of Communication and Information at the University of Kentucky. Her work focuses on health behavior change, message design, and mass media campaigns.

Matthew W. Savage (Ph.D., Arizona State University) is an Assistant Professor in the Department of Communication at the University of Kentucky. His scholarship focuses on the design, implementation, and evaluation of health communication campaigns that aim to change behavior among adolescents and young adults.

Allison M. Scott (Ph.D., University of Illinois at Urbana-Champaign) is an Assistant Professor in the Department of Communication at the University of Kentucky. Her research focuses on how the quality of people's interpersonal communication affects their end-of-life health decisions.

Timothy L. Sellnow (Ph.D., Wayne State University) is a Professor of Communication and Risk Sciences at the University of Kentucky, where he teaches courses in risk and crisis communication. Dr. Sellnow's research focuses on bioterrorism, pre-crisis planning, and communication strategies for risk management and mitigation in organizational and health settings.

Sara Shaunfield (M.S., University of North Texas) is a doctoral candidate studying health communication in the College of Communication and Information at the University of Kentucky. Her work addresses interpersonal health communication regarding family caregiving in the context of end-of-life hospice and palliative care.

Shari R. Veil (Ph.D., North Dakota State University) is an Associate Professor in the Department of Communication and Associate Dean for Undergraduate Affairs in the College of Communication and Information at the University of Kentucky. Her research interests include organizational learning in high-risk environments, community preparedness, and communication strategies for crisis management.

Melinda Villagran (Ph.D., University of Oklahoma) is a Professor and Chair of the Department of Communication Studies at Texas State University. Her research focuses on strategic communication related to health and organizational communication, with a special emphasis on how clinical interactions can positively impact quality of life for patients and their families.

Sarah C. Vos (M.A., University of Kentucky) is a doctoral student in the College of Communication and Information at the University of Kentucky. Her work examines mass media, social media, health communication campaigns, and health disparities.

Melinda R. Weathers (Ph.D., George Mason University) is an Assistant Professor in the Department of Communication Studies at Clemson University. Her work addresses health behaviors and communication in a variety of contexts, including between doctors and patients, caregivers and older adults, and in heterosexual dating relationships, to better understand how effective communication relates to the mental and physical well-being of persons and society.

Elaine Wittenberg-Lyles (Ph.D., University of Oklahoma) is an Associate Professor in the Division of Nursing Research and Education at City of Hope Comprehensive Cancer Center in Duarte, California. With a focus on hospice and palliative care, she is co-author of a communication curriculum that assists interprofessional healthcare staff with difficult and sensitive discussions.

Acknowledgments

Writing and editing a book takes a village, so I have tons of people to thank. First, I want to thank my excellent chapter authors. I appreciate your willingness to share your expertise and the tremendous effort you put into writing and revising your chapters, as well as your flexibility and responsiveness to my nearly incessant feedback. You have been a joy to work with. To Allison Scott, thank you for pilot testing this book in your health communication class, allowing me to gather helpful feedback from real, live undergraduate students, and thank you for developing the materials for this book's companion website. Your work is outstanding, and I am lucky to have you as a colleague. To the students in Allison's class, thank you for answering the same questions about what you liked, what you didn't like, what you found confusing, and what you would change over and over again for all 16 chapters. I did consider all of your feedback, and we did make several changes based on it (except we didn't jettison our attention to metatheory; sorry). To Rachael Record, my dedicated doctoral assistant on this project, thank you for cheerfully helping me with countless details and bringing your enthusiasm and creativity to the book. It was wonderful always being able to count on you. To everyone who wrote an entry for chapter sidebars—too many names to list here—I appreciate your willingness to share your experiences from your lives and your work. Your narratives clearly convey how health communication does affect each and every one of us, often in very profound ways. To Regan Hatfield, the amazingly talented artist who did the cover art for the book, thank you for sharing your talent. It is said that people shouldn't judge a book by its cover, but in this case, I hope they do. And to Connie Moore, the amazingly talented photographer who shot the image of the original painting so it could actually become a book cover, I thank you, as well. If it weren't for you, we only would have been able to publish one giant book, and that would have been awkward. To my publisher, Linda Bathgate, and her assistant editors, I offer my sincere gratitude for supporting this project in the first place and then seeing it through to fruition. Your enduring patience was priceless. I also offer my sincere gratitude to the faculty and staff in the Department of Communication at the

University of Kentucky. You guys aren't just colleagues and friends, you are family. I am happy so many of you are a part of this book. I also thank my husband, Troy, who is the most supportive and patient husband in the world. I promise the next holiday break won't be spent working 24/7 making final edits on a book. And finally, to you, the readers of this book, thank you for taking the time to read these acknowledgments, all of the chapters, and even the epilogue. I hope you find the book informative, engaging, and motivating; I hope you share in my excitement about health communication; and I do truly hope you never get attacked by zombies.

Foreword

My passionate interest in health communication has remained constant since 1980 when I was part of a team presenting a paper at the International Communication Association's annual convention in Acapulco. The scholarly area of health communication has grown precipitously since that time in both the number of professionals who study it, and more importantly, in the body of knowledge constituting its essence. *Health Communication: Theory, Method, and Application* edited by Dr. Nancy Grant Harrington is an important part of that knowledge base, and the chapters congregated within it make unique contributions in many areas relevant to scholars and students of health communication, health behavior, public health, health services research, behavioral medicine, provider–patient communication, and many others. In many ways *Health Communication* represents a form of fermentation of the research focused on communication and healthcare. For years I wondered if we would get to a point where our knowledge base demonstrated the maturity necessary to advance better health. This book is a testament of those efforts. Moreover, at the time of this writing (January 2014) effective communication in healthcare contexts could not be more important. We are witnessing the implementation of the Affordable Care Act that places importance on communication-intensive activities and procedures such as health navigators, wellness incentives, electronic medical records, and patient-centered care. It is also a time of incredible advances in technology for the healthcare context with daily headlines touting the roll-out of products such as electronic aspirin (migraines), needle-free diabetes care, robotic check-ups, mobile apps for tailored messages, electronic medical records (EMRs), and 3D printed drugs (printing any kind of drugs that contain patented molecules at home). Bionic ears and other organs can be printed at the patient's bedside. Fully understanding how patients will adapt to new technologies will require transformative communication research.

Health Communication provides a solid orientation to the field of study by ensuring consistency across chapters that highlight some of the newest trends in healthcare while also including staples of the field that are emphasized through the latest research. Contextually, Harrington organized the book into three areas that group individual chapters into coherent sets: people and their perspectives, challenges and complexities in health communication, and technology, media, and eHealth. The chapter authors are an impressive collection of seasoned and respected communication scientists who understand health communication from theoretical, methodological, and translation perspectives. The versatility of the book offers the potential for multiple uses whether by students and faculty as a textbook, by researchers as a reference, or by practitioners and policy makers as a guide. I would suspect think tanks, NGOs, and elected government officials will find the book valuable as a source for ideation and innovation. I was particularly drawn to the features embedded in each chapter, including the meta-theoretical treatment of the chapters' topics, attention to methods of conducting research in the particular area, and sections drawing practical implications where the research of interest could be applied to naturalistic conditions. The chapter endings are a special feature of the book with a section devoted to future research directions. Some of these I found particularly insightful and recommend the following:

- The need for proof of concept studies in innovation and technology areas to demonstrate effectiveness and promote use (Chapter 15). I would go even further to recommend that "proof of concept" ought to be employed for a wide range of studies in the health communication area.
- Additional research should focus on how new eHealth technologies (e.g., mobile apps) can interface with other technologies such as electronic medical records (Chapter 15).
- Additional campaign research is needed for examining how subsequent interpersonal interaction affects campaign results (i.e., two-step flow; Chapter 14).
- How can more interest be generated in the ethical choices facing decision makers about divulging or withholding information from audiences when the level of uncertainty is high (Chapter 16)?
- Future work should expand to determine how to leverage communication strategies with patients (and providers) who are managing serious or terminal illness (Chapter 3).
- Certainly a neglected issue in the literature, but more prevalent as an ongoing phenomenon, is understanding how multiple patients in a household manage and influence one another's illness conditions (Chapter 2).
- An important insight is often overlooked—the need for professional journalists and researchers to work collaboratively to improve health conditions. Too often, players in this arena leverage one another's work independently when efforts toward true collaboration could produce unique and meaningful results (Chapter 13).

- Has technology outpaced our ability to balance good judgment with disciplined practice? Can we recognize patients' right to privacy in the face of extraordinary opportunities to make a difference in health status? Does patient-centered practice pre-empt advances in healthcare delivery (Chapter 12)?
- As we become a more diverse society, can we keep up with the needs for intercultural care, especially as language interpreters assume a more prominent role in healthcare deliberations? Do we assume that interpreters maintain a neutral position between provider and patient? Should they favor one role over another for the cause of effective healthcare delivery (Chapter 11)?
- How can new approaches to health communication research address the stigma of mental health and associated disparities? Will the Affordable Care Act open new windows of opportunities? How can findings from this type of research be broadly disseminated so that mental health patients seek care for their conditions rather than obscure its existence (Chapter 10)?
- Several authors requested expanded and improved research efforts that contribute to public policy deliberations about health communication. This is a call I have voiced for years. Until such time when policy makers include communication as part of their agenda, research in the area will not attract the priority status it so richly deserves.
- Investigators need to coordinate efforts to expand research programs that connect health outcomes with health communication studies. Greater collaboration is required among communication researchers and epidemiologists, health services researchers, and other data scientists.
- Through what mechanisms can we encourage temporal-based studies, especially longitudinal ones, to demonstrate the unique qualities of time as a factor in healthcare communication (Chapter 5)? One such factor would be how time is recorded in the ER and then discussed by patients and practitioners. Time's healing qualities would be ripe for discussion, as well.
- As technology improves health status and allows providers more time to concentrate on patient-centered care, what types of new education and training programs can be developed and tested for improving interpersonal communication with patients (Chapter 4)?

These calls for new research are highly compatible with assumptions made by those of us who are constantly trying to peer around the corner of change and transition. With traditional and online media coverage heavily investing their resources on healthcare coverage, and with healthcare issues being one of the most searched topics on the Internet, *Health Communication* can serve as a difference maker for those seeking additional information on the topics represented in the contents. This book serves to focus new perspectives on traditional challenges (e.g., provider–patient communication, health literacy), but simultaneously functions as a trusted source of ideas and methods for emerging issues. Implicit in its approach and content are ever-present urgencies for healthcare delivery: multidisciplinary study and application, technology as a disruptive influence, transferrable and scalable ideas and processes, and entrepreneurial thinking that bends the light toward measurable progress in preventing disease and mending the body and mind.

A few decades have passed since my first engaged experience with health communication at that Acapulco convention, and we know a lot more now than we did then. Decades more will pass before we feel satisfied with our knowledge base in health communication. However, I feel certain that this book will serve as a framework for the next generation of theorists, methodologists, and practitioners of health communication who expect to make a difference. It stands as a testament to the fact that health communication research is an essential enterprise and that better-informed students, scholars, and practitioners are needed to improve the health conditions of a rapidly health-centered society.

H. Dan O'Hair
Dean and Professor
College of Communication and Information
University of Kentucky

Preface

The field of health communication is one of the most vibrant, complex, and significant areas of research and practice in contemporary society. With its foundation anchored in the communication discipline, the field simultaneously is informed by multiple disciplinary and meta-theoretical perspectives, with research being conducted across the social and behavioral sciences, health practice communities, the humanities, and the critical-cultural domain. As many scholars have noted, health communication affects all persons throughout their lives, whether through interpersonal conversations about health, exposure to health images and information through the media, or involvement in the healthcare system. As health issues become more pressing in society, including the omnipresent threat of a zombie apocalypse, attention to health communication is certain to increase. That attention is reflected in higher education and communication departments that offer courses in health communication. The question becomes what books are available to use in these courses.

Of course, there are multiple options on the market. At the graduate level, *The Routledge Handbook of Health Communication* is the go-to text. At the undergraduate level, though, it gets more complicated. There's at least one book that works really well for lower-division courses. It's comprehensive and offers all of the features of a textbook, but it takes a primarily descriptive approach to presenting information, which is not necessarily suited for upper-division courses. For upper-division courses, there are several books that could work, but either they're not really textbooks or they're topic specific (so teachers may require multiple books—which tends not to go over so well with students). What seems to be missing in the field is a textbook that can work for upper-division courses. That's the gap that *Health Communication: Theory, Method, and Application* is meant to fill.

On the one hand, unlike topic- or perspective-specific books, *Health Communication: Theory, Method, and Application* provides comprehensive coverage of multiple areas of interest (e.g., interpersonal, organizational, media). On the other hand, unlike current textbooks, it takes a more in-depth approach to health communication by analyzing and critically evaluating research conducted across multiple paradigmatic perspectives. In addition, it offer several features important to undergraduate texts, such as sidebars, summary boxes, suggestions for in-class activities, and discussion questions.

Chapters are written by leading scholars in health communication. As much as possible, each chapter follows an outline to promote a consistent reading experience, presenting a state-of-the-science review of research in the particular content area and considering research from multiple disciplines and paradigms. Authors address both theory and method and provide in-depth reviews of exemplar studies. Critical analysis reveals to what extent conflicting results appear in the literature, which lays a foundation for stimulating class discussion. Chapters also provide directions for future research, which will be useful if teachers choose to assign research projects in their courses. Finally, I asked authors to try to write in an engaging, even humorous style. Where they succeeded, I believe the book is a better read for it.

ORGANIZATION AND FEATURES OF THE BOOK

The book begins with an introductory chapter that provides an orientation to the field of health communication; presents information on theory, research, and metatheory; and offers the perspectives of four of the discipline's leading scholars. After that, the book is organized into three major sections, and each section has five chapters addressing important aspects of the topic area. The first section, *People and Their Perspectives*, offers chapters on the perspectives of patients, family members and caregivers, and healthcare providers; it also covers patient-provider communication and interprofessional communication. The second section, *Challenges and Complexities in Health Communication*, contains chapters that address factors affecting the patient, such as health literacy and health disparities, socio-cultural factors, risky health behavior, mental health and illness, and ethical issues, such as informed consent and organ donation. The third section, *Technology, Media, and eHealth*, features chapters on new technologies and approaches to healthcare, media effects, campaigns and interventions, the Internet and eHealth, and risk and crisis communication. Finally, in a brief epilogue, I offer some final observations and share some additional thoughts from our group of scholars.

STUDENT EVALUATIONS

One of my colleagues, Allison Scott, and I were in the unique position to pilot test a draft of the book with real, live undergraduate students. We collected evaluations on each chapter. We asked students what they liked most and least about the chapter, what they found confusing, what parts they thought should be longer or shorter (that feedback was fun), and if there was anything they would change. We also asked students on a 1–7 scale how much they disagreed or agreed with several statements about the chapter (e.g., it was interesting, the writing style was easy to follow, it provided clear examples of research application). Qualitative evaluations were positive overall, although students did offer several suggestions across chapters to improve clarity and streamline information. Quantitative evaluations were positive, as well, with mean scores ranging from 5.30 to 6.51 on the 7-point scale. These evaluations provided substantive feedback that guided chapter revisions. Thus, as is good practice, this book is based on formative research. ☺

COMPANION WEBSITE

Routledge hosts a companion website for the textbook. There is a section for students and instructors (password protected). The student section includes a list of additional resources for each chapter, such as websites of interest and additional readings beyond those included in the chapters. We also include a list of popular films that relate to almost all of the chapters. There's nothing like a movie day in class, and these films offer excellent fodder for discussion. (*Wit* is one of my favorites.) There are also "flash cards" to help students prepare for exams. For instructors, we have sample syllabi, PowerPoints for all chapters, sample assignments, and sample exams.

AUDIENCES FOR THE BOOK

As I already mentioned, this book is designed to be used in upper-division health communication courses, although it may be of interest for master's level courses, as well. I anticipate that programs in communication will be most likely to adopt the book; however, other social science disciplines such as health education and public health may also find the book to be of interest. Of course, avid health communication folks of any background may be interested in the book. And my husband wants a copy.

As you adopt *Health Communication: Theory, Method, and Application* for your courses, I hope you find it engaging and easy to use. I hope your students like it, as well. If you have any feedback you'd like to share, I'd love to hear from you. You can reach me through email or the feedback page on the book's website. Best wishes for a successful class!

N. G. H.

1

Health Communication

An Introduction to Theory, Method, and Application

Nancy Grant Harrington

WELCOME TO HEALTH COMMUNICATION

Pop quiz: You're reading this book right now because . . .

A. There's been a zombie apocalypse, and you no longer have access to social media.
B. You have an interest in health communication and thought this book looked good.
C. You're a student in a health communication class, and this book is your text.
D. You're a health communication teacher, researcher, or practitioner, and you can't get enough of this stuff.
E. None of the above.

If principles of multiple choice test construction hold true, the answer is most likely C. Of course, it's possible that B or D is true, and if so, that's great. E has to be there just in case. And if the answer is A, well, I'm really, really sorry. Good luck to you. I hope no one eats your brains.

But back to C. Let's go with probability and say that you're a student in a health communication class. You're reading this book because your teacher assigned it. You're hoping that it will be interesting, engaging, and not a painful waste of your

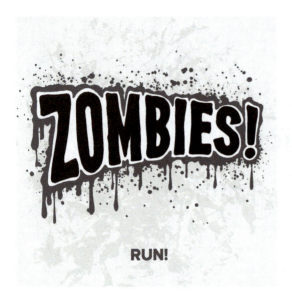

RUN!

limited time. That's what I'm hoping, too. I have certain goals for this book, not the least of which is making it a good read. If you get halfway through and start hoping for zombies, I have not done my job.

But what else do I want for this book? Several things. I want it to offer you a cutting edge, comprehensive presentation of health communication research from multiple disciplinary and paradigmatic perspectives. I want it to reveal the challenges and complexities inherent in the field and the kinds of contributions our research can make to society. I want it to make you question how we know what we know about health communication and what it means for us in our everyday lives. I want it to help you appreciate that while health communication is ubiquitous, it also is highly personal, affecting each of us in unique ways.

Studying health communication is not merely an academic endeavor; it has meaning for our lived lives. Think about this for a second: Most of the illness, injury, and premature death in our nation can be prevented. Prevented—as in it didn't happen. Although the well-timed stomach bug might be useful when midterms roll around and "chicks dig scars" (or so I've heard), I think we can all agree that illness (especially chronic), injury (especially serious), and premature death (just plain especially) are

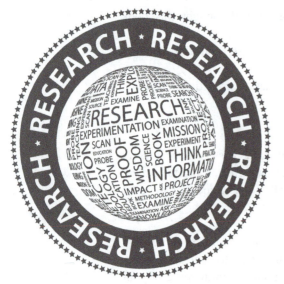

bad things. So when you consider the central role of health communication in the prevention of illness and premature death, you know we have a crucial role to play.

I asked four of our discipline's leading scholars to answer this question: "If you had to highlight one thing about the field of health communication, what would it be?" As you'll see in their answers, all four of them emphasized health communication's ability to have an impact on people's lives. As you consider their answers, ask yourself these questions: "How has health communication had an impact on your life?" And, "Can you see a role for yourself in health communication—perhaps as a researcher, teacher, practitioner, or some combination thereof—that would let you have an impact on others' lives?"

Dr. Teresa Thompson, Professor at the University of Dayton and editor of our field's premier journal, *Health Communication*

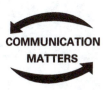

If I had to highlight one thing about the field of health communication, I would focus on the unique opportunity that we have in this area of study to examine real world, bottom-line impacts of communicative processes as they relate to health outcomes. I moved into the study of health communication from an earlier focus on communication and disability issues, prompted by my personal interest in the topic due to my younger brother's severe disabilities and my observations of the strongly negative impact that they had on how others approached (or did not approach) him. This desire to DO something about a social problem has also prompted my interest in the broader area of health communication, and my focus on impacting social justice issues is not unique amongst health communication scholars. My early reading within health communication led me to research that indicated that pre-operative communication from anesthesiologists affects post-operative vomiting, for instance. Other research has indicated that, even prior to anti-retroviral treatments for AIDS, those individuals who were more assertive in their communication with care providers lived longer. Communication matters—and affects health and healthcare delivery.

The U.S. government, in its *Healthy People* initiative (Healthy People 2020 Framework, n.d.), has identified four health-related goals for our nation:

1. Attain high quality, longer lives free of preventable disease, disability, injury, and premature death.
2. Achieve health equity, eliminate disparities, and improve the health of all groups.
3. Create social and physical environments that promote good health for all.
4. Promote quality of life, healthy development, and healthy behaviors across all life stages.

To achieve these goals, we need work on several fronts: We need individuals to modify their health behavior to reduce risk and promote well-being; we need legislation, regulation, and social sanctions to make the physical and social environment healthier; and we need healthcare providers to promote health and prevent, not just treat, diseases and conditions that lead to premature death and chronic illness and disability. Furthermore, we need everyone—patients, healthcare providers, health professionals, and policy makers—to understand and appreciate the principles of competent communication and to put those principles into practice.

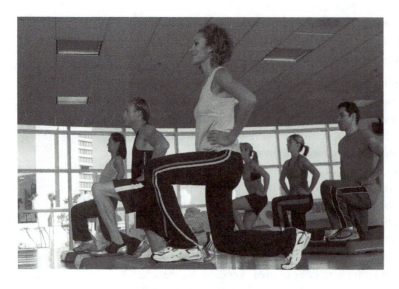

At the center of all of this is health communication. So if this book can raise your awareness of health communication scholarship, increase your understanding of how it operates in our daily lives, and help you take an active role in the promotion of health and prevention of disease, then I will have done my job.

A tall order? You bet. That's why I'm not doing it all by myself! When surviving a zombie apocalypse, there is safety in numbers. So, I've recruited a group of leading scholars in health communication to write chapters for us. I'll give you a preview of the chapters in just a bit. For now, let me provide a brief orientation to our field. (♪ Hot Pockets . . . ♪)

A BRIEF ORIENTATION TO HEALTH COMMUNICATION

Although the 1970s as a decade has taken a lot of flak, quite possibly because of leisure suits and frighteningly bad hairstyles, a lot of good things came out of that

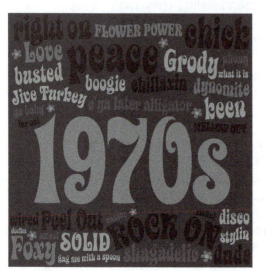

decade. Stephen Hawking discovered the second law of black hole dynamics. AC/DC released "Highway to Hell." Microwave ovens became commercially available, paving the way for Hot Pockets. And most notably, for our purposes, health communication was established as a distinct subdiscipline in communication.

The year was 1975. The location, Chicago, Illinois. Communication scholars from around the world were convening for the 28th annual convention of the International Communication Association (ICA). Large professional organizations like ICA usually have divisions to facilitate scholarly interaction among members with similar research interests. A small group of scholars had been getting together at ICA since 1972, calling themselves the "Therapeutic Communication" interest group. At the 1975 meeting, these folks decided to change their group's name to "Health Communication" to reflect a broader scope of interest in health. And thus our field was born.

THE BEGINNING OF HEALTH COMMUNICATION

Health communication officially became a subdiscipline of communication in 1975 at the annual convention of the International Communication Association.

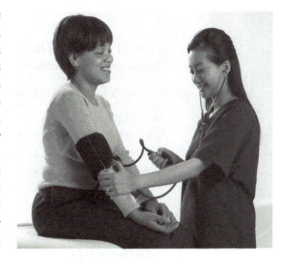

Maybe the stars were aligned just right. Maybe there was something in the water. Maybe it was simply an idea whose time had come. But health communication took hold and took off. Today, health communication is one of the most vibrant, complex, and significant areas of research and practice in contemporary society. As many scholars have noted, health communication affects all persons throughout their lives, whether through interpersonal conversations about health, exposure to health images and information through the media, or involvement in the healthcare system. As health issues become more pressing in society, the interest in health communication and the roles for health communication scholars and practitioners are certain to increase.

Health communication has division status in both ICA and the National Communication Association (NCA); three out of four regional organizations have health communication interest groups; and there are health communication focused organizations and initiatives peppering the scholarly landscape the world over. With its foundation anchored in the communication discipline, the field simultaneously is informed by multiple disciplinary and metatheoretical perspectives, with research being conducted across the social and behavioral sciences, health practice communities, the humanities, and the critical–cultural domain.

There at least five journals dedicated to publishing health communication scholarship: *Health Communication, Journal of Health Communication, Journal of Communication in Healthcare, Communication & Medicine*, and *Journal of Health and Mass Communication*; scores of journals with broader scope also publish health communication research. The *Routledge Handbook of Health Communication* is in its second edition. Numerous top research universities offer graduate and undergraduate programs in health communication. There are several conferences that focus on health communication, including the Kentucky Conference on Health Communication (KCHC) and its partner conference, the DC-area Health Communication Conference (DCHC). And health communication scholarship has attracted hundreds of millions of dollars in extramural funding from government agencies and private organizations.

Table 1.1 provides a sample of universities that offer graduate programs or certificates in health communication, conferences that feature health communication research, and federal agencies that support health communication research. This is an A-list by any standard.

Table 1.1 A Sample of Graduate Programs, Conferences, and Federal Agencies Supporting Health Communication Research

University Graduate Programs[a]

Boston University, College of Communication
Chapman University, College of Science & Technology
Colorado State University, School of Public Health
Cornell University, College of Agriculture & Life Sciences
East Carolina University, School of Communication
Emerson College, Department of Communication Sciences & Disorders
George Washington University, School of Public Health & Health Services
George Mason University, College of Humanities and Social Sciences
Johns Hopkins University, School of Public Health
Michigan State University, College of Communication Arts & Sciences
The Ohio State University, School of Communication
Penn State University, College of Health and Human Development
Purdue University, College of Liberal Arts
Texas A&M University, College of Liberal Arts
Tufts University, School of Medicine
University at Buffalo, SUNY, College of Arts & Sciences
University of Georgia, College of Arts & Sciences
University of Illinois at Urbana-Champaign, College of Liberal Arts & Sciences
University of Iowa, College of Public Health
University of Kentucky, College of Communication & Information
University of North Carolina-Chapel Hill, School of Journalism & Mass Communication
University of North Carolina-Charlotte, College of Liberal Arts & Sciences
University of Oklahoma, College of Arts & Sciences
University of South Carolina, School of Public Health

University of Texas-Austin, Department of Communication Studies
University of Utah, Department of Communication

Conferences

American Public Health Association (APHA) annual meeting (APHA) sponsors the Health
   Communication Working Group as part of the division of Public Health Education and Health
   Promotion (http://www.apha.org/membergroups/sections/aphasections/phehp/HCWG)
Association for Education in Journalism and Mass Communication Annual Meeting (AEJMC)
   sponsors a Communicating Science, Health, Environment and Risk Division
   (http://communication.utexas.edu/push/comsher)
DC-area Health Communication conference (DCHC), sponsored by George Mason University's
   Center for Health & Risk Communication (http://chrc.gmu.edu/DCHC.html)
Global Conference on Health Promotion, sponsored by the World Health Organization
   (http://www.who.int/healthpromotion/conferences/8gchp/en/index.html)
International Communication Association (ICA) convention programs Health Communication
   Division research presentations (http://www.icahdq.org/divisions/index.html#DIVISION8)
International Conference on Communication in Healthcare (ICCH), sponsored by the American
   Academy on Communication in Healthcare (http://www.aachonline.org) and the European
   Association for Communication in Healthcare (http://www.each-conference.com)
Kentucky Conference on Health Communication (KCHC) sponsored by the University of
   Kentucky?s Department of Communication (http://comm.uky.edu/kchc)
National Communication Association (NCA) convention programs Health Communication Division
   research presentations (http://www.natcom.org/interestgroups/#HCD)
Society of Teachers of Family Medicine (STFM) sponsors an annual meeting on medical
   education, which includes a focus on interpersonal and instructional aspects of health
   communication in the medical/clinical setting (http://www.stfm.org)

Federal Agencies

Centers for Disease Control & Prevention (CDC), in particular the National Center for
   Chronic Disease Prevention and Health Promotion (NCCDPHP)
Office of Disease Prevention and Health Promotion, Department of Health & Human Services (DHHS)
National Institutes of Health (NIH), in particular the following institutes:
National Cancer Institute (NCI)
National Heart, Lung, and Blood Institute (NHLBI)
National Institute on Aging (NIA)
National Institute on Alcohol Abuse and Alcoholism (NIAAA)
National Institute of Arthritis and Musculoskeletal and Skin Diseases (NIAMS)
National Institute of Dental and Craniofacial Research (NIDCR)
National Institute of Diabetes and Digestive and Kidney Diseases (NIDDK)
National Institute on Drug Abuse (NIDA)
National Institute of General Medical Sciences (NIGMS)

National Institute of Mental Health (NIMH)

National Institute on Minority Health and Health Disparities (NIMHD)

National Institute of Neurological Disorders and Stroke (NINDS)

National Institute of Nursing Research (NINR)

---

[a]To learn more about these graduate programs, visit the Coalition for Health Communication website: http://healthcommunication.net

WHAT IS HEALTH COMMUNICATION ANYWAY?

At this point, I think it's important for us to stop and ask what we really mean when we say "health communication." Earlier, I described it as ubiquitous and highly personal. So is body odor. Clearly, we need a more precise definition.

If you scan the literature, you will find a cornucopia of definitions for health communication. These definitions range from the concise to the comprehensive, from the superficial to the substantive. For example, Rogers (1996) gives us a basic definition: "Health communication is any type of human communication whose content is concerned with health" (p. 15). A more detailed definition comes from Schiavo (2007):

> Health communication is a multifaceted and multidisciplinary approach to reach different audiences and share health-related information with the goal of influencing, engaging, and supporting individuals, communities, health professionals, special groups, policymakers and the public to champion, introduce, adopt, or sustain a behavior, practice, or policy that will ultimately improve health outcomes.
>
> (p. 7)

We also have definitions of health communication from the divisions of our professional organizations. The health communication division of NCA tells us that health communication is "The study of communication as it relates to health professionals and health education, including the study of provider-client interaction, as well as the diffusion of health information through public health campaigns." And the health communication division of ICA offers this definition: "Health communication is primarily concerned with the role of communication theory, research and practice in health promotion and health care. Areas of research include provider-patient interaction, social support networks, health information systems, medical ethics, health policy and health promotion."

We should also consider definitions from government agencies. Here is a definition of health communication that is shared by the Centers for Disease Control and Prevention

(CDC) and the National Cancer Institute (NCI): "The study and use of communication strategies to inform and influence individual decisions that enhance health." Here's one from the Office of Disease Prevention and Health Promotion (ODPHP): "Health communication is the study and use of communication strategies to inform and influence individual and community decisions that affect health." And let's not forget the important *Healthy People* initiative, which presents this definition of health communication in its 2010 edition:

> The art and technique of informing, influencing, and motivating individual, institutional, and public audiences about important health issues. The scope of health communication includes disease prevention, health promotion, health care policy, and the business of health care as well as enhancement of the quality of life and health of individuals within the community.
>
> (Healthy People 2010, pp. 11–20)

We have a lot of ideas swirling around in all of these definitions. We have purposes such as information dissemination, persuasion, and education. We have people such as patients, providers, professionals, and policy makers (yeah, that's too many "p"s). We have goals such as disease prevention, health promotion, policy development, and business operations/management. And we have channels such as interpersonal communication, mediated campaigns, and information systems. It's too much! So let's dial it back and break it down.

At the core of health communication, we have health and communication. From NCA, we can be assured that communication is the study of "how people use messages to generate meaning within and across various contexts, cultures, channels, and media." Central to this definition is the idea that we use messages to generate meaning. Messages and meanings constitute the heart of communication. Now, from the World Health Organization (WHO), we have the definition of health: "Health is a state of complete physical, mental and social well-being and not merely the absence of disease or infirmity" (WHO, 1948). So . . .

DEFINITION OF HEALTH COMMUNICATION

Health communication is the study of messages that create meaning in relation to physical, mental, and social well-being.

Health communication is the study of messages that create meaning in relation to physical, mental, and social well-being. Handy, no? Of course, we can branch out in all directions from here, and that's what we're going to do with this book. We'll consider health messages across a variety of contexts, channels, and purposes, and we'll cover the physical, mental, and social aspects of health. In doing so, we're going to be presenting a lot of what we know about health communication from basic and applied research and from multi- and interdisciplinary perspectives. We'll also be delving into how we know what we know. That is, we're going to be considering the theory and method we use to conduct the research that leads to new knowledge. And we're going to be considering the metatheoretical paradigms from which our research stems so that we can develop a deeper understanding of our scholarship. Let me explain more what I mean by all of this.

THE NATURE OF HEALTH COMMUNICATION RESEARCH

You may have heard tell of the "ivory tower." This is a mythical place in which pampered professors pursue esoteric research questions simply out of intellectual interest. They teach large lecture classes of students who sit quietly with rapt attention, and they have teaching assistants to do all of their grading (and pick up their dry cleaning). I also hear they drink tea at 4:00 pm every afternoon and wear lots of tweed. In the real world, there really (truly) is no such place. However, there is something called an "academic silo." This is a nasty place where myopic professors cling rigidly to their disciplinary centers, believing that their discipline is the "be all-end all" of the universe. And to make matters worse, these people don't play well with others. Health communication doesn't have time for that! Although this book certainly is emphasizing the communication in health communication, I want to be very clear that health communication research is informed by many disciplines.

THE NATURE OF HEALTH COMMUNICATION RESEARCH

Health communication research is multidisciplinary, interdisciplinary, and transdisciplinary. Research can be conducted from scientific, interpretive, or critical–cultural paradigmatic perspectives. Research results can be translated to have positive impact on the health and well-being of society.

Roxanne Parrott and Matt Kreuter, two renowned health communication scholars, describe in detail how research can be characterized as multidisciplinary, interdisciplinary, and transdisciplinary (Parrott & Kreuter, 2011). **Multidisciplinary research** in health communication involves researchers from multiple disciplines *independently* investigating the communication dimension of a health problem. For example, researchers from nursing, medicine, public health, and communication may each study how to persuade girls and young women to receive the human papillomavirus (HPV) vaccine to prevent cervical cancer. In doing so, they'll bring their unique disciplinary knowledge to bear on the research question. These days we understand that such an independent approach, especially for complex questions regarding human health behavior, can easily lead to the classic "describe the elephant" problem: Different people focusing exclusively on different aspects of the same problem can develop radically different impressions and be nowhere close to reality. Thus, the importance of interdisciplinary research.

Interdisciplinary research involves researchers from multiple disciplines *collaboratively* investigating multiple dimensions of either a health problem in general or the communication aspect of a health problem. As in the previous example, they may study separate questions or the same question. The important difference is that they're doing so in teams whose members bring different types of expertise to the problem and who can learn from one another to more fully inform the problem.

A terrific example of interdisciplinary health communication research is a project conducted by researchers at the University of Kentucky. The project is designed to encourage young women in rural areas of the state to fully adhere to the HPV vaccination series. For the HPV vaccine to be effective, women need to receive three injections over a six-month time period. Some women who get the first injection never return for the second and third and, therefore, remain at increased risk of contracting HPV.

A team of researchers from communication, public health, and medicine worked together to design an intervention to increase vaccine adherence. From medicine, there was expertise in HPV transmission and vaccine effectiveness; from public health, there was expertise in rural communities, health clinics, and health behavior; and from communication, there was expertise in message and intervention design. Together, these researchers designed a DVD-based intervention that led women who watched the DVD to be more than twice as likely to complete the vaccination series as those who did not watch the DVD (Vanderpool et al., 2013).

One particularly cool aspect of health communication research—and one that is exemplified by the HPV vaccination project—is that such research is translatable. I'm not talking about going from English to French. I'm talking about taking research results and translating them from an experimental context to an actual community setting. For far, far, far too long, academic researchers have been "advancing the frontiers of knowledge" only to have that knowledge end up in a journal on a bookshelf. Sharing our knowledge with other researchers through journals is absolutely fine and part of what establishes disciplines and advances science. However, publication should not necessarily be just an ending point; it should often be a starting point.

Translating knowledge to practice is what allows health communication research to make contributions to the promotion of health and well-being. In fact, DCHC, one of the health communication conferences I mentioned earlier, offers an award for **translational research**: the Charles K. Atkin Translational Health Communication Scholar Research Award. To date, there have been two winners. I'll briefly describe their work so you can see what I mean about translational scholarship.

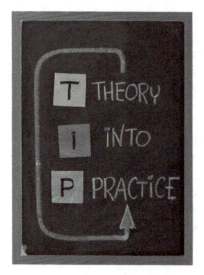

David Gustafson, Professor of Industrial Engineering and Preventive Medicine at the University of Wisconsin in Madison, won the Atkin award in 2011 for his work in developing and evaluating the Comprehensive Health Enhancement Support System, a.k.a. CHESS. CHESS is a computer system designed to help people who are ill find information and sources of support to better manage their illness. CHESS has expanded from its initial focus on breast cancer to include issues related to aging, obesity, emergency medical services, and substance use. CHESS can be used through a personal computer in a person's home or accessed through select community centers, health centers, college dorms, and workplaces. Evaluation studies show use of CHESS is related to improved patient quality of life, reduced use of physician time, and reduced healthcare costs in some cases. You can learn more about CHESS here: http://chess.wisc.edu/chess/projects/about_chess.aspx

The second winner, Linda Neuhauser, is Clinical Professor in the Division of Community Health and Human Development in the School of Public Health at the University of California at Berkeley. Dr. Neuhauser won the 2013 Atkin award not only for her own translational research but also for being a leader in advancing translational scholarship. Her work has included developing a parenting education program for new parents, which has benefited millions of new parents in the United States and is being adapted for use in Australia, and developing a multilingual mass communication intervention for older adults and people with disabilities to help improve their ability to navigate the Medicaid system. Further, through decades of international health intervention research, Dr. Neuhauser has identified and refined collaborative research methods that promote a systematic approach to translational research that helps to bridge research, practice, and policy. The Health Research for Action (HRA) center that she co-created at Berkeley attracts researchers and practitioners worldwide who are interested in research translation. You can learn more about HRA here: http://www.healthresearchforaction.org

This kind of interdisciplinary translational research is inspiring for the impact it has on improving people's health. It's also exciting from an academic perspective because of its potential to develop into what is called transdisciplinary research. **Transdisciplinary research** is research that spans disciplinary boundaries to create new theories and methods that integrate knowledge from multiple disciplines to address complex social problems. According to Parrott and Kreuter (2011), "The broad aim of transdisciplinary research relates to removing barriers to thought about what might be possible if we harnessed all knowledge, without regard to disciplinary borders, in generating solutions to health issues" (p. 11).

Although examples of true transdisciplinary research are rather rare, an exemplar is the Centers of Excellence in Cancer Communication Research (CECCR) funded by NCI. Each of these centers brings together researchers who have expertise from several disciplines, including communication, psychology, behavioral science, engineering, and social work. All of the CECCR research is obviously cancer related, but each center pursues its own emphasis. For example, researchers at the Health Communication Research Laboratory at Washington University in St. Louis bring their expertise to bear on eliminating cancer disparities among low-income and minority populations. Researchers at the Annenberg School for Communication at the University of Pennsylvania focus their work on cancer-related decision making. Researchers at the University of Michigan's Center for Health Communications Research devote their efforts to tailored health behavior interventions. The work by researchers at the University of Wisconsin-Madison CECCR will sound familiar to you: The mission is to advance interactive cancer communication systems (ICCS) to improve the quality of life of cancer patients and their families; one of the ICCSs is CHESS. You can learn more about all of the CECCRs here: http://cancercontrol.cancer.gov/hcirb/ceccr/ceccr_i/about.html

Let me take a moment to apologize for all of the abbreviations I've been using, only some of which are acronyms. Academics tend to like really long, informative names for projects, and we also love to abbreviate. I've seen colleagues spend hours trying to come up with titles for grant applications that form catchy acronyms. No, I'm not kidding. Now, back to business.

Beyond all the levels of disciplinarity, another important distinction to consider is the difference between basic and applied research. **Basic research** is designed to test and refine theoretical models, whereas **applied research** is designed to solve a problem (Frey, Botan, & Kreps, 2000). Both are important to health communication, and they need not (and probably should not) be mutually exclusive. In fact, in cases of programmatic research, researchers often begin with basic research and build toward applied research.

One excellent example of basic to applied programmatic research comes from the University of Kentucky (UK), where researchers have investigated how sensation seeking, a biologically based personality trait, influences response to message design. Lewis Donohew and Phil Palmgreen, professors in the UK Department of Communication, used an activation model of information exposure (Donohew, Palmgreen, & Duncan, 1980) to explore how high and low sensation seekers (HSS and LSS) responded to high and low sensation value messages (HSV and LSV). These researchers wanted to know what message characteristics would attract and hold the attention of HSS and LSS television viewers.

They first conducted laboratory-based research to learn about characteristics of messages that appealed differentially to HSS and LSS. Once this basic research revealed message characteristics that could differentiate viewer response, the research became more applied in nature. The target audience was HSS adolescents and young adults, the folks much more likely to engage in risky health behavior. Several media campaigns testing the impact of HSV messages on audience response revealed that properly designed and targeted messages could result in reduced marijuana use and increased safer sex behavior in targeted populations (Palmgreen, Donohew, Lorch, Hoyle, & Stephenson, 2001; Zimmerman et al., 2007). This work ultimately influenced national policy on drug abuse prevention campaigns (Palmgreen, Lorch, Stephenson, Hoyle, & Donohew, 2007).

As you read subsequent chapters in this book, pay attention to who's doing the research and if it can be characterized as multi-, inter-, or even transdisciplinary. Ask yourself if there's evidence of research translation. Finally, see if you can distinguish the extent to which the research appears to be basic or applied.

Now, I have just one more foundational aspect to cover before I get to the good stuff and preview the rest of the book for you. It's time to talk about theory, method, and metatheory.

THEORY, METHOD, AND METATHEORY (HANG IN THERE, GUYS. IT'S OKAY!)

Before you start hoping for a zombie attack, let me assure you that I'm going to be as concise as possible here. My goal is not to provide an in-depth review of theory, method, and metatheory but rather to provide an orientation that will be helpful to you as you read subsequent chapters. Now many students would just as soon ignore these aspects of research because they can be, frankly, meaty. But if you really are to develop an understanding of the scholarship of health communication, and not merely skim the descriptive surface, you should tackle this information. It's what separates the men and the women from the boys and the girls.

Okay, theory. It's the Rodney Dangerfield of terms. It don't get no respect! Quite possibly, people are leery of the theoretical because they consider it to be the opposite of the practical. But Kurt Lewin, a noted psychologist who has been identified as one of the "forefathers" of the communication discipline (Schramm, 1997), is known for having said, "There is nothing so practical as a good theory."

Why is a good theory practical? Because it helps to guide our research. Sure, we could just decide to study some communication phenomenon with no theoretical guidance whatsoever. But how do we know where to begin? How do we know what questions to ask? How do we know what's important to look for? How do we make sense of the data we gather? How do we even know what kind of data to gather?

One of my favorite quotes about theory, besides Lewin's, comes from DaVinci: "He who loves practice without theory is like the sailor who boards ship without rudder or compass and never knows where he may cast." That kind of sailing is highly impractical (and downright dangerous). You have no idea where you're going, so unless you are extremely lucky, chances are that you'll just be adrift at sea or possibly shipwrecked. That's what doing atheoretical research is like. So for now, let's just all agree that theory plays an important role in research, and let's be familiar with a basic definition: "**Theory** is an organized set of concepts and explanations about a phenomenon" (Littlejohn, 2001, p. 19).

Next, methods. Methods are simply the strategies researchers use to study the phenomena of interest. Methods are often grouped broadly into the quantitative and qualitative. **Quantitative methods** require data in numerical form so that the data can be analyzed through statistical techniques. The goal of quantitative research usually involves making generalizations about groups of people or phenomena. Alternatively, **qualitative methods** require data that allow for in-depth analysis of the socially constructed meaning of language and behavior. The goal of qualitative research usually involves developing a rich understanding of particular experiences.

Remember the academic silos I mentioned earlier and the myopic professors who inhabit them? Some of these folks not only will engage in vociferous debate about their disciplines but also sometimes come to blows (I'm not kidding) over the relative merits of quantitative versus qualitative methods. "We must do experiments, you idiot!" "No, we must do in-depth interviews, you pompous jerk!" "POW!" "BAM!" Sigh . . .

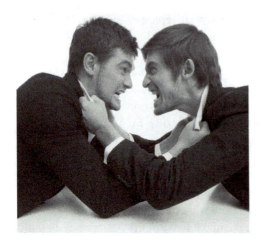

Let me be clear: The "best" method isn't quantitative or qualitative; it's the one that fits your research question, pure and simple. A classic concept called "the law of the instrument" says something to this effect: If your only tool is a hammer, everything you see looks like a nail. So the goal is to have a well-stocked toolbox so you can have the right tool for the right job. Pretty simple, huh? Good. Because now I'm going to mess it all up.

Metatheory! If you think people get bent out of shape over quantitative and qualitative methods, you should see them when they start talking about metatheory. Meta is a prefix that means "about," so metatheory is pretty much theory about theory. In essence, **metatheory** encompasses a paradigmatic perspective, or a way of "looking at the world." It makes assumptions about the nature of reality (**ontology**), the nature of knowledge (**epistemology**), and the role of values in research (**axiology**). These assumptions matter because they influence the way you do your research.

In this book, we'll be considering three paradigmatic approaches to health communication research: scientific, interpretive, and critical–cultural. Depending on the area of inquiry, health communication research may primarily emphasize one paradigmatic approach over another or there may be work representing two or even all three paradigms. Let me briefly describe each approach and review one exemplar study for each to make matters a little clearer. (By the way, an exemplar is simply a typical instance of something, so an exemplar study is one that stands out as a typical example of the kind of research done in an area.)

Scientific Paradigm

According to the **scientific paradigm** (a.k.a., post-positivist, objectivist), there is one objective "Truth" that is out there to be discovered. (Cue Mulder and Scully, please.) This "Truth" is independent of the researcher, who can work objectively and without bias to reveal said "Truth." It doesn't matter that human behavior is complex and each person is a unique individual; there are regularities underlying who we are and what we do, and research conducted from the scientific perspective is out to identify them. As you might expect, the scientific paradigm embraces quantitative methods, although qualitative methods also can play a role.

One of my favorite examples of research that represents the scientific paradigm is a study that investigated the effect of physician word choice on patient communication

---

Dr. Lewis Donohew, Professor Emeritus at the University of Kentucky

Health Communication is a field in which we can develop theories and test propositions deduced from them in real-life settings to find answers to real-life problems— all in one project, much like what has come to be called Pasteur's quadrant. In other words, we can do both basic and applied research and, when it is all done, know if we have contributed something worthwhile to humanity. Pasteur invented a theory of germs that were spoiling milk (basic research), found support for the theory through his research, then set out to find a way to solve the problem it caused (applied research). We invent theories, some of them very informal, about communication between doctors and patients or about message processing and behavior change, for example, then work to solve the problems that led to the theory building in the first place. Not many researchers get to do that.

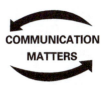

COMMUNICATION MATTERS

(Heritage, Robinson, Elliott, Beckett, & Wilkes, 2007). The study is informed by conversation analysis, which falls within the interpretive paradigm, but its research design and analysis fall firmly within the scientific paradigm, so I'm discussing it here. The theoretical underpinnings for this study came from linguistics and a concept called polarity. Certain words have what is called negative or positive polarity, which relates to how words are used in sentences. For example, you probably would say, "I don't have any" but wouldn't say, "I don't have some." Alternatively, you probably would say, "I do have some" but not "I do have any." Because *do not* goes with *any, any* has negative polarity, and because *do* goes with *some, some* has positive polarity. The researchers were interested in learning if this word polarity would have an impact on patient communication.

The researchers designed an experiment to test the effect of *some* versus *any* on patient communication. They trained one group of physicians to ask patients, "Is there something else you want to address in the visit today?" and another group of physicians to ask, "Is there anything else you want to address in the visit today?" Before patients entered the exam room, the researchers asked them to list not only the primary reason for their visit that day but also other "issues, problems, or concerns" they wanted to talk to the doctor about. (You know how you go to the doctor because you think you have strep throat, but you also happen to be worried about dizzy spells you've been having?) Then the researchers videotaped the office visits so they could count the number of the "unmet concerns" that patients brought up in response to the doctor's question and determine whether there were differences in patient behavior based on physician word choice.

Results showed that if physicians asked about "something else," patients were significantly more likely to mention "unmet concerns," but if physicians asked about

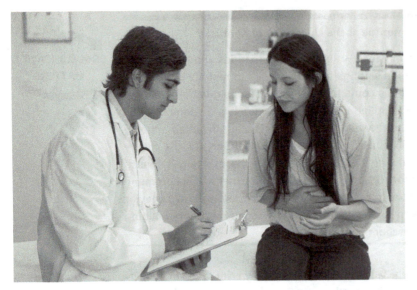

"anything else," it didn't affect patient behavior in a statistically significant way. In other words, word choice affected behavior in a predictable (and therefore potentially controllable) way. That's a very scientific perspective. And very important from a practical and translational point of view: The office visits didn't last significantly longer regardless of how the doctors asked about other concerns.

Interpretive Paradigm

The **interpretive paradigm** (a.k.a., humanistic) has little interest in conducting experiments and counting words or doing anything that attempts to make generalizations or predict or control behavior. Instead, the real interest lies in uncovering and understanding the subjective, situated meanings of human behavior. According to the interpretive paradigm, there are multiple subjective "truths" that are socially constructed by humans in everyday interaction. The researcher plays an active role in constructing these "truths," and the research, therefore, can be biased by the perspective of the researcher; of course, good qualitative research recognizes the potential for such bias and takes steps to minimize it. Interpretive researchers employ qualitative methods such as interviewing and participant-observation, gathering detailed, descriptive data that they can mine for meaning.

An intriguing example of research from the interpretive perspective is a study by Alan DeSantis (2002). In this study, DeSantis explored how cigar smokers who hang out together at a cigar shop construct arguments to counter anti-smoking messages from the media and their doctors, friends, and family members. He was an active participant in this cigar-smoking group before he decided to do the study. That membership status gave him the access he needed to observe this group in its real-life context. Once DeSantis began his ethnographic research, he spent nearly three years and more than 600 hours doing participant observation at the cigar shop and interviewing group members. He was sensitive to the potential impact his new role as researcher might

---

Dr. Barbara F. Sharf, Professor Emeritus at the Texas A&M University

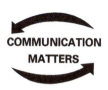

COMMUNICATION MATTERS

A few years ago, I invited health communication scholar Lynn Harter to present in my department. Lynn showed her wonderful documentary film, *The Art of the Possible*, featuring families with a child being treated for cancer. Even though Lynn's talk had been well advertised with flyers that described her work, I received angry feedback afterward from a few graduate students who inadvertently cried, and complained that they had not been adequately warned about the nature of the presentation. "Welcome to health communication," I thought to myself. "These are the kinds of issues we deal with all the time." The incident got me thinking about why students from other areas of study would be so taken aback. It is likely that those of us who do narrative and ethnographic work are more likely to come into contact with emotions head on, but health communication scholars of every methodological stripe deal with fear, risk, pain, loss, and/or grief in our studies. Many health communication researchers chose their professional focus because of personal or familial encounters with serious health problems. I think health communication scholarship is distinguished by its close and necessary ongoing involvement with profound, even mortal, human experiences.

---

have on the group's behavior, so he did not participate in any conversations about the health effects of cigar smoking.

The theoretical framework that informed this study was peer cluster theory (Oetting & Beauvais, 1986). This theory recognizes the role of communication in constructing social and psychological reality among members of a small group. Data for the study consisted of written field notes, dictations of observations DeSantis made, and audio recordings of group conversations and interviews. DeSantis transcribed the data, identified statements about health issues related to cigar smoking, and organized the statements into dominant themes, which he called arguments. He found that the "regulars" at the cigar shop co-created six pro-smoking arguments: (a) all things in moderation, (b) health benefits of cigars, (c) cigars are not cigarettes, (d) flawed health effects research, (e) life is dangerous anyway, and (f) the "Greg" argument. (Greg was a cigar shop regular who died of a heart attack; the "Greg" argument was that it was stress and alcohol—not cigar smoking—that killed him.) Whenever there was a threat from anti-smoking rhetoric, the cigar smokers would invoke one or more of the pro-smoking arguments as defense. That way, they could keep smoking the cigars in the cigar shop without any of that nasty cognitive dissonance getting in the way.

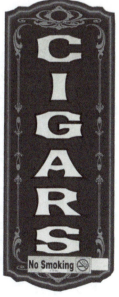

Critical–Cultural Paradigm

And now for something completely different. The **critical–cultural paradigm** is similar to the interpretive paradigm in its orientation to ontology, epistemology, and axiology, but it distinguishes itself by its focus on power: the social, political, economic, and cultural means of oppression by the haves of the have-nots. Its methods strive to give voice to people who have been marginalized and to empower them to create social change. In the health communication context, the critical–cultural perspective forces us to question the assumptions we make about what it means to be healthy or sick and who has the authority to say what counts as health promotion or disease prevention behavior (Dutta & Zoller, 2008). Further, it encourages us to find ways to change the system to promote greater fairness and equality.

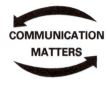

COMMUNICATION MATTERS

Dr. Mohan Dutta, Head of the Department of Communications and New Media at the National University of Singapore

What strikes me the most about health communication is the continual negotiation of theory and practice that health communicators work through. After all, a key element of health communication is rooted in understanding, explaining, critiquing and applying concepts of communication within health settings. In this sense then, the field is always working to find better ways of communication, which hopefully relate to improved health experiences of communities, families, relationships, and individuals. That health is the basis of measurement also means that health communicators are pushed to engage with profound questions related to meanings of health, disparate frameworks of healing and curing, etc.

Against this backdrop, the practice of communicating health works through theory to reflect on what works and what does not work, and what can be improved. The scope of what works and what does not work however is not static; rather, it is constituted in an uncertain, complex, and dynamic web, thus suggesting the need for continual reflection and humility to guide the engagement with theory.

Especially as health communicators work with difference in culturally situated arenas of health, they are challenged to interrogate their own assumptions about health and communication, examining their long held beliefs about healing and curing systems, and the science underlying them. In this sense, immersion in health communication becomes an opportunity for learning, for revisiting received versions of knowledge, and for working through these received versions in dialogues with one's own experiences, dialogues with communities, and dialogues within the self.

An excellent example of health communication research from the critical perspective is work by Laura Ellingson (2008). This research involved a case study of communication between healthcare providers and patients at a dialysis clinic. Ellingson noted that the medical model that is firmly entrenched in our healthcare system was established under now questionable assumptions: that patients have acute illnesses and that physicians are all-knowing and all-powerful. The dialysis clinic she investigated saw patients with chronic illness, of course, and the hands-on healthcare providers at the clinic were patient care technicians.

Ellingson (2008) spent more than 100 hours observing patient and staff interactions at the clinic, taking notes, transcribing conversations, and conducting informal interviews; she also conducted more formal interviews with 17 staff members and 20 patients. Noting her identity as a feminist ethnographer, she reported being "highly cognizant" of power in the clinic setting: "who had it, how they got it, how it was invoked and resisted, what it did, how it was revealed and obscured in discourse, and how I, as a researcher, both participated in it and resisted it" (p. 298).

The theoretical perspective informing Ellingson's (2008) study came from Goffman's work on the presentation of self, which emphasizes how people constantly play one or more "roles" as they go through their lives. Different contexts, such as organizations in which we work, will constrain the ways we can enact our roles. The healthcare context presents all sorts of constraints, including how different providers may interact (or not) and how they are to communicate with 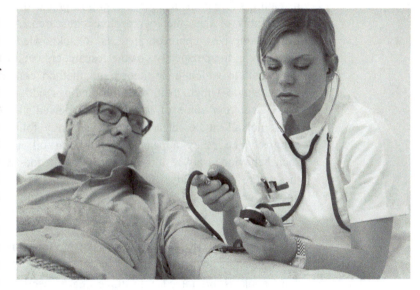 patients. Ellingson used a grounded theory approach for data analysis, which means she did not use a particular theory to guide analysis but instead let meaning emerge from the data. Through an extensive coding process, she ultimately developed categories to describe the communication behavior she witnessed in the dialysis clinic.

Ellingson's (2008) results revealed that the staff engaged in what she called two "competing performances," routinization and adaptation, and she identified several behaviors that comprised each performance, such as "on/off rituals" for beginning and ending dialysis sessions and "coordination" for helping staff adapt to changes in routine. She discussed how routinization and adaptation represented a dialectical tension in which each day always had tremendous repetition but also always brought something new. In keeping with the critical perspective, Ellingson (2008) also offered suggestions for resisting the "repressive cycles that reinforce hierarchy of providers over patients and professionals over paraprofessionals" (p. 308).

Oil and Water and . . . Acid?

What do you make of these three paradigmatic approaches to health communication study? Each arguably offers an internally coherent, valid approach to the study of human communication. Each also questions the metatheoretical assumptions of the others (particularly scientific versus interpretive and critical–cultural), revealing substantial, meaningful philosophical differences that call into question the validity of the other perspective's research. Although I love a good debate, I think our best approach here is to acknowledge the differences, identify as best we can the perspective of the researchers conducting the studies, and consider the extent to which their theory and method comport with their paradigms and the extent to which their research findings add to our body of knowledge. As you'll see from some of the studies reviewed in the remaining chapters of this book, not all studies clearly and consistently follow a well-defined paradigmatic approach (i.e., they appear to be mixing oil and water and acid). Although such behavior rarely results in explosions, it does raise legitimate concerns about the nature and quality of the scholarship and its ability to contribute to our knowledge base.

ORGANIZATION AND FEATURES OF THIS BOOK

This book is organized into three major sections, and each section has five chapters addressing important aspects of the topic area. The first section, *People and Their Perspectives*, offers chapters on the perspectives of patients, family members and caregivers, and healthcare providers; it also covers patient–provider communication and interprofessional communication. The second section, *Challenges and Complexities in Health Communication*, contains chapters that address factors affecting the patient, such as health literacy and health disparities, socio-cultural factors, risky health behavior, mental health and illness, and ethical issues, such as informed consent and organ donation. The third section, *Technology, Media, and eHealth*, features chapters on new technologies and approaches to healthcare, media effects, campaigns and interventions, the Internet and eHealth, and risk and crisis communication. Finally, in a brief epilogue, I offer some final observations and share some additional thoughts from our group of leading scholars.

To provide some structure and consistency across chapters, I asked authors to follow, as much as possible, a template when writing their chapters. I asked them to review what we know about the topic area and from what multiple perspectives we know it (across disciplines and paradigms). Obviously, authors had to be selective in reviewing their literatures or else they would be writing an entire book instead of a chapter! So the content in each chapter reflects these experts' opinions on the research that should be highlighted in their areas. Also, authors took different approaches to addressing paradigmatic aspects of research, sometimes devoting segments of their chapters to particular paradigms and sometimes embedding paradigmatic observations within their reviews. I think this variety will make the overall book more engaging.

Specifically in terms of reviewing the literature, I asked authors to address theory and method as they reviewed research studies and to provide reviews of exemplar studies. I also asked them to identify, when possible, to what extent research results conflict within or across disciplines and paradigms. Research results don't always conflict, but when they do, it provides a great opportunity to take a closer look at the impact of theory and method on the development of knowledge. With an eye to translational research, I asked authors to address how research in their area has been applied in real world settings. Finally, I asked them to provide directions for future research in their areas. What questions haven't been asked yet? What questions need to be answered?

Each chapter offers pedagogical features to facilitate this book's use as a textbook. We have summary boxes in each chapter to identify the main points of the chapter, and **key terms** are bolded throughout the text. Sidebars provide information to complement the chapter text, such as the perspectives of persons in the field (e.g., in this introductory chapter, Drs. Thompson, Donohew, Sharf, and Dutta), examples of scales, brief case studies, descriptions of important concepts, and so on. Each chapter also offers discussion questions, suggestions for in-class activities, and, under recommended readings, three publications to supplement the chapter if your teacher so desires. The text's companion website includes a list of additional resources for each chapter.

CONCLUSION

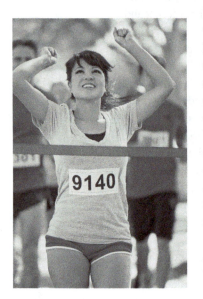

I hope that this introductory chapter has given you a good sense of what a complex, vibrant, and exciting field health communication is. From its beginnings in the early 1970s until today, health communication has benefited from the research contributions of scholars from communication and other social, behavioral, and health-related disciplines, all of whom have made extensive contributions to our knowledge of health communication across a multitude of contexts. We have learned so much about the experiences and perspectives of patients, their families, and their healthcare providers; the challenges and complexities that people encounter in health promotion and disease prevention; and the impact of new technologies and mass mediated communication on health behavior. Yet there is so much more to know.

As health communication scholars continue their work, our knowledge will be enriched through multidisciplinary, interdisciplinary, and trans-disciplinary research. When we translate our research into practice, our potential to improve the health and well-being of society will be monumental. Although all of us have been and inevitably will be participants in the healthcare system, my hope is that the knowledge gained and shared by health communication scholars will help us manage these experiences skillfully and effectively and come out winners.

DISCUSSION QUESTIONS

1. What is your opinion of the various definitions of health communication? Do you have a preferred definition? Which aspects of communication and health do you think are important to emphasize? Can you develop a definition that you think is superior to any of those presented in the text?

2. Consider the examples of research studies presented from the scientific, interpretive, and critical paradigmatic perspectives. Is there one approach that is most interesting to you? Is there one that you think would be most informative or useful to the research community? To the practice community? If so, why?

3. What do you think are some pressing questions for health communication researchers to investigate?

IN-CLASS ACTIVITIES

1. Select several issues of *Health Communication* or the *Journal of Health Communication*. In small groups, do a content analysis of the articles in your sample of issues. What research topics are included? What paradigmatic perspectives are represented? Are the authors communication scholars, or do they represent other disciplines? Are teams of authors from the same or multiple disciplines? Is there evidence of research application or translation?
2. Put the students in small groups. Have each person share a story of how health communication has affected their lives in some way. It could be a particularly memorable conversation with a healthcare provider, or maybe something they saw on television made a strong impact, or maybe they're using a new communication technology to promote their health. Have each group pick one story to share with the rest of the class. Throughout the rest of the term, keep these stories in mind to see if the research presented in the remaining chapters shed any light on them.

RECOMMENDED READINGS

Edgar, T., & Freimuth, V. S. (2006). Introduction: 10 years of health communication. *Journal of Health Communication, 11*(1), 7–9.

This article, the introduction to the 10-year anniversary issue of the *Journal of Health Communication*, provides a general introduction to health communication scholarship.

Thompson, T. L., & Zorn, M. (2010). Welcome to the 100th issue of *Health Communication! Health Communication, 25*, 483–486.

This article, the introduction to the 100th issue of *Health Communication*, provides a general introduction to health communication scholarship.

Dutta, M. J. (2007). Communicating about culture and health: Theorizing culture-centered and cultural sensitivity approaches. *Communication Theory, 17*, 304–328.

This article addresses the critical–cultural approach to health communication scholarship.

REFERENCES

DeSantis, A. (2002). Smoke screen: An ethnographic study of a cigar shop's collective rationalization. *Health Communication, 14*(2), 167–198.

Donohew, L., Palmgreen, P., & Duncan, J. (1980). An activation model of information exposure. *Communication Monographs, 47*, 295–303.

Dutta, M. J., & Zoller, H. M. (2008). Theoretical foundations: Interpretive, critical, and cultural approaches to health communication. In H. M. Zoller & M. J. Dutta (Eds.), *Emerging perspectives in health communication: Meaning, culture, and power* (pp. 1–27). New York: Routledge.

Ellingson, L. L. (2008). Changing realities and entrenched norms in dialysis: A case study of power, knowledge, and communication in health-care delivery. In H. M. Zoller & M. J. Dutta (Eds.), *Emerging perspectives in health communication: Meaning, culture, and power* (pp. 293–312). New York: Routledge.

Frey, L. R., Botan, C. H., & Kreps, G. L. (2000). *Investigating communication: An introduction to research methods* (2nd ed.). Boston: Allyn and Bacon.

Healthy People 2010: Understanding and improving health. (n.d.). http://www.healthypeople. gov/2010/Document/tableofcontents.htm#volume1

Healthy People 2020 Framework. (n.d.). http://www.healthypeople.gov/2020/about/default. aspx

Heritage, J., Robinson, J. D., Elliott, M. N., Beckett, M., & Wilkes, M. (2007). Reducing patients' unmet concerns in primary care: The difference one word can make. *Journal of General Internal Medicine, 22*(10), 1429–1433.

Littlejohn, S. (2001). *Theories of human communication* (7th ed.). Belmont, CA: Wadsworth.

Oetting, E. R., & Beauvais, F. (1986). Peer cluster theory: Drugs and the adolescent. *Journal of Counseling Development, 65*, 17–22.

Palmgreen, P., Donohew, L., Lorch, E. P., Hoyle, R. H., & Stephenson, M. T. (2001). Television campaigns and adolescent marijuana use: Tests of sensation seeking targeting. *American Journal of Public Health, 91*(2), 292–296.

Palmgreen, P., Lorch, E. P., Stephenson, M. T., Hoyle, R. H., & Donohew, L. (2007). Effects of the Office of National Drug Control Policy's marijuana initiative campaign on high-sensation-seeking adolescents. *American Journal of Public Health, 97*(9), 1644–1649.

Parrott, R., & Kreuter, M. W. (2011). Multidisciplinary, interdisciplinary, and transdisciplinary approaches to health communication: Where do we draw the line? In T. L. Thompson, R. Parrott, & J. Nussbaum (Eds.), *The Routledge handbook of health communication* (2nd ed., pp. 3–17). New York: Routledge.

Rogers, E. M. (1996). The field of health communication today: An up-to-date report. *Journal of Health Communication, 1*(1), 15–23.

Schiavo, R. (2007). *Health communication: From theory to practice.* San Francisco: Jossey-Bass.

Schramm, W. (1997). *The beginnings of communication study in America: A personal memoir.* Thousand Oaks, CA: Sage.

Vanderpool, R. C., Cohen, E. L., Crosby, R. C., Jones, M. G., Bates, W., Casey, B. R., & Collins, T. (2013). "1-2-3 Pap" intervention improves HPV vaccine series completion among Appalachian women. *Journal of Communication, 63*(1), 95–115.

World Health Organization. (1948). *Definition of health.* http://apps.who.int/gb/bd/PDF/bd47/ EN/constitution-en.pdf

Zimmerman, R. S., Palmgreen, P., Noar, S. M., Lustria, M. L. A., Lu, H. Y., & Horosewski, M. L. (2007). Effects of a televised two-city safer sex mass media campaign targeting high sensation-seeking and impulsive decision-making young adults. *Health Education & Behavior*, *34*(5), 810–826.

People and Their Perspectives

CHAPTER 2

The Patient Experience

Gretchen Norling Holmes and
Nancy Grant Harrington

> Illness is the night-side of life, a more onerous citizenship. Everyone who is born
> holds dual citizenship, in the kingdom of the well and in the kingdom of the sick.
> Although we prefer only to use the good passport, sooner or later each of us is
> obliged, at least for a spell, to identify ourselves as citizens of that other place.
>
> Susan Sontag, *Illness as Metaphor*

As Sontag (1978) notes, everybody gets sick. Sure, some of us seem to get sick a lot
more often than others, but unless you're Bruce Willis in *Unbreakable* (or Chuck
Norris in real life), suffering illness or injury is just a part of life. And while some of
you reading this textbook will protest, "Hey, I never get sick!" sooner or later we bet
something happens—flu, sprained ankle, bad gas station sushi—that leads you to seek
medical care and, therefore, become a patient.

The experience of being a patient is the focus of this chapter. As you might imagine,
there has been an enormous amount of research done to explore and understand this
experience. In deciding what information to include, we've focused on what we think
is the most relevant and representative. We're also drawing on some of our own experiences. Not only have we both had the usual run-ins with the medical system like
most people but we also both have had life-threatening illnesses, although the experiences were vastly different. By reviewing the research and sharing our experiences,
we hope to provide you with a rich and nuanced understanding of what it is like to be
a patient, emphasizing, obviously, the communicative aspects of the experience.

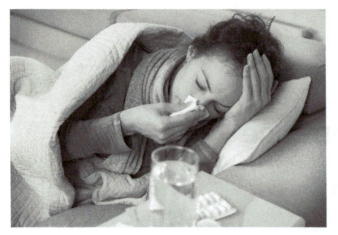

Throughout this chapter, we want to impress upon you the importance of understanding the patient perspective. After all, the patient is at the center of healthcare, even though some providers may tend to forget that from time to time. The patient also is often a member of a family, and the patient's illness can affect the family, too. Furthermore, the nature of patient experiences and how those experiences affect their responses to healthcare can sometimes mean the difference between life and death.

We've chosen to organize the chapter around the major metatheoretical paradigms. Within the scientific paradigm, we're going to focus on research that looks at aspects of patient participation. From the interpretive perspective, we will consider patient illness narratives, uncertainty management (also see Chapter 7), and decision making. Within the critical paradigm, we will explore a feminist perspective on breast cancer and then present a famous case of one patient's control over his healthcare. Once we have presented the research, we will take a more in-depth look at one of the areas of study to reveal some of its complexities and nuances. We'll also look at the application of research in the real world, and we'll discuss what we think are some of the pressing questions for future research on the patient perspective. Let's get started, shall we?

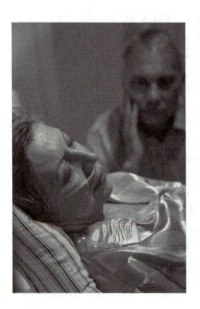

PARADIGMATIC PERSPECTIVES

Research that explores the patient experience from the scientific paradigm is interested in variables that have an impact on how patients experience the medical encounter. Different models help us to understand and appreciate the variety of variables that may come into play. Research that investigates the patient perspective from the interpretive paradigm seeks to understand the meaning of illness in people's lives. Illness narratives provide insight into the patient experience and can be studied using semi-structured interviews, participant-observation, ethnography, and textual analysis. Research that considers the patient experience from the critical–cultural paradigm focuses on issues of power, voice, and control. The goal is to work toward making changes to improve the systems that marginalize patients and their experiences.

Gretchen's Experience

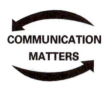

COMMUNICATION MATTERS

When I was 29 years old and getting ready to graduate with my bachelor's degree from New York University, I found a lump at the base of my neck. Being a student, I went to student health services. They told me I needed to eat more salt. I wasn't convinced. I then went to a doctor who told me that, yes, there was a mass on my thyroid but I "wasn't sick." It was her job to determine if I was sick, she said, and "you're not sick." At some point I began to wonder if I was imagining it all but I could see the mass and I was having trouble swallowing so I knew something was wrong! Finally, I went to a well-known specialist who did a biopsy and determined that the mass had to come out. Tests confirmed a follicular-papillary variant of thyroid cancer. The diagnosis certainly explained my need to sleep 10–12 hours a day, my inability to concentrate, my fast weight gain (over 80 pounds in six months), and all of the joint pain I was experiencing!

During spring break I had surgery to remove half my thyroid (not my favorite way to spend spring break, but it was memorable). Six months later (after doctors at a nearby cancer center observed tissue taken from my thyroid), I found out for certain it was cancer, and I had to have the rest of my thyroid removed. I was presented with the option to do radioactive iodine treatment right away or wait. I asked each of my doctors what they would do: They both said they couldn't tell me what to do, it was my decision. I decided I would wait as I was newly married and wanted to have children. That decision would be a huge mistake.

Five years later, I found myself dealing with a reoccurrence and a diagnosis of stage IV thyroid cancer; it had spread to my lungs. How did this happen? Well, I had just moved to a new town and needed to find a new thyroid cancer doctor (because I had to have ongoing check-ups). One morning it became very clear I needed to get to the doctor. It's hard to explain but I just knew something was wrong. I had no physical symptoms; I felt fine. But something was wrong. I went to the doctor and found out that I was one of a few patients who didn't respond to the blood tests I'd been having done all these years to make sure the cancer hadn't returned. The reality of it was devastating: Had I not gone to see my new doctor, I would have died. I endured intensive treatment, multiple stays in isolation in the hospital where I had to take radioactive iodine pills (the person who delivered my medicine was always dressed in a hazmat suit), and months of recovery after each treatment. Ten years later I'm still cancer free. I'm one of the lucky ones.

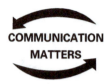

COMMUNICATION MATTERS

Nancy's Experience

When the patient is a young child, the parent is the one who must communicate with the healthcare providers and make decisions. This was my experience. I was 18 months old when I contracted spinal meningitis. This is an infection of the fluids and membranes surrounding the brain and spinal cord. It spreads very rapidly, and without treatment, it can cause death in 24 hours.

My mother knew something was seriously wrong with me when (forgive the ugly visual) I threw up and the vomit hit the far wall of the bathroom 20 feet away. It was either demonic possession or a very serious illness. She chose to call the doctor and not a priest. The problem was that it was a Thursday. Pediatrician's day off. (You know how doctors like to golf?) Now, some parents may have let that deter them. They'd be intimidated and convince themselves that maybe it was just a stomach bug; they'd call the doctor in the morning if the baby was still sick. Ordinarily, my mother was a non-assertive person, so she easily could have fallen into that camp. I'm really happy she didn't. Probably like with Gretchen's experience, she *just knew* something was seriously wrong. She insisted that she be put in touch with the doctor. When she reached him, she conveyed my symptoms. He told her he'd meet her in the emergency room. He later told her that had she waited until the next day to call him, I would not have survived.

This experience has stuck with me for obvious reasons. While I don't directly recall one minute of it, I heard my mother tell the story enough that I know all the details. The experience highlights the importance of assertiveness and trusting your experience and the absolutely crucial role that parents play in their children's health, as well as the impact that a child's illness can have on the family. Apparently, anyone who'd been in contact with me had to take prophylactic antibiotics! Sorry, guys.

UNDER THE MICROSCOPE: THE SCIENTIFIC PERSPECTIVE

Research that explores the patient experience from the scientific paradigm is interested in variables that have an impact on how patients experience the medical encounter. Different models help us to understand and appreciate the variety of variables that may come into play. For example, Rick Street's ecological model considers variables that can influence patients' and healthcare providers' communication behavior across five contexts: interpersonal, organizational, cultural, media, and political–legal (Street, 2003). Likewise, a shared decision-making model that Street developed in collaboration with Mary Politi, a clinical psychologist who is an assistant professor of surgery (how's that for interdisciplinary?), identifies the patient and provider characteristics and behaviors that influence decision outcomes (Politi & Street, 2011).

How do we conceptualize the patient experience from a scientific perspective? When we're considering quantifiable variables, which ones capture the patient experience in a meaningful way? In answer to these questions, we think it's important to consider how much a patient actually gets to be an active participant in the medical visit. We're first going to look at research that explores the factors that promote patient participation during the office visit, and then we're going to consider research on physician behavior that can get in the way of patient participation.

Promoting Patient Participation

Patient participation can be considered along several dimensions, including the extent to which patients have medical knowledge and engage in self-care. For our purposes, however, we are concerned with the communicative aspect of patient participation. We share the definition presented in Chapter 7 of this text, where you will find a more comprehensive review of the topic: Patient participation is "the extent to which patients produce verbal responses that have the potential to significantly influence the content and structure of the interaction as well as the health care provider's beliefs and behaviors" (Street & Millay, 2001, p. 62).

Now, there is a multitude of ways to categorize "verbal responses." We could easily devote an entire chapter to all of the coding systems that are out there to slice, dice, and organize patient (and healthcare provider) verbalizations. And in fact, Chapter 5 discusses coding systems that researchers have used to study verbal interaction. For our purposes, though, we need to emphasize the kinds of responses that can "significantly influence" content, structure, beliefs, and behaviors. Don Cegala, one of the most prominent patient–provider communication researchers in our discipline, offers us just such a list.

Cegala (2011) argues that patient participation has four components: **information seeking**, which includes asking medically related questions and attempting to verify information the doctor has provided; **assertive utterances**, in which patients state an opinion, preference, suggestion, recommendation, disagreement, or request; **information provision**, which involves patients responding to questions from the doctor or volunteering medically related information on their own; and **expression of concern**, in which patients express fear, anxiety, or worry in relation to their medical condition. Cegala took advantage of one of his datasets on physician–patient communication to investigate the extent to which various components of Street's (2003) ecological model were related to patient participation. If we know which components are positively related to increases in patient participation, and if those components are malleable, then we can design interventions to improve them.

PATIENT PARTICIPATION

Patient participation has four components:

Information seeking – when patients ask medically related questions and attempt to verify information the doctor has provided

Assertive utterances – when patients state an opinion, preference, suggestion, recommendation, disagreement, or request

Information provision – when patients respond to questions from the doctor or volunteer medically related information

Expression of concern – when patients express fear, anxiety, or worry about their medical condition

---

Cegala's (2011) dataset allowed him to investigate three of the five contexts in the ecological model: cultural (patient ethnicity, physician ethnicity, and patient–physician ethnic concordance), organizational (appointment length, wait time, clinic type, and patient participation in a communication skills intervention), and interpersonal (12 variables categorized into physician predisposing variables, patient predisposing variables, and cognitive–affective variables). He used hierarchical linear

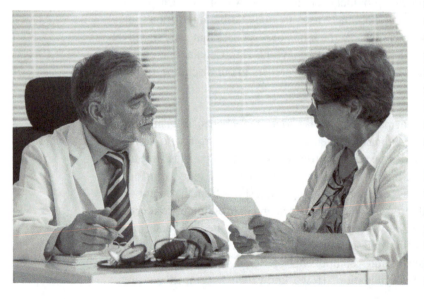

modeling to analyze the extent to which the 19 ecological variables predicted patient participation, and he found that three organizational variables and five interpersonal variables (but no cultural variables) were significant.

In terms of the organizational variables, Cegala (2011) found that if patients had participated in communication skills training (his PACE program, actually), they were more likely to participate in the medical visit. This is a reassuring finding. Likewise, the longer the appointment lasted, the more likely patients were to participate. We do want to point out, of course, that a longer visit is not necessarily a requirement for more involved patient participation (that would be a deal breaker for any intervention research). In fact, although some studies have shown that having more involved patients leads to longer visits, plenty of others show no such relationship. Cegala also found that the longer patients had been waiting for their appointment, the *less* likely they were to participate. Perhaps a long wait time makes a patient feel rushed or crabby.

In terms of the interpersonal level variables, patients whose physicians were more patient-centered were more likely to participate. Older patients and patients who perceived their medical condition to be painful and physically limiting were more likely to participate. Finally, patients whose physicians perceived their medical condition to be severe/complex and whose physicians perceived them as desiring information and involvement were more likely to participate. This seems to suggest that patients are sensitive to their doctors' perceptions.

As Cegala (2011) pointed out in the rationale for this study, "Extensive research has identified numerous variables that potentially impact and shape physician-patient communication, *but relatively little is known about what combinations of variables exert the most powerful influence on communication in the medical interview*" (p. 427, emphasis added). In real life, there are a multitude of variables that come into play in any given interaction. Identifying what those variables are and how important they are when operating simultaneously is crucial to advancing our scientific understanding of any outcome.

Cegala's (2011) analysis of multiple variables from the ecological model revealed a combination of eight that explained about 40% of the variance in the regression model (in other words, about 40% of the difference in patient participation was accounted for by differences in these variables). The strength of an analysis like this is that it reveals which variables "matter most." If you study a variable in isolation, it may appear to have an impact; but if you study it with additional variables, then its impact may change and your understanding, therefore, improve. For example, Cegala found that patient minority status had a small significant negative correlation with patient participation when considering just those two variables. This is something previous studies have found. However, when he included patient minority status in the multivariate model, its impact was no longer significant. In other words, other variables mattered more.

Of course, we need additional research to confirm Cegala's (2011) overall findings. And it would be nice to have a similar study that included variables from all five contexts of Street's model. But this study still makes an important contribution because discovering which variables don't matter so much is as important as discovering which variables do matter. This is especially true when the variables that do matter are ones we can change—like whether or not someone participates in a communication training program and, with some effort on the part of the clinic, whether or not a patient's wait time is reasonable!

How Rude?

In one of the relatively early studies of physician–patient communication, Beckman and Frankel (1984) investigated how physicians' behavior influences their patients' ability to describe their reasons for making an office visit. It's kind of a "no duh," but physicians really should know why patients come to see them before they proceed with the visit. What Beckman, an MD, and Frankel, a sociology Ph.D., found was startling, however: In only 23% of the visits they studied were patients able to fully state the reasons for their visits before the physician interrupted them, and of the patients who were interrupted ($n = 51$), only one of them was able to get back on track and actually finish what he/she had started to say before the interruption. Oh, and on average, patients were able to speak for only 18 seconds before the doctor interrupted. The researchers expressed serious concerns that physicians' interruptions would compromise their ability to fully understand the reasons for their patients' visits and, therefore, could ultimately compromise care. What's really frustrating about the situation is that of the patients who were able to finish their statements ($n = 17$), most took less than a minute to do so, and none took longer than two and a half minutes.

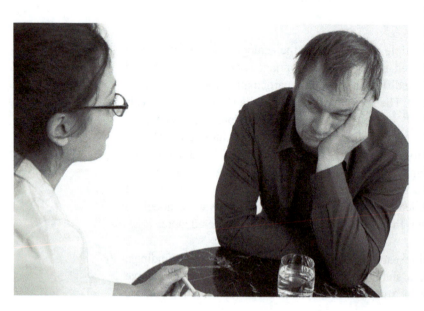

Like any study, Beckman and Frankel's (1984) had some limitations. Most of the physicians in their sample were internal medicine residents (i.e., pretty new docs); their sample size was small, with only 74 patients; and data were collected in one inner-city practice. To improve upon these limitations and also to see if the interruption situation had improved any over time, Marvel, Epstein, Flowers, and Beckman (1999) replicated the study with a larger, more diverse sample. Before we share what they found, let's delve a little deeper into their research design and method. (And let's also point out that Dr. Marvel has one of the coolest names ever.)

Marvel et al. (1999) recruited 29 board-certified family physicians from three different locations in the United States and Canada; nine of them had training in communication skills. Over a one-year period, the researchers audiotaped 300 office visits, striving to get 10 patients per physician. Of the 300 visits, 264 provided usable data. The researchers transcribed and then coded the data in three steps. First, they coded the physician's open-ended question used to determine the reason for the patient's visit and whether it was asked at the beginning of the visit or later in the visit, if indeed it was asked at all (sometimes the physicians didn't ask!). Second, they determined whether or not patients were able to complete their response; if patients said something like "That's all," if they asked a question about their concern (e.g., "Is it serious?"), or if they said "No" in response to the physician's asking "Anything else?" then their response was coded as completed. Finally, in the case of non-completed concerns, the researchers coded how physicians interrupted. Following Beckman and Frankel's (1984) categories, they coded for (a) closed question (when the doctor asks specific questions about what the patient just said), (b) elaborator (when the doctor asks for more details about what the patient just said), (c) recompleter (when the doctor repeats or paraphrases what the patient just said), and (d) statement (when the doctor comments on the patient's previous statement). Of course, the researchers also measured how long each patient spoke along with some other related variables.

Marvel et al.'s (1999) results were quite similar to what Beckman and Frankel (1984) found 15 years earlier. In only 28% of the visits were patients able to fully state the reasons for their visits before the physician interrupted them, and of the patients who were interrupted, only 8% of them were able to finish what they had started to say before the interruption. The average amount of time patients were able to speak before being interrupted increased to 23 seconds, which does show *some* improvement. The patients who were able to finish their statements, however, took on average only 32 seconds to do so. So if doctors only showed their patients a little more patience (ha?), they would be more likely to hear the whole story. Finally, physicians who had training in communication skills were more likely to allow their patients to speak without interruption (44%) than physicians who did not have the benefit of such training (22%). Seems that training can work.

We're going to revisit this research on how doctors determine patients' medical concerns later in the chapter, taking a look at some additional studies that provide further insight into the issue. For now, we want to turn our attention to research that considers the patient experience from the interpretive paradigm.

THE LIVED PATIENT EXPERIENCE:
THE INTERPRETIVE PERSPECTIVE

> Illness has meaning; and to understand how it obtains meaning is to understand
> something fundamental about illness, about care, and perhaps about life generally.
>
> Arthur Kleinman, *The Illness Narratives*

Research that investigates the patient perspective from the interpretive paradigm seeks to understand the meaning of illness in people's lives. According to Kleinman (1988), "Illness refers to how the sick person and the members of the family or wider social network perceive, live with, and respond to symptoms and disability" (p. 3). This means that illness encompasses all aspects of being sick, not just the physical, and that illness doesn't just affect the patient but also those who are close to the patient. Illness is, as Kleinman argues, a "lived experience," not just what test results reveal. One of the most prominent ways to approach the lived experience is through the stories that patients tell about their illnesses—their illness narratives.

Illness Narratives

Human beings are storytellers. Although biologists call human beings homo sapiens, Walter Fisher (1984) calls us homo narrans (storytelling man). No matter what you call us, we share information and make sense of what happens to us by telling stories. This especially applies when we are sick.

Eliciting and Analyzing Patient Narratives. Vanderford, Jenks, and Sharf (1997) encourage researchers to use the following methods to elicit and analyze patient narratives: (a) semi-structured interviews, (b) participant-observation, (c) ethnographic studies of illness and the patient experience, and (d) textual analysis. Semi-structured interviews encourage patients to tell their stories in response to open-ended questions that the researchers pose; researchers also encourage patients to go beyond the interview questions if they want and talk about what is important to them about their illness experience. Participant-observation is especially useful when studying self-help or support groups, where researchers gain access to how patients talk with others about their experiences and feelings. Ethnographic fieldwork involves studying people in their natural environments through observation or immersion, with special attention to what shared understandings are necessary to be a member of a specific group; this work allows researchers to gather highly contextualized and rich descriptions of the patient experience. Finally, a textual analysis allows researchers to analyze written texts and personal accounts of the illness experience. All of these methods are useful to gain insight into the challenges, nuances, and emotions of patients.

Types of Illness Narratives. Arthur Frank, a well-known sociologist who writes about illness and storytelling, suggests that illness narratives fall into three categories: the restitution narrative, the chaos narrative, and the quest narrative (Frank, 1998). The **restitution narrative** is a popular and favored narrative in our culture. This narrative describes how a person gets sick, suffers, receives treatment, and then is restored to health. As a culture, we like this narrative because it has a happy ending and it discourages sick people from dwelling on their illness. The problem, Frank suggests, is when restoration isn't possible. That happens not only in cases of very serious or terminal illnesses but also in cases of chronic illness such as diabetes and heart disease.

Such illness experiences may be better reflected in the **chaos narrative**. In this narrative, the condition continues to get worse, pain and suffering increase, relationships and jobs suffer, patients are dragged into healthcare bureaucracies that cause frustration and anxiety, stress increases, family and work responsibilities cannot be met, and the people around the ill person become less supportive, more demanding, and less patient. In other words, in the chaos narrative, chaos reigns. As a culture, we are uncomfortable with this narrative and its focus on suffering, despair, and hopelessness; we prefer stories of triumph and cures. However, to deny the telling of these stories is to negate the experience for the ill person. Every story needs a listener, and not allowing the patients to tell their stories, no matter how

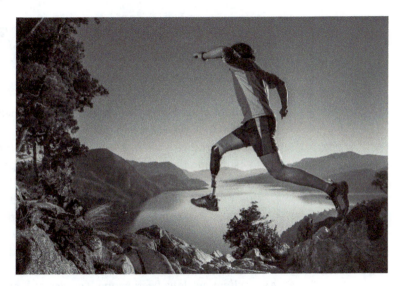

uncomfortable it may be for the listener, makes the patients' illness experience worse. A breast cancer patient put it this way: "What I really needed was people who relieved me of the job of making *them* feel better, and who were able to listen to both my bad and good feelings" (Kahane, 1995, p. 18). It's hard enough being sick. Having to worry about how other people are feeling about your being sick makes it even harder.

Perhaps somewhere in between the restoration and chaos narratives is the **quest narrative**. We often hear stories about people who have suffered serious or debilitating illnesses who go through the journey and face it head-on with the belief that something positive will come of the experience, even if the illness is chronic or debilitating. For example, in Mathieson and Stam's (1995) study, a woman who had had breast cancer surgery found the positive in her experience: "I think what cancer does is it smartens you up. I [*sic*] makes you look at yourself; it makes you look at your life . . . your perception changes . . . it has to" (p. 299). Similarly, a study by Mosack, Abbott, Singer, Weeks, and Lucy (2005), which involved semi-structured interviews with 60 low-income, urban HIV+ minority drug users about what it meant to them to be HIV+, found that one theme that emerged emphasized the *benefits* of having HIV. A 53-year-old woman summed it up:

> [Having HIV] doesn't mean I am going to die today. It would have meant I could have died tomorrow or a week from now if I didn't change my life around. If I had continued to use drugs and not try to go and see what AIDS is all about and the treatment that is needed—yeah, I would have died.

(p. 7)

ILLNESS NARRATIVES

Illness narratives fall into three categories:

Restitution narrative – when someone gets sick, suffers, receives treatment, and then is restored to health

Chaos narrative – when someone gets sick, the condition worsens, pain and suffering increases, jobs and relationships suffer, and support decreases for the ill person

Quest narrative – when someone gets sick and faces the issue head-on with the belief that something better will come of the experience, even if the illness is chronic or debilitating

---

As a culture, we love hearing about stories of how people persevere and turn a devastating health event into a life's passion. These illness sufferers come to realize how short life really is, and they make changes for the better. This message from the quest narrative is compelling, and listeners want to hear it. Not every patient is able to triumph over illness, however, and that can introduce added tension to the illness experience.

Uncertainty in Disease and Illness

Uncertainty is a common part of everyday life, affecting everything from work to relationships. Brashers (2001) wrote, "Uncertainty exists when details of situations are ambiguous, complex, or probabilistic; when information is unavailable or inconsistent; and when people feel insecure in their own state of knowledge in general" (p. 478). As you can imagine, this description suggests that uncertainty is particularly relevant to the illness experience. Indeed, although some conditions are simple and relatively easy to diagnose and cure, many are not, and that thrusts patients into the realm of uncertainty. Mishel (1984), who explored uncertainty in illness theory, agrees that uncertainty is an integral part of being sick and said that uncertainty occurs when "the decision-maker is unable to assign definite value to objects and events and/or is unable to predict outcomes accurately" (p. 163).

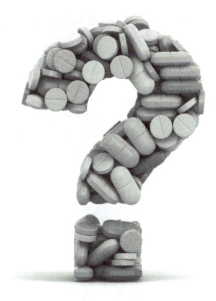

If we asked you to brainstorm a list of diseases that are rife with uncertainty, we're sure you could come up with a long list. At the top would probably be diseases like HIV/AIDS and cancer, diseases that are complex and unpredictable and that often require patients to make difficult decisions quickly, often with limited knowledge. Mathieson and Stam (1995) reported the experience of one woman with breast cancer who was asked to make a choice about her post-surgical cancer treatment. This woman challenges everyone:

> I defy anybody, after having an operation for cancer, first of all, be logical, or whatever, to be that much in control of themselves to say, "Oh, sure, I'll take chemo, because I know all about it." You know nothing about anything . . . I just became so doubtful of everything, and I'm not that kind of person.
> (p. 298)

Brashers et al. (2003) explored uncertainty with HIV patients. In this study, the researchers conducted focus groups with newly diagnosed and more advanced HIV+ men and women. They used open-ended questions to explore medical, personal, and social causes of uncertainty. What they found was that there is a lot of uncertainty when you are HIV+. From a medical perspective, participants reported insufficient information about diagnosis, ambiguous symptom patterns (leading one participant to ask, "How do you tell the difference between 'different' and 'wrong'?" [p. 504]), complexity of treatment and care, and unpredictable disease progression or prognosis. Personal forms of uncertainty included complex or conflicting roles (e.g., having to balance receiving and providing care) and unclear financial impact of the disease (medication and treatment for HIV/AIDS can be very costly, even with insurance). Social uncertainty focused on issues of stigmatization, concerns about acceptance versus rejection, and unclear relational implications (e.g., when and if to disclose HIV status to a potential sexual partner). As you can see, this population has a lot of uncertainty about a lot of issues.

Decision Making

All illnesses involve **decision making**, including whether or not to seek medical treatment in the first place. When patients do decide to seek medical treatment, there may be several treatment options or options may be limited, depending on the diagnosis (which, itself, might be uncertain!). When there are options, the question then is to what extent the patient becomes involved in the decision making. Outdated **physician-centered communication** practices privileged the doctor in decision making; the patient had little to say and was expected to simply follow the "doctor's orders." Today, however, **patient-centered communication** and **patient autonomy** have become the norm, and patients can expect to be active participants in medical decision making.

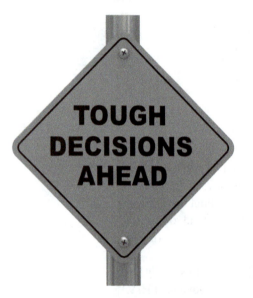

What exactly is involved in making a sound medical decision? Politi and Street (2011) list four components that should be considered: (a) the best clinical evidence, (b) the patient's values and preferences, (c) the patient's desire to be involved in the decision-making process, and (d) the feasibility of the treatment decision. Let's consider each of these components briefly.

First, sometimes clinical evidence is clear-cut; other times, there is considerable uncertainty. Plus, medical knowledge is continually accruing, so best practices evolve over time. In other words, the state of clinical evidence can complicate decision making. Second, a patient's values and preferences should come into play when there are treatment options. Some women with breast cancer, for example, opt for full mastectomies even when less radical treatment is an option because they want to reduce the risk of recurrence as much as possible. Third, sometimes being patient-centered involves recognizing that the patient may prefer not to be integrally involved in the decision-making process. The process can be taxing and intimidating, and some patients, especially those who are very ill, may prefer not to deal with such pressures. Even if patients are very involved during the decision-making process, they often defer the actual decision to the doctor (Politi & Street, 2011). Finally, sometimes treatments just are not feasible in a particular situation. For example, a patient may want to participate in a clinical trial that's testing a promising new drug. But if the drug requires administration every other day by a physician, and the clinical trial is going on in a large city two hours away from the patient's rural community where she raises three small children, works two part-time jobs, and drives an unreliable car, her participation just may not be possible. All four of these components need to be considered in medical decision making. Ultimately, we need to remember that decision making is, at heart, a communicative process that involves doctors and patients talking together to come to the "best" decision.

DECISION MAKING

There are four components that should inform decision making:

- the best clinical evidence
- the patient's values and preferences
- the patient's desire to be involved in the decision-making process
- the feasibility of the treatment decision

Decision aids can help with decision making along with improving provider–patient communication and patient involvement.

What do we know about the processes and outcomes of medical decision making? A recent Cochrane review (Stacey et al., 2011) assessed the literature on **decision aids** that physicians and patients use to help guide decisions about medical treatment and screening. The researchers reviewed the literature and identified 86 studies involving more than 20,000 participants that met their inclusion criteria. They considered decision attributes (knowledge, risk perception, and value-based choices) and decision process attributes (feeling informed and feeling clear about values). They found that decision aids increase knowledge, improve accurate risk perceptions, and result in decisions that are both informed and consistent with patients' values. They also found that decision aids improve physician–patient communication and, no surprise, increase patient involvement in decision making. (A quick note: If you are thinking this section on decision aids sounds scientific, you would be right. In a blatant act of organizational heresy, we've comingled the scientific and interpretive. Mea culpa.)

It might interest you to know that there is an international conference series on shared decision making! As we were writing this chapter, the International Shared Decision Making (ISDM) conference was getting ready to host its seventh conference in 2013 in Lima, Peru (we sort of wished we were going). The fifth conference, held in 2009 in Boston, Massachusetts, resulted in the publication of a special issue of the journal *Health Expectations* (Barry, Levin, MacCuaig, Mulley, & Sepucha, 2011). The issue contains articles that address basic issues of what defines a shared medical decision; how to implement (translate) patient decision aids, particularly considering the needs of special populations (underserved, chronically ill, multicultural); how to measure the effects of shared decision making; and how to teach shared decision-making skills to healthcare providers. In addition, there is a professional organization dedicated to advancing evidence-based practice in decision making, the Informed Medical Decisions Foundation (http://www.informedmedicaldecisions.org). The level of academic and professional interest in this topic is heartening and suggests how important shared decision making has become to the patient and practice community.

CHALLENGING THE STATUS QUO: THE CRITICAL–CULTURAL PARADIGM

A third perspective used to explore health and illness is the critical–cultural approach. This approach identifies **power imbalances**, challenges the **status quo**, and gives voice to **marginalized populations** who otherwise go unheard.

The Breast Cancer Experience

A good example of research from this paradigm is the case study of Ellen, a woman diagnosed with breast cancer. Ellen's story is reported by Ford and Christmon (2005), who argue that there is no one "true" breast cancer story and each narrative is "rooted in a specific political cultural context" (p. 157). In Ellen's case, her story highlights how we as a culture talk about breast cancer.

Ellen challenges what many take for granted, down to the pink dressing room where she changed into a pink hospital gown before having her mammogram. She writes, "The room was so pink, five or six different shades of pink. How many shades of pink

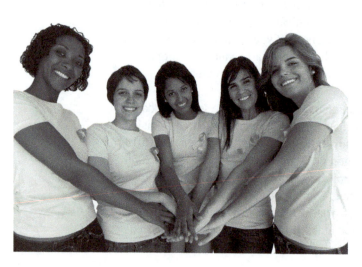

can there possibly be? I was suffocating in pink, right down to the pink-flowered gown they gave me to wear as I prepared to bare my chest" (Ford & Christmon, 2005, p. 163). Later, she realizes that all of the pink décor, including the "kitsch posters," was her introduction to "the tension between trivialization and the valorization of women with breast cancer" (p. 163).

Ellen describes how when she joined a support group, she found a very strong mythical story and expectation of behavior surrounding breast cancer and learned that every woman is expected to follow it. The myth encompasses hope and encouragement, not discussions about causes of cancer, treatments for cancer, or the corporatization of breast cancer, which is what she wanted to talk about. Ellen wonders if the corporatization of breast cancer is suppressing women's anger out of fear of losing corporate sponsorship. She questions the emphasis on survivors of breast cancer and what she calls the marginalization of those who die, who at breast cancer events are rarely mentioned, with the emphasis on the living. Additionally, Ellen questions the "relentless cheerfulness" and the expectation that those who are part of the breast cancer culture must have a positive attitude. Finally, she wants to talk about the use of pink ribbons and the language of war used to describe cancer. "Why," she asks, "Why can't we talk about these issues?"

"What a Jerk!"

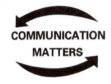

COMMUNICATION MATTERS

Ellen found herself mired in a system that refused to acknowledge her concerns about how breast cancer has been overtaken by pink cheeriness. There are other power struggles women face in the medical setting, such as being taken seriously by physicians. Here's one example from one of the interviews that Gretchen did for her dissertation:

> I had been having these episodes of getting really weak and shaky and sweating and really nervous and I decided that, and several people had told me, too, that I probably had low blood sugar and I knew it was when I hadn't eaten in a while so I went to him and told him what my symptoms were and stuff. And, he said, "Tell me something, do you subscribe to Redbook, Cosmopolitan, any of those women's magazines?' I said, "What does that have to do with anything?" He said, "You know, every time they publish a story about low blood sugar or whatever, I get 10 women in the next day who have it." I was so angry. What a jerk.

Patient Command and Control

You may have heard the story of Norman Cousins, a prominent American journalist, editor, and liberal political activist who became very, very (very!) ill after a grueling diplomatic mission to Russia in 1964. During the trip, he not only endured a great deal of work-related stress but also was exposed to excessive amounts of diesel exhaust from trucks that constantly drove by his hotel and from a jet at the airport that spewed exhaust at him at "point-blank range." He started feeling sick when he got home and was hospitalized within a week. What started as a slight fever rapidly progressed to severe stiffness throughout his body. He was eventually diagnosed with "ankylosing spondylitis," a degenerative collagen disease that was

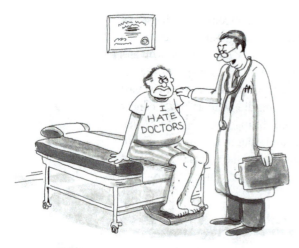

"I'm happy to see you, too."

making his connective tissue disintegrate (good grief!). Specialists gave him a 1 in 500 chance at recovery. That's when he decided he needed to take charge.

Being a journalist, Cousins was no stranger to research, so he delved into the medical literature and put together a logical, albeit extremely unconventional, treatment strategy. First, he asked to be moved out of the hospital, which he had concluded "was no place for a person who was seriously ill" (Cousins, 1976, p. 1458):

The surprising lack of respect for basic sanitation, ... the extensive and sometimes promiscuous use of x-ray equipment, the seemingly indiscriminate administration of tranquilizers and powerful painkillers, more for the convenience of hospital staff in managing patients than for therapeutic needs, and the regularity with which hospital routine takes precedence over the rest requirements for the patient ... all these and other practices seemed to me to be critical shortcomings of the modern hospital.

(p. 1458)

Second, he asked to be taken off his prescribed medications, which he determined were making him sicker. "The history of medicine is replete with instances involving drugs and modes of treatment that were in use for many years before it was recognized that they did more harm than good" (p. 1460). Third, he requested massive doses of vitamin C to combat his collagen breakdown, and, positing that positive emotions may produce positive chemical changes in the body, arranged to watch lots and lots of entertaining television (e.g., *Candid Camera* episodes).

Fortunately, Cousins' doctor, who had been a close friend of his for more than 20 years, was an early adopter of patient-centered medicine and fully supported Cousins in his efforts. Blood tests after his doses of vitamin C and laughter showed continuous and cumulative improvements. Cousins also discovered that laughter was highly effective pain medicine: "10 minutes of genuine belly laughter ... would give me at least two hours of pain-free sleep" (p. 1461). Although it took a while, Cousins did recover.

This story captures a lot of what we've been discussing in this chapter, including aspects of the illness narrative (Cousins actually wrote a whole book on his experience, and Hollywood made a movie about it), uncertainty and decision making, and patient participation. We highlight it in this section on the critical paradigm because we believe Cousins' experience reveals the positive outcomes that can result from "bucking the system." We're not advocating that people totally ignore medical advice, obviously. But in Cousins' case, the healthcare system was not helping him and, instead, was actually hurting him. Had he not taken matters into his own hands, he may not have recovered.

CONFLICTS IN RESEARCH

Earlier in this chapter, we reviewed research showing that physicians tend to interrupt patients when patients try to present the reason(s) for their medical visits. We reviewed two studies, published 15 years apart, that pretty much showed the same results: Physicians stink at keeping their mouths shut. So why are we bringing this up again under a section on conflicting research? Because we want to show you some of the other ways researchers have considered interruption behavior and how those findings add complexity to our understanding and the implications of the results. Specifically, we'll present studies that further explore the impact of physician interruptions and consider patient interrupting behavior, as well. (A quick note: Research in shared decision making also provides a rich opportunity to consider conflicting results; see Guadagnoli and Ward [1998] for a start.)

Does It Really Matter?

Dyche and Swiderski (2005) wanted to explore the impact of physician interruptions in greater detail. They acknowledged the importance of patients being able to get their medical concerns on the table, but they noted that some of the behaviors Beckman and Frankel (1984) counted as interruptions may actually help patients express their concerns (e.g., elaborators), and they emphasized how Marvel et al. (1999) found that some physicians were able to solicit patient concerns even after interrupting them. Their main research question was "whether physician interruption compromises physician understanding of patient concerns" (p. 267).

Dyche and Swiderski (2005) developed a measure they called an index of under-standing (IOU), which was the percentage of agreement between the concerns that patients listed and the concerns that doctors said the patients had. So, if you were in this study and told the researcher that you were concerned about an upset stomach and a headache, and your doctor had no clue what your concern was or told the researcher that you were concerned about a rash, the IOU would be 0%; if the doctor said upset stomach, the IOU would be 50%; if the doctor said upset stomach and headache, the IOU would be 100%.

What Dyche and Swiderski (2005) found was that it mattered <u>not</u> whether or not doctors interrupted patients when patients were expressing concerns: the IOU scores did not differ significantly. Specifically, the average IOU score for the physicians who did not interrupt patients (n = 18, 26%) was 84.6%; the average IOU score for the physicians who did interrupt their patients (n = 26, 37%) was 82.2%. What <u>did</u> matter was whether physicians solicited patients' concerns at all. In total, 26 physicians (37%) did not bother to solicit patient concerns in the first five minutes of the visit; those wannabe psychics had an average IOU score of only 59.2%, significantly lower than the other two groups. So the lesson here is that—for physician understanding of patient concerns—it doesn't matter whether or not they interrupt the patient, but it does matter if they ask about patient concerns to begin with!

Who's Interrupting Whom?

So far, the picture we have painted of the patient's experience is one of patients being interrupted by physicians. Turns out, though, that patients do their fair share of interrupting, as well. That's what Irish and Hall (1995) found in their study designed to consider the impact of participant role (physician or patient), physician status, and gender on interrupting behavior and how interruptions may reflect dominance.

These researchers' definition of what counts as an interruption was much more detailed than earlier definitions. For example, Beckman and Frankel (1984) defined an interruption as "Any response that physically disrupted the speech stream or inhibited further topical development" (p. 693), and they identified four types of interruptions: closed question, elaborator, recompleter, and statement. Irish and Hall (1995) used a 17-category system that allowed them to consider the extent to which interruptive speech was successful at actually interrupting, and they distinguished successful, partially successful, and unsuccessful interruptions. They also coded cases of simple "overlapping" speech, which happens when one person starts to speak right before the other person finishes but doesn't stop the other person from finishing. They also considered whether the speaker was asking a question or making a statement. Findings were quite revealing.

Irish and Hall (1995) found that there were <u>no</u> differences in the overall frequency of successful interruptions by physicians and patients. However, when you considered what participants were saying, there were huge differences. Physicians interrupted patients successfully more with questions, whereas patients interrupted physicians successfully more with statements. The same held true for partially successful interruptions. For unsuccessful interruptions, patients had more unsuccessful attempts with statements; there were no differences for questions. Finally, patients overlapped with physicians more overall and more with statements, whereas physicians overlapped more with questions. The picture we're getting from this study is that there's plenty of interrupting going on, whether successful or not, and that patients tend to interrupt with statements and physicians tend to interrupt with questions. (In case you're interested, neither physician status nor participant gender had any consistent impact on interrupting behavior.)

What Really Matters Here

The take-home message we'd like you to get from this section of the chapter is that there are many, many ways to consider the same question and that it is crucial to know both what you're asking and what you're answering. Beckman and Frankel (1984) and subsequently Marvel et al. (1999) looked at four types of interruptions and whether the interruptions prevented patients from completely expressing their concerns. What's easy to miss in these studies is that physician "interruptions" may not have been actual interrupting speech at all. Each speaker could have taken non-overlapping turns at talk. The crux was whether or not what the physician said took the patient off course. Indeed, Marvel et al. (1999) argued for use of the term "redirection" instead of "interruption" to emphasize the outcome of the behavior over the process.

Irish and Hall (1995) were interested in actual interrupting speech, concerned with its relationship to participant role and status. They focused more on interruptions as a sign of dominance, which certainly has implications for effective physician–patient communication but steers attention away from the focus on the patient's medical agenda. Dyche and Swiderski (2005) were interested in the patient's agenda and discovered that it didn't matter if physicians interrupted patients but it did matter if they asked about patient concerns in the first place.

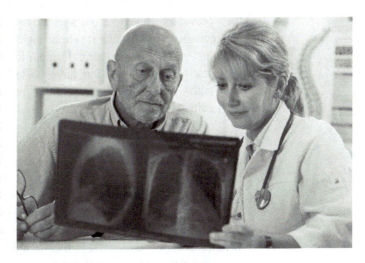

What all of this tells us is that there is great opportunity here to improve the patient experience if we keep what matters most in mind. Patients must be able to express their concerns. If doctors don't ask, patients should tell. And when patients are sharing their concerns, especially in the give-and-take of conversation, physician interruption may not matter so much. But if physician interruption starts to steer patients off track, patients need to get right back on track. Patient communication training programs like Cegala's PACE can go a long way to empowering patients to be active and successful participants in their own medical visits.

ARE WE HAVING AN IMPACT?

By now you should sense that health communication scholars do a lot of research and we publish it in a lot of academic journals. You also may be asking, "So, what? How does any of it make a difference in my life?" That's a good question. Let us give you two examples of research put into practice.

One project that is putting research into practice is Don Cegala's PACE program. We've mentioned PACE a few times in this chapter, but what is it exactly? PACE is a program designed to train adult patients to communicate more effectively by *P*resenting detailed information about how they feel, *A*sking their physicians questions, *C*hecking their understanding of information their doctor gives them, and *E*xpressing any concerns they have about the recommended treatment. The program has been tested many times and has been found to enhance information exchange, patient control, and patient adherence. The patient program currently is being used in British Columbia, Canada to teach patients how to better communicate with their providers and to encourage informed decision making. It's also being used in the United Kingdom to assist diabetic patients in communicating with their providers. Beyond those specific programs, PACE is available on the Web for anyone who wants to use it (either visit http://www.comm.ohio-state.edu/PACE or Google PACE and Cegala). In addition, the American Heart Association and American Lung Association have posted a version that hospitals can download and tailor for distribution to their patients: http://hearthealth.aha-krames.com/RelatedItems/77,AHACOM3. Pretty cool, right?

A second example is an innovative project called "Let's Talk Health." The goal of this project is to share health and health communication information with the listeners of WUMR 92 FM, the University of Memphis radio station. This interdisciplinary collaboration involves researchers in the Department of Communication and the Lowenberg School of Nursing. The two-minute radio spots translate important health information and patient-centered health communication research into vignettes that are broadcast to more than 70,000 listeners in the Memphis area. The communication spots focus on both patients and providers. Spots directed at patients provide relevant information that patients can use to enhance their healthcare experiences, such as preparing for their doctor's appointment by writing down their questions to take to the office visit or making sure they understand what their doctor is saying by letting them know if something is unclear. Spots directed at providers focus on issues related to rapport and speaking in language patients can understand. If you would like to hear one of the spots, the podcasts are available at http://www.memphis.edu/communication/letstalkhealth.php

PACE

In order to get more out of your medical visit, be prepared to follow PACE guidelines:

P = **Present** detailed information about how you are feeling.

- Be specific: Are you experiencing pain? If so, is it a sharp pain or a dull ache? Does it come and go or is it constant? Has anything helped alleviate the pain? What have you tried?

A = **Ask** questions.

- Thinking about what you want to ask *before* your office visit and writing it down will make sure you ask what is important to you. You may want to ask, "How serious is my condition? What should I do if it gets worse? How long before I start feeling better?"

C = **Check** for understanding.

- It's really important that you understand everything the doctor is telling you about your condition, the treatment, and any medications that are prescribed. It's your responsibility as a patient to speak up if you don't understand something.
- Ask the doctor to repeat or clarify any information that is unclear. Then repeat or paraphrase what he or she told you to make sure you understand.

E = **Express** concerns about the recommended treatment.

- If you have concerns about the recommended treatment (for example, difficulty swallowing pills), speak up. Be honest with your doctor by explaining how you are following the treatment (for example, taking all, some, or none of your medication or doing all, some, or none of your at home physical therapy). If you are having trouble, be sure to explain why and offer to work with your doctor to find a modified or alternative treatment.

Before your next visit, answer the following questions:

What is the purpose of your visit? _____

What are your symptoms? Be specific: _____

What do you hope to get out of your doctor's visit? _____

What questions/concerns do you have? _____

List of medications:

_____   _____   _____

_____   _____   _____

DIRECTIONS FOR FUTURE RESEARCH ON THE PATIENT EXPERIENCE

While we know a lot about the patient experience, there's much more we need to know. We think there is opportunity to learn more about how having multiple illnesses

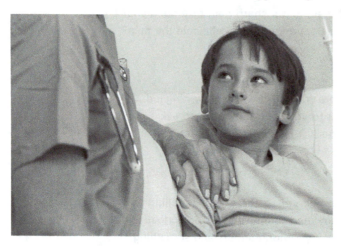

within a family influences the patient experience. With the extent of chronic illness and disability in our society these days, it is not unique to have more than one patient in a household. How do the healthcare experiences of one patient affect the other? We also could learn more about the experience of child patients. Children have largely been neglected in health communication research, in part due to the difficulty of gaining access to them because they are considered an especially vulnerable population. The perspective of children, however, may give us unique insight into the patient experience.

We also think we need to learn more about the good experiences of patients and learn more about the patient experience through the lens of humor. A number of comedians either weave illness experiences into their routines or build entire acts around them (e.g., Mike Birbiglia, Tig Notaro, Maysoon Zayid). Maybe laughter is the best medicine. Finally, we need to keep our eyes open for how changes in the healthcare system and advances in health information and communication technology affect the patient experience. Chapters 7, 12, and 15 address these topics, but our point here is that change happens so rapidly these days, we must be vigilant to ask the pressing research questions.

CONCLUSION

Our goal for this chapter was to provide you with a window into patients' experiences, to give you a glimpse into what it means to be a patient through a sampling of scientific, interpretive, and critical–cultural research. We wanted you to understand the complexity of the patient experience: trying to communicate with healthcare providers, managing uncertainty and decision making, sharing their own stories while trying to comfort their friends and families, dealing with pink ribbons and pink hospital gowns while fearing for their lives.

Being a patient isn't easy. It takes courage. The fear, isolation, and pain can be over-whelming. Illness is complicated and people are complicated and sometimes it takes a while to understand what is going on, if you ever do. We hope that you've begun to appreciate these complexities somewhat. We also hope that when you find yourself or a close friend or family member experiencing an illness, you now have greater insight into some of the communication concerns that play a role in the patient experience.

DISCUSSION QUESTIONS

1. How does studying the patient experience differ when looking at it from a scientific perspective? An interpretive perspective? A critical–cultural perspective? Which perspective are you most comfortable with? Why?
2. How do you think being seriously ill (e.g., having cancer, HIV/AIDS) would affect your relationships with family? With friends? With students? With co-workers? Are there different effects depending on the type of relationship?
3. How do you view people who are sick? Does talking to someone who has a serious illness make you uncomfortable? Why or why not?
4. Ellen's narrative from the case study cited in the chapter talks about the "tension between trivialization and the valorization of women with breast cancer." What does she mean? Do you agree with her? Why or why not? Can you identify other tensions associated with breast cancer or other diseases and the messages that surround them?
5. Do you think there are social pressures for patients to focus on the positives and to not talk about the negatives when diagnosed with serious illnesses? Why or why not? If you believe there are such pressures, why do you think this is?

IN-CLASS ACTIVITIES

1. Read an illness experience blog from the Internet. (There are several listed on this text's companion website or you can find one on your own.) Answer the following questions:

    (a) What stands out about this particular patient's experience?
    (b) What most surprised you?
    (c) Is the description representative of what you thought the experience would be like?
    (d) What would you like to ask the blogger if you could? Why?

2. Find a patient experience on YouTube and watch it in class. Discuss the following questions:

(a) How is this patient's experience different from or similar to the experiences of patients described in this chapter?

(b) What role did communication play in the patient's illness experience?

(c) What did the video make you think about? Why?

3. Talk to someone who has been a patient about their illness experience. What questions did you ask? Why? What did you want to ask but didn't? What did you find out? How does that change your preconceived ideas about what it means to be ill?

RECOMMENDED READINGS

Anderson, J., & Martin, P. (2003). Narratives and healing: Exploring one family's stories of cancer survivorship. *Health Communication, 15,* 133–158.

This article explores the cancer experience from the patient and the family perspectives, highlighting the struggles with coping, support, and identity.

Helitzer, D., LaNoue, M., Wilson, B., de Hernandez, B., Warner, T., & Roter, D. (2011). A randomized controlled trial of communication training with primary care providers to improve patient-centeredness and health risk communication. *Patient Education and Counseling, 82,* 21–29.

This article reports on a successful simulated patient-centered communication training focused on behavioral risk factors that showed long-term effects.

Middleton, A, LaVoie, N., & Brown, L. (2012). Sources of uncertainty in Type 2 diabetes: Explication and implications for health communication theory and clinical practice. *Health Communication, 27,* 591–601.

This article reports interviews with 49 Type 2 diabetic patients, revealing causes of uncertainty in the context of dealing with their disease.

Politi, M., Clark, M., Ombao, H., Dizon, D., & Elwin, G. (2011). Communicating uncertainty can lead to less decision satisfaction: A necessary cost of involving patients in shared decision making? *Health Expectations, 14,* 84–91.

This article explores how provider communication about uncertainty may lead to less decision satisfaction for patients.

REFERENCES

Barry, M., Levin, C., MacCuaig, M., Mulley, A., & Sepucha, K. (2011). Shared decision making: Vision to reality. *Health Expectations, 14,* 1–5.

Beckman, H. B., & Frankel, R. M. (1984). The effect of physician behavior on the collection of data. *Annals of Internal Medicine, 101*, 692–696.

Brashers, D. E. (2001). Communication and uncertainty management. *Journal of Communication, 51*, 477–497.

Brashers, D., Neidig, J., Russell, J., Cardillo, L., Haas, S., Dobbs, L., . . . Nemeth, S. (2003). The medical, personal, and social causes of uncertainty in HIV illness. *Issues in Mental Health Nursing, 24*, 497–522.

Cegala, D. J. (2011). An exploration of factors promoting patient participation in primary care medical interviews. *Health Communication, 26*, 427–436.

Cousins, N. (1976). Anatomy of an illness (as perceived by the patient). *The New England Journal of Medicine, 295*, 1458–1463.

Dyche, L., & Swiderski, D. (2005). The effect of physician solicitation approaches on ability to identify patient concerns. *Journal of General Internal Medicine, 20*, 267–270.

Fisher, W. (1984). Narration as a human communication paradigm: The case of public moral argument. *Communication Monographs, 51*, 1–22.

Ford, L. A., & Christmon, B. C. (2005). Every breast cancer is different: Illness narratives and the management of identity in breast cancer. In E. B. Ray (Ed.) *Health communication in practice: A case study approach* (pp. 157–170). Mahwah, NJ: Lawrence Erlbaum.

Frank, A. (1998). Just listening: Narrative and deep illness. *Families, Systems, & Health, 16*, 197–212.

Guadagnoli, E., & Ward, P. (1998). Patient participation and decision-making. *Social Science & Medicine, 47*(3), 329–339.

Irish, J. T., & Hall, J. A. (1995). Interruptive patterns in medical visits: The effects of role, status and gender. *Social Science & Medicine, 41*(6), 873–881.

Kahane, D. (1995). *No less a woman: Femininity, sexuality & breast cancer.* Alameda, CA: Hunter House.

Kleinman, A. (1988). *The illness narratives: Suffering, healing & the human condition.* New York, NY: Basic Books Publishers.

Marvel, M. K., Epstein, R. M., Flowers, K., & Beckman, H. B. (1999). Soliciting the patient's agenda: Have we improved? *Journal of the American Medical Association, 281*(3), 283–287.

Mathieson, C., & Stam, H. (1995). Renegotiating identity: Cancer narratives. *Sociology of Health and Illness, 17*, 283–306.

Mishel, M. (1984). Perceived uncertainty and stress in illness. *Research in Nursing and Health, 7*, 163–171.

Mosack, K., Abbott, M., Singer, M., Weeks, M., & Lucy, R. (2005). If I didn't have HIV I'd be dead now: Illness narratives of drug users living with HIV/AIDS. *Qualitative Health Research, 15*(5), 586–605.

Politi, M., & Street, R. L. (2011). Patient-centered communication during collaborative decision making. In T. L. Thompson, R. Parrott, & J. F. Nussbaum (Eds.), *The Routledge handbook of health communication* (2nd ed., pp. 399–413). New York: Routledge.

Sontag, S. (1978). *Illness as metaphor.* Toronto, Canada: Farrar, Straus & Giroux.

Stacey, D., Bennett, C. L., Barry, M. J., Col, N. F., Eden, K. B., Holmes-Rovner, M., . . . Thomson, R. (2011). Decision aids for people facing health treatment or screening decisions (Review). *Cochrane Database of Systematic Reviews*, Issue 10. Art. No.: CD001431.

Street, R. L. (2003). Communication in medical encounters: An ecological perspective. In T. L. Thompson, A. M. Dorsey, K. I. Miller, & R. Parrott (Eds.), *Handbook of health communication* (pp. 63–89). Mahwah, NJ: Lawrence Erlbaum Associates.

Street, R. L., & Millay, B. (2001). Analyzing patient participation in medical encounters. *Health Communication, 13*(1), 61–73.

Vanderford, M., Jenks, E., & Sharf, B. (1997). Exploring patients' experiences as a primary source of meaning. *Health Communication, 9,* 13–26.

3

Understanding Caregiver Challenges and Social Support Needs

*Elaine Wittenberg-Lyles,
Joy Goldsmith, and Sara Shaunfield*

There are only four kinds of people in the world—those who have been care-givers, those who are currently caregivers, those who will be caregivers, and those who will need caregivers.

Rosalyn Carter

By age fourteen, Ty began looking like his dad—a concave chest and an acute kyphotic curve in the upper spine. They looked so much the same in their faces that their now-similar silhouette seemed to be a family trait passed from father to son.

This is your first look at Ty. Something is changing about his body. He is a typical teenager with friends, and there is disagreement with his parents and younger brother. But how will his family and school friends know how to provide or locate support as Ty barrels toward receiving a devastating diagnosis? As we share his unfolding story throughout this chapter, we examine the state of the research on social support, share support interventions taking place across the country, and consider what is ahead for some of you who might contribute to the growing research and practice of communication in the healthcare system.

We begin our chapter with some background information on the extent of lay caregiving in the nation, research on caregivers and caregiver needs. Then we provide

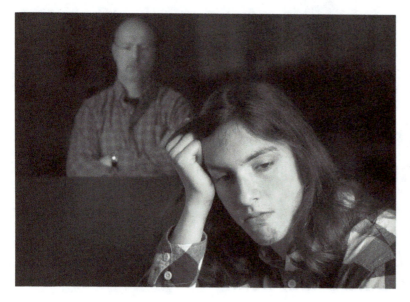

further information on social support and applied interventions. We follow that with research conducted through the lens of scientific, interpretive, and critical–cultural research, highlighting how the approach you take to investigate social support determines whom you will talk to about patient support (patient, caregiver, and/or healthcare professional), what part of the communication process you will focus on (e.g., sources of support, supportive messages, perceptions of support), and how you study it (i.e., research method). Finally, we address conflicting findings and directions for future research.

THE LAY OF THE CAREGIVER LAND

Approximately 20–30% of U.S. households include a **lay caregiver** providing unpaid patient care, with one in five caregivers working over 40 hours weekly to assist with

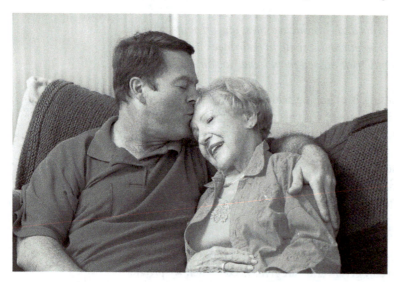

patient medication, activities of daily living (i.e., toileting, dressing, eating, feeding, walking, moving), transportation needs, and scheduling clinical visits (National Alliance for Caregiving and AARP, 2004). In 2009, unpaid caregiving services and contributions were estimated to represent $450 billion (American Association of Retired Persons Policy Institute, 2011). The demand to supply care and support for our families and friends is predicted only to increase as the population increases and grows older and as medical interventions proliferate. Social support needs and deficits are crucial concerns for us all.

Odds are that your current class, virtual or otherwise, includes three or four people who are part of a household providing care to a loved one. This chapter highlights the role of people who provide patient support, namely family members and primary family caregivers. We will describe the complex communication processes that comprise the caregiver journey of anxiety, depression, distress, and fear. For many, the caregiving experience can result in a loss of social connections, activities, and even a career. Although a lay caregiver can lose so much in the caring process, there are unique and priceless experiences that can benefit the caregiver, as well. These experiences require our consideration from a communication perspective to further understand those who support the patient, the impact of caregiving on their own health, and how research can contribute to the development and delivery of resources to aid in caregiver coping, information seeking, and the acquisition of services that can ease the supportive role.

THE ROLE OF CAREGIVERS

As a result of an increasing aging population and a shortage of healthcare professionals in our hospitals, friends and family members of patients (often called informal or lay caregivers) are providing unpaid patient care in the home. Caregiving duties often involve scheduling clinical visits, participation in clinical interactions with healthcare staff, overseeing pain management medication and administration, and providing assistance with activities of daily living. Given their role as liaison between patient and healthcare staff, caregivers have a variety of communication responsibilities. They are responsible for sharing the patient's medical history with providers, engaging in information-seeking about treatment and placement options, and facilitating communication between the healthcare team and other members of the family.

A considerable amount of research on patient support, with specific attention to the role of family caregivers, has been conducted in the field of nursing (Bakas, Li, Habermann, McLennon, & Weaver, 2011; Gebhardt, McGehee, Grindel, & Testani-Dufour, 2011; Parker, Teel, Leenerts, & Macan, 2011). According to the National Institute of Nursing Research, lay caregivers (also referred to as informal caregivers or family caregivers) are considered nurse-extenders, providing uncompensated nursing care to the majority of elderly in the United States (Reinhard, Given, Petlick, & Bemis, 2008). With patient support so frequently coming from within the family, healthcare professionals identify a primary family caregiver who serves as the main contact for patient

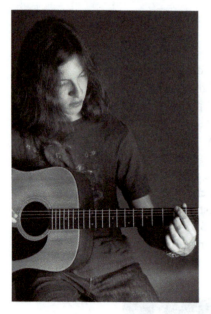

support needs and care coordination with staff. Additional lay caregivers can emerge from extended family, friends, members of religious or social organizations, and the local community.

Ty began having trouble holding and fingering the frets on his guitar, so much so that he regularly complained about this to his mom and dad. His mom, Estelle, shuttled him to and from their family doctor to see if he was practicing too hard with his band or if there were other explanations. The visit to the physician yielded no clear answers, and Ty was placed on a low dose regimen of Ibuprofen and was told to reduce his practice time. For Ty, this was frustrating as his band was the most committed and satisfying part of his life. Estelle, in particular, was alone in her worry. She knew her son's body was changing in a way that reminded her of Ty's dad. Plus, their family had moved to a rural southwestern town the previous year—thousands of miles from her family and well-established circle of friends.

Family caregivers have been referred to as **second order patients** because they share in the intimate suffering of patients and experience their own profound personal losses as a result of providing patient care (Sherman, 1998; Wittenberg-Lyles et al., 2013). For both the patient and the caregiver, there are intrapersonal concerns about coping with their own suffering and the suffering of the other person (Ferrell, 1996). The intimate relationship of caregiving can begin with the caregiver's involvement in the diagnosis/prognosis and subsequent healthcare decision

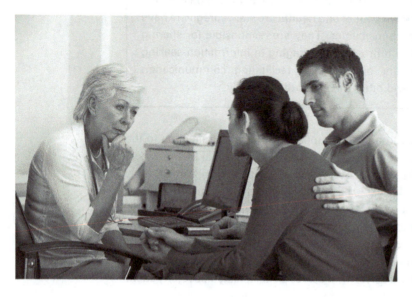

making (Wittenberg-Lyles, Goldsmith, Ragan, & Sanchez-Reilly, 2010). Caregivers routinely attend clinical visits to collaborate with the patient and healthcare staff about treatment options. A study of outpatient oncology clinics revealed that 92% of cancer patients had at least one companion accompany them to the visit; some patients had up to five companions come along (Eggly et al., 2006).

The impact of administering lay care can be described as **caregiver burden**; this accounts for caregiving tasks that are often highly time consuming, overwhelming, and likely unanticipated or sudden in nature. Some caregivers sacrifice social identity and personal relationships, and they curtail social activities and experiences to provide care (Gonyea, Paris, & de Saxe Zerden, 2008). Caregiving duties often interfere with work responsibilities, which can create an unsupportive work environment and add more social and emotional stress (Swanberg, 2006). Although most caregivers adjust well to their role, up to 30% experience significant psychological distress and depression (Given et al., 2004; Rivera, 2009). Caregivers also experience loneliness as an integral part of their patient's compromised health (Rokach, Matalon, Safarov, & Bercovitch, 2007).

Communication with providers is quintessential to the caregiving role. During serious illness, approximately 70% of a patient's prior medical history is shared orally by family members (Bevan & Pecchioni, 2008). Commonly, complex medical words and abbreviations are used to describe medications, medical treatments, procedures, and disease processes during inpatient and outpatient consultations with patients and families (Maniaci, Heckman, & Dawson, 2008). The clinician's use of medical words can obstruct the shared decision-making process as patients and family members fear appearing ignorant and thus become reluctant to ask what medical terms mean (Roter,

---

Betty Ferrell, Ph.D., M.A., FAAN, FPCN

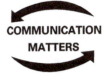

COMMUNICATION MATTERS

In cancer care, family caregivers are often neglected during treatment, although they play a critical role providing patient care and support. Oncology caregivers are often sleep-deprived, anxious, depressed, and have trouble coping with worries about the future, finances, and spiritual questions. Dr. Betty Ferrell, a Professor and the Director of Nursing Research and Education at City of Hope Medical Center, a leading research, treatment, and education center for cancer, diabetes, and other life-threatening diseases, has devoted the past three decades to understanding the experiences and needs of the oncology family caregiver. Dr. Ferrell and her research team focus their work on family caregivers in oncology, conducting many studies and educational projects to support a family from diagnosis through long-term survivorship or end-of-life care. Dr. Ferrell's team has been funded by the National Cancer Institute to test a model of support for family caregivers of patients with lung cancer. The intervention uses an interdisciplinary assessment and care planning process accompanied by education in four quality of life domains: physical, psychological, social, and spiritual well-being. Although the intervention is still being tested, Dr. Ferrell expects that it will help support family caregiver quality of life and add to their knowledge and skills in providing care. Dr. Ferrell highlights a need for future interventions and research that focus on family caregivers' need of information and support for both the physical and emotional aspects of caregiving.

2011). Poor communication between providers and caregivers can impede the understanding of prescription instructions and impact the quality of care delivered by the caregiver (Lau et al., 2010).

THE NEEDS OF CAREGIVERS

Caregivers are "second order patients" who experience suffering and anxiety alongside the patient. The stress and burden of caregiving, called caregiver burden, takes a toll on caregivers. Many caregivers experience the loss of career or employment, face social isolation, and report psychological distress and depression. Social support research can contribute to the development of resources to aid in caregiver coping. Depending on the approach, this research may involve measuring caregivers' social networks (scientific approach), describing caregivers' understanding of social support (interpretive approach), or giving voice to a disadvantaged caregiving population (critical approach). While social support research has predominantly portrayed social support as positive, several studies reveal that there are instances where social support contributes to caregiver burden.

Information needs remain high for caregivers who need and want information about the patient's illness, patient resources, and caregiver support (Hauser & Kramer, 2004). Nationally, about 79% of caregivers have access to the Internet, with the majority seeking health information about treatment options, hospital ratings, and end-of-life decision making (Fox & Brenner, 2012). Issues related to health literacy, which encompasses visual (graphs/charts), computer (Internet/search), information seeking, numeracy (calculations/statistical reasoning), oral (interpersonal), and other components needed to navigate the healthcare system, are crucial to caregivers and their task (Nielsen-Bohlman, Panzer, & Kindig, 2004). Prior research establishes that health literacy barriers include providers' frequent use of medical jargon, language discordance, purposeful ambiguity, and cultural insensitivity (The Joint Commission, 2009). For the caregiver all of these factors can and do lead to an ineffectiveness, and worse, an inability to navigate the healthcare system. The biggest cost is that of the patient's quality of care and decision making (Ragan, Wittenberg-Lyles, Goldsmith, & Sanchez-Reilly, 2008).

Given that family members are a primary resource for patients, family communication and family conflict can compromise patient care and goals of care. In the caretaking context, family conflict can erupt when one or more of five areas of disagreement emerge: (1) a perception unfolds that one or more family members are not supporting the caregiving effort with enough resources, (2) family members cannot agree on care coordination, (3) the patient's care needs are not being met, (4) there is disagreement about the nature of the illness or prognosis, or (5) historic conflicts from within the family are drawn out and magnified in light of the health situation (Kramer, Boelk, & Auer, 2006).

By Ty's senior year of high school, his body had significantly changed. His upper arms were skin and bone with almost no strength and significantly reduced movement. His thriving band had moved on without him. A new family nurse practitioner had arranged for a pediatric neurology visit for Ty in a research hospital two hours away. Estelle was frustrated with Hugh, Ty's dad. He was passive about Ty's medical situation and interacted less and less with the family.

The diagnostic news for Ty and his family was like a bomb exploding. One neurologist turned into a team of pediatric neurologists. After three days of testing, the diagnosis of Facioscapulohumeralis Muscular Dystrophy was delivered. Muscular Dystrophy (MD) is a group of inherited diseases in which the muscles that control movement (the voluntary muscles) progressively weaken. In Ty's type of MD, the muscles that move the face, shoulder blades, and upper arm bones are rendered useless. Ultimately, his walking, chewing, swallowing, and speaking will also become problematic. Ty, his mom and dad, and his younger brother were all completely at a loss in knowing how to process this tragic news or even begin to know how to plan for a life in the face of this destructive disease.

SOCIAL SUPPORT AND APPLIED INTERVENTIONS

Imagine all of the changes facing Ty's family. Imagine all of the loss. Imagine all of the need. Research that identifies active and translatable interventions for a patient like Ty and his family is a growing and developing area of work for communication scholars. Communication researchers have demonstrated that seeking and receiving support is a complex communicative process (Albrecht & Goldsmith, 2003). **Social support** is based on mutual reciprocation within the interpersonal relationship (Egbert, Koch, Coeling, & Ayers, 2006). The support patients receive from family members can enhance or undermine efforts to improve patient outcomes and overall quality of life (Rosland, Heisler, & Piette, 2012). Due to the hardships lay caregivers face when providing informal care to their loved ones, interventions have been developed to provide support to family caregivers and improve patient outcomes (Reinhard et al., 2008).

Many supportive interventions are provided to patients and caregivers individually; however, several now involve the patient and caregiver dyad by including content like patient care, relational maintenance, and self-care (Northouse, Katapodi, Song, Zhang, & Mood, 2010). Interventions aimed at supporting family caregivers of patients with chronic illnesses are often provided through psychoeducational, skills training, or therapeutic counseling approaches. The majority of caregiver intervention research, however, is delivered through a psychoeducational approach that simultaneously provides psychological and educational support and treats caregivers as secondary patients (Reinhard et al., 2008).

While tailored interventions yield significant improvement in caregiver and patient outcomes, today's caregiver support interventions are provided to caregivers in a standardized format rather than customized to meet their specific needs (Stoltz, Udén, & Willman, 2004). While supportive caregiver interventions significantly improve quality of life, coping skills, and self-efficacy and reduce caregiver burden, stress, and anxiety, the success of the intervention is dependent upon a host of factors that include who received it (caregiver only versus caregiver and patient), number of intervention sessions and duration of session, and medium of delivery (face-to-face or via technology; Northouse et al., 2010). Below are some key findings in caregiver and patient intervention research.

Family Communication

Family communication patterns and behaviors impact patient and caregiver outcomes in several ways. The patient outcomes influenced by family communication and behaviors include mortality, glycemic control, joint inflammation, blood pressure, and heart disease (Rosland et al., 2012). The diagnosis of an illness is disruptive to family functioning, and the family can react positively or negatively, which influences patient health. For example, family behaviors that demonstrate critical, overprotective, controlling, and distracting responses to illness are associated with negative patient outcomes (Rosland et al., 2012). Unresolved conflicts regarding the illness and illness management often result in angry responses, which decreases patient health (Rosland et al., 2012). Similar to patients, caregivers in a discordant family environment experience health deterioration in the form of depression, distress, burden, fatigue, and mortality (Reinhard et al., 2008). Reduced caregiver health and functioning can lead to poor patient health as a result of neglect, inadequate pain management, abuse, improper feeding, infection, and dehydration. New research exploring concrete practices that health professionals can employ for specific caregiver types is an exciting new extension of family communication patterns research (Wittenberg-Lyles, Goldsmith, Parker Oliver, Demiris, & Rankin, 2012).

Barbara Jones, Ph.D., MSW

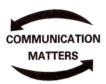

COMMUNICATION MATTERS

Not only do family support interventions address the needs of adult patients and family members, clinicians have also begun to focus on the children in these families. Dr. Barbara Jones, Associate Professor, Co-Director of the Institute for Grief, Loss, and Family Survival at the University of Texas at Austin School of Social Work, provides an intervention designed to support parental caregivers of children diagnosed with chronic illnesses. Family caregivers need honest, timely, and sensitive information to assist them in making the best medical decisions for their child. In pediatrics, the parents, grandparents, and family members are caregivers of children with cancer. Dr. Jones and her team work to guide family members by helping them to understand and support their child's emotions and experiences by (a) asking them to be open to the wide range of "normal" expressions of feeling from sick children and/or their siblings, (b) encouraging them to listen without judgment and to reassure the child that the parent will be there and will love them no matter what happens, (c) encouraging them to remind the child that nothing that has happened to them is their fault, and (d) supporting caregivers in having fun even in the midst of illness. Through her work, Dr. Jones has learned that children often protect their parents from their deepest feelings, especially when there is illness in the family.

Benefits of Support Interventions

The family environment and patient–caregiver communication behaviors significantly influence patient outcomes (Reinhard et al., 2008). Families who use problem-focused coping strategies and open communication help to improve patient and caregiver well-being (Rosland et al., 2012). Supportive family communication and behaviors that demonstrate illness attentiveness and symptom responsiveness,

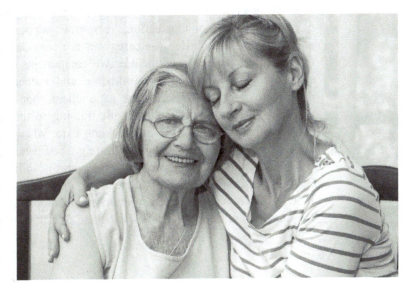

encourage self-reliance, and foster a cohesive family environment have been linked to improved patient outcomes (Rosland et al., 2012). These findings illustrate the importance of supportive intervention research. Caregivers who receive psychosocial interventions report decreased levels of depression and burden, and when patient and family relational issues are addressed, caregivers report decreased levels of anxiety (Martire, Lustig, Schulz, Miller, & Helgeson, 2004).

Interventions designed to improve family communication patterns and behaviors not only improve caregiver outcomes but also result in patient benefits such as improved self-management, adherence, and health outcomes (Rosland et al., 2012). When caregivers do not have adequate family support, they may receive interventions designed to improve their quality of life, which in turn protects the patient from an ill-equipped or emotionally distressed caregiver (Reinhard et al., 2008). Family interventions that attend to the caregiver and patient reveal significant findings in terms of decreased patient mortality (Martire et al., 2004). Notable reductions in patient depressive symptoms and caregiver anxiety result from interventions that focus on the relational dynamics between spouses/partners. The success of these family support interventions may be a result of the fact that spouses begin to provide more support and become less critical and because the act of participating in the intervention may be perceived as support in itself (Martire et al., 2004).

Design of Caregiver Interventions

Existing interventions that take a psychoeducational approach are designed to improve patient–caregiver communication, reciprocal support, illness management, and emotional well-being. Because caregivers are considered secondary patients, effective caregiver interventions include two components (Reinhard et al., 2008). First, efforts to improve caregiver well-being and reduce distress must be provided directly to support the caregiver as a client, not as an afterthought. Second, caregiver interventions should provide training so the caregiver can become more confident and competent when providing care, which indirectly reduces caregiver burden and improves patient health (e.g., self-esteem, depression, burden) and self-efficacy (e.g., confidence, mastery, control, ability to adapt; Reinhard et al., 2008; Zulman et al., 2012). Caregiver support interventions can be delivered individually or via group interventions; both modalities have been shown to lead to improvement in caregiver well-being and patient health outcomes (Reinhard et al., 2008).

CAREGIVER INTERVENTION RESEARCH

Caregiver intervention research has grown over the last two decades. During this time intervention approaches have consisted of psycho-education, skills training, and therapeutic counseling. A variety of media for the delivery of supportive materials have been tested, ranging from dyadic face-to-face sessions to larger support groups, and future research is beginning to explore the use of technology to facilitate social support. Although this work has shown improvement to caregiver quality of life and coping and has shown to reduce caregiver burden, it is not clear how social support and health are connected. Interventions vary in approach (patient and caregiver dyad or caregiver only), medium (in person or via technology), and duration (total hours, number of visits). Researchers have yet to explore race/ethnicity, cultural beliefs, and other communication factors that may predispose caregivers to accept or reject social support interventions.

Interventions are expensive, so in an effort to increase the cost-effectiveness and geographical dissemination to rural communities and families with lower socioeconomic status, supportive interventions originally provided face-to-face are now being adapted to interactive web-based formats (Reinhard et al., 2008; Zulman et al., 2012). Preliminary results of web-based interventions have revealed that caregivers and patients perceive the experience as positive, regardless of prior technological knowledge (Zulman et al., 2012). Similar to face-to-face formats, web-based interventions have resulted in improved health outcomes for both patients and caregivers (Demiris et al., 2012; Reinhard et al., 2008).

THE SCIENTIFIC APPROACH TO SOCIAL SUPPORT

In the scientific paradigm, social support is considered present and measurable. Overall, social scientists view social support as a mediating variable that positively influences health outcomes. The underlying assumption within this research approach is that social support improves health outcomes, thus increased social support results in better health. This approach focuses on the predictive nature of communication variables and their association with health outcomes, and it tests theory related to communication processes. With a focus on health outcomes related to social support, a great deal of empirical research investigates the patient or caregiver perspective of support and their health. Several measures have been created to assess social support

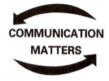

COMMUNICATION MATTERS

Debra Parker Oliver, Ph.D., MSW

Technological advancements continue to enhance channels through which caregivers can obtain support. While a significant amount of research focuses on facilitating online communities to support family caregivers and patients, Dr. Debra Parker Oliver, Professor at the University of Missouri, Department of Family and Community Medicine and members of the Telehospice project use video-based technology to enable hospice participation in routine hospice interdisciplinary team meetings. Hospice care is provided to terminally-ill patients and emphasizes quality of life. An interdisciplinary team composed of nurses, social workers, a chaplain, a medical director, and often a nutritionist work together to address the patient's and family's needs. To support hospice caregivers in their specific needs, Dr. Parker Oliver developed an intervention that equips hospice caregivers with tele-health technology to improve their quality of life, lower anxiety and depression, and assist them in pain management for their loved one in hospice. Hospice caregivers are linked via web conferencing software to their hospice caregiving team in order to participate in plans of care for their loved one, ask questions, and obtain emotional and informational support. The intervention has revealed promising results: Communicating with the hospice team has significantly lowered anxiety and depression and has changed caregiver perceptions and increased confidence related to pain management. To allow caregivers more frequent communication with the team and ongoing communication and support with other hospice caregivers, Dr. Parker Oliver plans to add a social media component to the intervention in her future work.

and social networks, and each is designed to collect a person's perception of social support (see Additional Resources on this text's companion website).

To account for health outcomes, or consequences, associated with social support, researchers in nursing and social work have explored the influence of social support on the likelihood to seek and obtain treatment, decision making, information-seeking behavior, evaluation and assessment of supportive messages, caregiver burden, and caregiver quality of life (Glover et al., 2011; Pedersen, Olesen, Hansen, Zachariae, & Vedsted, 2011). Patient demographics, such as age, race, ethnicity, and gender, are key variables in further understanding how social support mediates health outcomes. Pedersen et al. (2011) found gender differences in social support effects, with women reporting shorter delay times between first symptom and clinic visit than men. Social support from extended family and peer groups has been shown to reduce the likelihood of treatment delays (Glover et al., 2011). Specific research on family caregiving has included the impact of social support on caregiver burden, caregiving experiences, caregiving mastery, and family attachment and structure. Lower levels of social support are significantly associated with caregiver burden (Majerovitz, 2007).

Given the increasing reliance on technology to facilitate supportive needs such as information and support, social network characteristics have also been extensively explored within the scientific paradigm. The size of the network, communication channels utilized to communicate with members of the social network, frequency

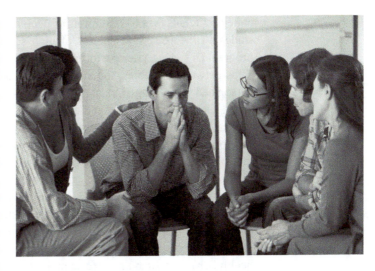

of contact, and duration of intervention/participation have all routinely been explored in computer-mediated social support such as online chat rooms, blogs, and social support groups (Rains & Young, 2009). Outcomes of social support that are associated with virtual contexts include coping, perceived significance in social support, and increased education or emotional support (Rains & Young, 2009). Additional research on sources of social support (Goldsmith & Albrecht, 2011) and differences in **weak-tie/strong-tie support networks** (Wright & Miller, 2010) reveal that computer-mediated contexts are changing the way we perceive, seek, and receive social support.

How is Social Support Related to Health?

Segrin and Passalacqua (2010) explored how and why social support is related to health. Using a theory of loneliness and health outcomes, they considered various functional mediators that might provide an explanation. A functional mediator is a variable that explains the relationship between an independent variable (social support) and an outcome variable (health). For this study, the presence of a social support network and frequency of contact with network members comprised the measure of social support. The goal of the study was to test the hypotheses that social support influences loneliness, that loneliness influences perceived stress and health behaviors, and all of these variables ultimately influence general health.

The researchers gave a survey that included measures of social network size and contact, loneliness, stress, social support, general health, health behaviors, and demographic items to 265 adults that they recruited from three settings: undergraduate college students ($n = 61$), referrals of people over 30 years of age from undergraduate students ($n = 163$), and parents of high school students enrolled in a youth sports program ($n = 41$). After performing a series of statistical tests to assess the relationships between variables, the authors found that the *number of close relationships* a person had was strongly and negatively associated with loneliness (i.e., more relationships, less loneliness) but that the *amount of contact* with social network members did not really matter. They found that social support from a significant other, from friends, and from family was all related to general health and, more important, that loneliness mediated those relationships. In other words, the more social support people had from their significant others, friends, and family members, the less lonely they were, and the less lonely they were, the more generally healthy they were. Further, they found that perceived stress mediated the relationship between loneliness and health: The lonelier that people were, the more perceived stress they felt, and the more perceived stress they felt, the less healthy they were. The researchers also found that specific health behaviors such as exercise and diet mediated the relationship between loneliness and health (less lonely, more healthy behaviors; more healthy behaviors, more general health).

THE INTERPRETIVE APPROACH TO SOCIAL SUPPORT

Placing yourself in another person's shoes is the aim of interpretive studies that investigate social support. So, from the point of view of participants enduring a particular context and experience, like Ty's story for instance, we go forward to pursue a subjective understanding of social support. The intent is not to impose the researcher's interpretation, but rather to capture the interpretations of understanding experienced and expressed by participants. Very common in this kind of research is to utilize, in some way, the language of participants themselves to better capture in-depth knowledge about social support in the context of illness.

A growing area of social support research has to do with how communication processes are used to manage **uncertainty**. Because gathering the experience of research participants is the priority of interpretive work, clinicians also play a substantial role in identifying the research problem, describing the elements and characteristics of a problem, and working with patients and caregivers to develop a solution. Interpretive work can advance what we know about social support as this research *contextualizes* health and social support by disease and values the subjectivity of persons or groups. This class of research emphasizes that humans have free will and choice, that social reality is produced in everyday life, and that theory is most productively engaged through the observation and interpretation of people's experiences.

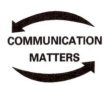

Christina Puchalski, MD, MS

One way to approach assessing social support is to consider the four quality-of-life domains. Dr. Christina Puchalski, a Professor of Medicine and Health Sciences at the George Washington University School of Medicine and Director of the George Washington Institute for Spirituality and Health (GWish), has devoted much of her career and research to integrating spiritual care into education across disciplines. Dr. Puchalski considers spiritual needs one of the most pressing communication and support needs in providing caregiver support. She has developed a spiritual assessment tool called FICA, which assesses patient and family spirituality along four dimensions (Faith, Importance/Influence, Community, Address/Application). FICA is a brief quantitative questionnaire that is used in a multitude of clinical settings to explore the spiritual beliefs and needs of caregivers and identify sources of support. The measure not only provides a quantitative score for spirituality needs but also can lead to discussions about care preferences and life goals and readily be incorporated into the flow of conversation. On the basis of her research, Dr. Puchalski believes that clinicians should be educated to recognize that spirituality is important to patient and caregiver care and learn to communicate with both patients and caregivers about spiritual beliefs, needs, and well-being.

Interpretive communication scholars Terry Albrecht and Mara Adelman proffered the first substantial research exploring and explaining social support and communication. Their work explored the dimensions and barriers inherent in communicating social support and the idea that "doing" support is a process inextricably woven into communication behavior (Albrecht & Adelman, 1987). Social support can aid family and caregivers in uncertainty management (Ford, Babrow, & Stohl, 1996). Interpretive research has established the social role for people struggling to navigate the changing identity and health of loved ones (Babrow & Mattson, 2011). Interpretive work in the areas of hospice and end of life gave rise to a further understanding in the social scientific community that families and caregivers are the "variables" of care that have the most impact on patient outcomes and clinical costs (Waldrop, Milch, & Skretny, 2005). This work not only paved the way for intervention and quality outcomes but

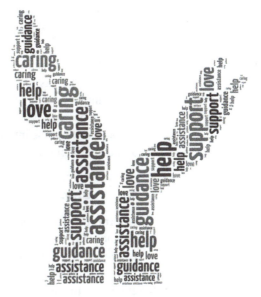

also established that health and illness are socially constructed by those involved in the communication surrounding health and illness. **Family communication patterns,**

problematic integration, communication privacy management, and **uncertainty management** constructs have been notably advanced by interpretive methods used in the pursuit of social support knowledge.

Because of interpretive work in health communication, our knowledge about social support has moved forward in ways not possible with other research approaches. The detailed understanding and focus on support experiences and how those experiences contribute to decision making and knowledge construction for caregivers are topics of growing study. Social support exploration has established a breadth of knowledge about health behaviors and challenges and barriers to social support in a variety of support contexts. This research has also expanded our understanding of relationship patterns and attributes that influence other's actions and beliefs that contribute to health actions/behaviors. Additionally, the caregiver's perceptions of healthcare and its practices, and the concerns of family, lay caregivers, and members of a patient's/ caregiver's social network, have been identified as key components to understanding social support.

Although work on **quality of life** has been ongoing in multiple disciplines using multiple perspectives, interpretive work showcases unique cases and understandings of the meaning of quality of life throughout illness. Studying the frequency and content of social support discussions has unlocked a wealth of knowledge about clinician patterns and family expectations, and it has similarly identified the factors central to illness coping strategies and caregiver roles.

Thanks to interdisciplinary research, a great deal is now known about clinical practice professional areas including allied health, mental health, medicine, social work, and chaplaincy (see Recommended Readings at the end of this chapter). Nursing, for instance, has elaborated on the challenges of patients, families, teams, and other populations thanks to the interpretive pathways offered through interviewing, focus groups, and ethnographies.

Communication in Families with Serious Illness

Communication avoidance is prevalent among families when a member has been diagnosed with a potentially terminal illness. Zhang and Siminoff (2003) qualitatively examined the decision-making experiences of Stage III and Stage IV lung cancer patients and their family members to learn more about family communication avoidance. Due to the significant time it takes to collect qualitative data, interpretive studies typically consist of small homogeneous samples; this study, however, examined a relatively large heterogeneous sample. Participants consisted of spouses, children, siblings, and other relatives, allowing a comprehensive definition of family, and the caregiver participants were either primary or secondary, encouraging a broad examination of caregiving experiences.

Initially, the researchers conducted focus groups with 13 participants; however, they changed the method for data collection to telephone interviews because the participants' fragile health kept many of them from attending focus groups. Overall, the researchers collected data from 77 participants from 26 different families (37 patients, 40 caregivers), which included caregiving triads (patient, primary caregiver, secondary caregiver) and dyads (patient, primary caregiver). The investigators questioned participants using a semi-structured interview protocol designed to resemble disease progression. They conducted follow-up interviews with 20 participants for further clarification. All focus group discussions and phone interviews were audio-recorded and later transcribed.

The analysis involved three steps. First, the authors read through each transcript and identified emerging themes within conversational paragraphs. Next, they used qualitative analysis software to create themes, and they sorted the conversational paragraphs into the corresponding nodes. Further analysis enabled the authors to collapse the themes into overarching hierarchal categories. After sorting transcripts into themes, the authors revisited the transcripts and identified issues specific to each theme. Finally, they defined the issues and used them for identifying the most common themes, substantiating evidence, and relationships among themes.

The results illustrated the lack of communication between caregivers and patients regarding specific issues related to the disease. The authors identified a "phenomenon of silence," which they defined as the absence of vocalized concerns among family members regarding cancer-related issues. Psychological distress, attempts at mutual protection, and an emphasis on positive thinking served to shape communication avoidance between family members. Overall, 65% of the families in the sample experienced communication difficulties. Psychological distress (e.g., depression, fear, anxiety, anguish) impacted caregiver and patient communication regarding

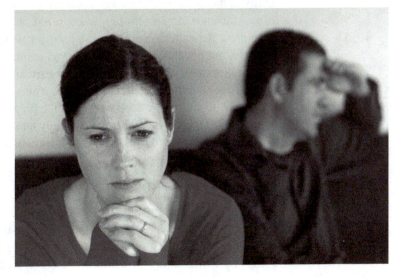

cancer, treatment options, and feelings. Participants reported a need to assuage both their own and the others' psychological distress, thus concealing concerns from one another.

This article illustrates the ways in which a person's health can impact family communication and related support efforts. It exemplifies how communication avoidance is used as a means of maintaining or even increasing uncertainty. For these families, to maintain or increase uncertainty means to hold on to hope. Gaining certainty, on the other hand, would involve acknowledging the fact that late-stage lung cancer often results in death and would emphasize the need to discuss the patient's end-of-life preferences. Indeed, results showed that only 26% of these families had discussed end-of-life issues and concerns, and only 12% had discussed hospice.

THE CRITICAL–CULTURAL APPROACH TO SOCIAL SUPPORT

Since the 1990s, a call has been made from voices in the subdiscipline of health communication to expand the role of critical and cultural guidance in the scholarship produced. This critique described health communication as disproportionately dominated by social psychological models of theory and behavior and as entrenched in sender-based examinations of response (Lupton, 1994). This awareness triggered further investigations into the practices of health education and launched ongoing debates about the connection between health literacy and health disparities.

As growing populations (the aged, the poor, the mentally ill, the chronically ill, the family of the ill) are finding ways to access healthcare, their health literacy and ability to pay for care are increasingly recognized as crucial to clinical communication. Examining the materials created and used for work with low health literacy groups, championing patient- and family-centered communication, and positioning patients and families as more active and powerful partners in care advances their role as more active owners of their health (Ishikawa & Yano, 2008). In this way, critical–cultural work in health and social support is essential for all people needing care as the climate of a managed care system changes radically and as progressively more stressors and demands are positioned back onto the patient and family.

The Needs of Young Caregivers

The phenomenon of young caregivers, those under age 18, is a global phenomenon that has, until recently, received little attention in the research literature. Many young caregivers find themselves in the caretaking role as very young children, often in the event of parental injury or catastrophic chronic illness. Caring activities can range from minimal assistance with the activities of daily living through sole responsibility for all activities of care. Life factors contributing to the level of care intensity that a young person might experience include socioeconomic status of family, support of family and friends, marriage status of parents, and the availability of access to a child-care provider in the home (Aldridge, 2006).

McAndrew, Warne, Fallon, and Moran (2012) sought to give voice to the children who have no platform and to share their caregiver needs. The researchers coordinated two events in which young caregiver representatives shared their caregiving needs and experiences with those professionals positioned to promote the lives of young caregivers faced with the care of seriously mentally ill parents or guardians.

The method of the piece exemplifies participatory action research. The researchers organized and hosted two large gatherings in the United Kingdom to bring together young caregivers and a multiagency audience to consider the scope of potential collaborations, as well as prioritize tasks for increasing support to young caregivers. The two large events began with formal presentations from young caregivers 13–17 years of age. These participants were identified as a result of their previous involvement in support groups for young caregivers. An invited audience of approximately 50 professionals representing education, foster care, youth detention, mental health, nurses, and social workers attended. Following the formal presentations, and on the basis of a brief question and answer session with the audience, the young caregiver participants along with the researchers identified topic areas for break out table discussions. Small groups at each table consisted of professionals from a mix of agencies (education, foster care, detention, etc.), as well as young caregiver participants. A flip chart and topics of discussion were available for each small group. Each group generated a network of ideas and shared their populated flip charts over a break, during which all attendees could circulate among other teams and add feedback. Networks of narratives were built, culminating in a final session with all groups combined. The data for this project resulted from the formal presentations delivered at the

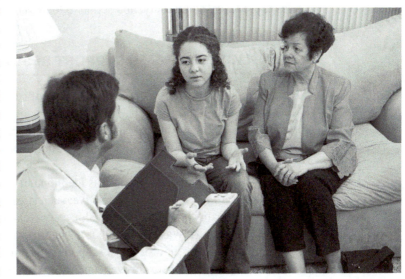

beginning of each of the two gatherings and corresponding question and answer periods.

Participants, along with the research team, identified themes of concern and need for young caregivers of the mentally ill. Themes included (a) exclusion from professional decision making, (b) ignoring the future of the young caregiver, (c) a lack of appropriate support for young caregivers, and (d) the recognition of young caregivers. In accord with the critical–cultural perspective, of central concern in this work was creating an opportunity to redistribute opportunity and power to a group—in this case child caregivers—who had a muted voice. The article comprehensively and effectively creates a picture of deficit and disparity for this group of children left to care for an adult without relief, support, or tools.

This piece is compelling and pulls strongly at the heart, despite the fact that it is written as a formal research artifact. The underserved nature of the young caregiver population is not only troubling but also compels us to want to immediately do something to relieve their plight. These are indications of an effective critical research effort. Quotes from the young caregivers' formal presentations are the launching point to the results section. The authors integrated short remarks to clarify the impact that caring for a mentally ill parent has had on these children's lives. For example, "I have no one to talk to; I look after him, but who will look after me" and "I hate my life, and I am 15" are chilling realities for the reader to face when it comes to the social isolation and low level of personal well-being these children endure. Since there are few structures and practices in place to identify and create support resources for them, this piece of research champions the young caregivers' concerns in a way that directly lends credence, community, and action to their needs.

CONFLICTING SOCIAL SUPPORT RESULTS

Where might your interests fit into this world of social support communication interventions? There are many challenges and areas of social support discovery for new researchers. Since we have examined each of the three research perspectives, we can now consider the differing results and opportunities for more learning.

Research about family caregiving has identified considerable stressors faced by those providing care for an ill or aging relative; such stressors can exact a significant toll on caregivers' quality of life, physical health, and psychological well-being (Wilder, Parker Oliver, Demiris, & Washington, 2008). The majority of research has led to an overwhelmingly positive view of social support (Goldsmith, 2004) and resulted in a body of research focused almost exclusively on the positive aspects of social support for family caregivers. Positive outcomes of supportive conversations and networks suggest that feedback encourages healthy behaviors, communication assists in seeking and acquiring health information, and communication can also influence tangible health support and coping assistance (Goldsmith & Albrecht, 2011). However, Goldsmith (2004) has noted that the term social support is often used as "an umbrella term" representing a general belief that social relationships are linked to well-being. The large body of social scientific research on social support accounts for this generalization within the literature.

When we take into account other research on support and relationships, it becomes clear that social support is not always perceived as supportive or helpful by those who receive the so-called support (Goldsmith, 2004), and potential dilemmas of social support result from the difference between a person's goals of support and those of support givers, resulting in an increase in stress and anxiety (Brashers, Goldsmith, & Hsieh, 2002). Likewise, social support findings in the computer-mediated context (e.g., text messaging, Facebook, blogs) have yielded mixed findings. For example, although researchers have commonly explored the impact of social support on a person's quality of life (physical and mental well-being), there has been little evidence for the benefits of participating in an online support group (see Rains & Young, 2009). While researchers have proposed higher social support benefits from strong tie support members, research has not clearly supported this conclusion (see Ackerson & Viswanath, 2009).

DIRECTIONS FOR FUTURE RESEARCH

The health professionals featured in this chapter represent the best of what social support research can offer: targeted and effective interventions of practical and emotional support for patients and families. Ty's family requires a variety of social support: physical, psychological, social, and spiritual. Despite these needs, findings on social ties and health communication are not clearly understood (Ackerson & Viswanath, 2009). Although research has concluded that family caregivers need instrumental (e.g., respite care), emotional (e.g., counseling services), and informational support (e.g., educational resources; Kutner et al., 2009; MacLeod, Skinner, & Low, 2012), a comprehensive review of the caregiving literature presents mixed results regarding social support benefits.

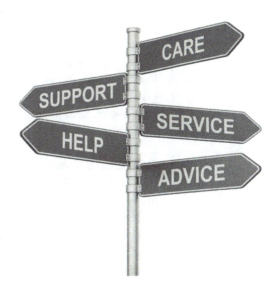

Although the "more is better" social support hypothesis is embedded in clinical practice approaches (i.e., clinicians offering a multitude of resources to all patients/families), research suggests that even well-intended acts of support may not be perceived as helpful by recipients and that an awareness of support receipt may, in fact, be harmful in some instances. Many studies have failed to consider whether received social support was provided without prompting by the person experiencing the stressor or whether the person solicited the support. This consideration segues into the literature on social support-seeking that paints an even less clear picture, with some research showing support-seeking to be an effective coping strategy and other research suggesting it is actually associated with higher levels of psychological distress (see Thoits, 1995, for a review).

Among the important factors that may impact social support are race/ethnicity, cultural beliefs, marital function, and predisposition to depressive symptoms (Rosland et al., 2012). Researchers should consider these and other specific factors such as variance in caregiver knowledge and skills, the caregiver–patient relationship, personality traits, caregiver health, stage of the disease, competing role demands, and hours of care when developing and testing interventions to support patients and caregivers (Reinhard et al., 2008; Rosland et al., 2012). Thus far, the majority of family communication research in our discipline has been scientific and atheoretical, with little research detailing the constraints within family relationships and changes in relationships over time, which may impede social support (Vangelisti, 2006).

Future research is needed to (a) understand the role of communication in nursing in serious, complex, and terminal illness, (b) identify pivotal points for healthcare provider communication training, and (c) develop undergraduate, graduate, and continuing nurse education curricula that address the communication exigencies at each level of education (Wittenberg-Lyles, Goldsmith, & Ragan, 2011). More research is needed to understand the perceived barriers between patients and caregivers that inhibit relational maintenance strategies during care (Wittenberg-Lyles, Demiris, Parker Oliver, & Burt, 2011), as well as further work to better understand the caregiver health literacy limitations of written and oral instruction on drug labels and administration of medications (Wittenberg-Lyles et al., 2013).

CONCLUSION

Six months following Ty's diagnosis, the trauma of his health situation and its impact on the family was made clear. Ty, along with a group of males from his high school, was arrested for breaking and entering into four homes in his small town. At the same time, his parents, married for 24 years, separated. Estelle was left to manage Ty's legal and medical matters alone. A clinical trial to slow the degradation of his muscle loss would start in one month. This opportunity would require a four-hour drive three times a week for the next year. Estelle wondered if she would have to once again feed her son all of his meals, bathe him, and assist him with his bathroom needs. These thoughts of loss for her young son were overwhelming. Her soon-to-be ex-husband had been diagnosed with a much milder case of MD when Ty was only 6. Hugh had passed this disease to Ty.

The needs of Ty, his parents, and his brother are profound as they all are thrown headlong into a crisis of health. The normalcy of life as they knew it is gone. They all now require social support, but how will they find it? Who will offer it? It is, in large part, the role of health-care professionals to find effective ways to relieve and comfort this patient and family. But without knowledge of family type, the coping tendencies of a patient—and in Ty's case a very young patient—and an understanding of the ongoing challenges of this family, health professionals are rendered impotent in finding appropriate support interventions to aid this family.

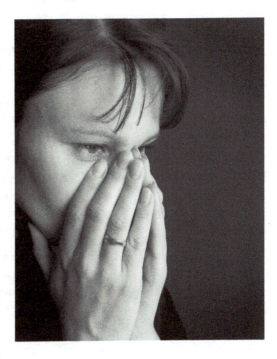

As part of the standard of care delivery in any healthcare context, social support plays an increasingly vital role. Productive experiences can emerge when communication with patients and family members emphasizes what can be done for symptom control and emotional support, realistic goals are set, and day-to-day living is the focus (Clayton, Butow, Arnold, & Tattersall, 2005; Ragan et al., 2008). Many resources must be presented to assist a family and patient with the instrumental requirements of coping with an advancing disease, as well as offering the emotional support necessary for the patient or family to persevere in times when they feel otherwise depleted of hope, esteem, identity, and normalcy.

DISCUSSION QUESTIONS

1. What social support needs for Ty and his family could be studied and identified?
2. What research perspective would you suggest in performing research about Ty and his family as they endure what will be decades of intensive medical care for Muscular Dystrophy?

3. Do you think that all research perspectives provide opportunities for translational research in social support? Can you create a list of potential social support research ideas/needs for each research tradition?

IN-CLASS ACTIVITIES

1. Split the class into groups of four to six and have them read the following passage:

   > *Mary is a 30-year-old single mother of two young boys, ages 8 and 12. In the last year, her mother, age 52, was diagnosed with early onset Alzheimer Disease, and she has deteriorated rapidly. Mary has had to take a second job working nights to be able to afford healthcare for her mother. In addition to taking care of her two sons, Mary is responsible for all of her mother's care at home. Mary is overwhelmed.*

   Within their groups, have the students discuss ideas for providing support to Mary. Have one student from each group share a strategy or two with the class.

2. Choose a caregiver experience blog from the Internet (you can find several here: http://www.rightathome.net/blog/8-great-caregiver-blogs). Read several posts. Answer the following questions:

   (a) What stands out about this particular caregiver's experience?
   (b) What most surprised you?
   (c) Is the description representative of what you thought the experience would be like?
   (d) What would you like to ask the blogger if you could? Why?

RECOMMENDED READINGS

Moore, C. D., & Cook, K. M. (2011). Promoting and measuring family caregiver self-efficacy in caregiver-physician interactions. *Social Work in Health Care*, *50*, 801–814.

From scholars in social work, this article introduces the Perceived Efficacy in Caregiver-Physician Interactions (PECPI) measure as a tool for social workers to promote caregiver self-efficacy.

Pedersen, A. F., Olesen, F., Hansen, R. P., Zachariae, R., & Vedsted, P. (2011). Social support, gender and patient delay. *British Journal of Cancer*, *104*, 1249–1255.

Patient delay, the time between first symptom and actual clinical visit, is explored in relation to perceived social support and gender; does the perception of social support and being female reduce patient delay?

Rosland, A., Heisler, M., & Piette, J. D. (2012). The impact of family behaviors and communication patterns on chronic illness outcomes: A systematic review. *Journal of Behavioral Medicine, 35*, 221–239.

A systematic review of published medical research is used to explore the connection between family communication patterns and patient outcomes.

REFERENCES

Ackerson, L. K., & Viswanath, K. (2009). Communication inequalities, social determinants, and intermittent smoking in the 2003 Health Information National Trends Survey. *Preventing Chronic Disease, 6*, A40. Retrieved from http://www.cdc.gov/pcd/issues/2009/apr/08_0076.htm

Albrecht, T., & Adelman, M. (1987). *Communicating about social support.* Thousand Oaks, CA: Sage Publishing.

Albrecht, T., & Goldsmith, D. J. (2003). Social support, social networks, and health. In T. Thompson, A. Dorsey, K. Miller, & R. Parrott (Eds.), *Handbook of health communication* (pp. 263–284). Mahway, NJ: Lawrence Erlbaum Associates.

Aldridge, J. (2006). The experiences of children living with and caring for parents with mental illness. *Child Abuse Review, 15*, 79–88.

American Association of Retired Persons Policy Institute. (2011). Valuing the invaluable: 2011 update. *The Growing Contributions and Costs of Family Caregiver.* Washington, DC: Author.

Babrow, A. S., & Mattson, M. (2011). Building health communication theories in the 21st century. In T. L. Thompson, R. Parrott, & J. F. Nussbaum (Eds.), *The Routledge handbook of health communication* (2nd ed., pp. 18–35). New York: Routledge.

Bakas, T., Li, Y., Habermann, B., McLennon, S. M., & Weaver, M. T. (2011). Developing a cost template for a nurse-led stroke caregiver intervention program. *Clinical Nurse Specialist, 25*, 41–46.

Bevan, J. L., & Pecchioni, L. L. (2008). Understanding the impact of family caregiver cancer literacy on patient health outcomes. *Patient Education and Counseling, 71*, 356–364.

Brashers, D., Goldsmith, D. J., & Hsieh, E. (2002). Information seeking and avoiding in health contexts. *Human Communication Research, 28*, 258–271.

Clayton, J. M., Butow, P. N., Arnold, R. M., & Tattersall, M. H. (2005). Fostering coping and nurturing hope when discussing the future with terminally ill cancer patients and their caregivers. *Cancer, 103*, 1965–1975.

Demiris, G., Parker Oliver, D., Wittenberg-Lyles, E., Washington, K., Doorenbos, A., Rue, T., & Berry, D. (2012). A non-inferiority trial of a problem solving intervention for hospice caregivers: In person vs. videophone. *Journal of Palliative Medicine, 15*(6), 653–660.

Egbert, N., Koch, L., Coeling, H., & Ayers, D. (2006). The role of social support in the family and community integration of right-hemisphere stroke survivors. *Health Communication, 20*, 45–55.

Eggly, S., Penner, L., Albrecht, T. L., Cline, R. J., Foster, T., Naughton, M., . . . Ruckdeschel, J. C. (2006). Discussing bad news in the outpatient oncology clinic: Rethinking current communication guidelines. *Journal of Clinical Oncology, 24*, 716–719.

Ferrell, B. (1996). *Suffering.* Sudbury, MA: Jones and Barlett.

Ford, L. A., Babrow, A. S., & Stohl, C. (1996). Social support messages and the management of uncertainty in the experience of breast cancer: An application of problematic integration theory. *Communication Monographs, 63*, 189–207.

Fox, S., & Brenner, J. (2012). *Family caregivers online.* Washington, DC: Pew Research Center. Retrieved from http://pewinternet.org/Reports/2012/Caregivers-online.aspx

Gebhardt, M. C., McGehee, L. A., Grindel, C. G., & Testani-Dufour, L. (2011). Caregiver and nurse hopes for recovery of patients with acquired brain injury. *Rehabilitation Nursing, 36*, 3–12.

Given, B., Wyatt, G., Given, C., Sherwood, P., Gift, A., DeVoss, D., & Rahbar, M. (2004). Burden and depression among caregivers of patients with cancer at the end of life. *Oncology Nursing Forum, 31*, 1105–1117.

Glover, R., Shenoy, P. J., Kharod, G. A., Schaefer, A., Bumpers, K., Berry, J. T., & Flowers, C. R. (2011). Patterns of social support among lymphoma patients considering stem cell transplantation. *Social Work in Health Care, 50*, 815–827.

Goldsmith, D., & Albrecht, T. (2011). Social support, social networks, and health. In T. Thompson, R. Parrott, & J. Nussbaum (Eds.), *The Routledge handbook of health communication* (2nd ed., pp. 335–348). New York: Routledge.

Goldsmith, D. J. (2004). *Communicating social support.* New York: Cambridge University Press.

Gonyea, J. G., Paris, R., & de Saxe Zerden, L. (2008). Adult daughters and aging mothers: The role of guilt in the experience of caregiver burden. *Aging and Mental Health, 12*, 559–567.

Hauser, J. M., & Kramer, B. J. (2004). Family caregivers in palliative care. *Clinics in Geriatric Medicine, 20*, 671–688, vi.

Ishikawa, H., & Yano, E. (2008). Patient health literacy and participation in the health care process. *Health Expectations, 11*, 113–122.

Kramer, B. J., Boelk, A. Z., & Auer, C. (2006). Family conflict at the end of life: Lessons learned in a model program for vulnerable older adults. *Journal of Palliative Medicine, 9*, 791–801.

Kutner, J., Kilbourn, K. M., Costenaro, A., Lee, C. A., Nowels, C., Vancura, J. L., . . . Keech, T. E. (2009). Support needs of informal hospice caregivers: A qualitative study. *Journal of Palliative Medicine, 12*, 1101–1104.

Lau, D. T., Berman, R., Halpern, L., Pickard, A. S., Schrauf, R., & Witt, W. (2010). Exploring factors that influence informal caregiving in medication management for home hospice patients. *Journal of Palliative Medicine, 13*, 1085–1090.

Lupton, D. (1994). Toward the development of critical health communication praxis. *Health Communication, 6*, 55–67.

MacLeod, A., Skinner, M. W., & Low, E. (2012). Supporting hospice volunteers and caregivers through community-based participatory research. *Health & Social Care in the Community, 20*, 190–198.

Majerovitz, S. D. (2007). Predictors of burden and depression among nursing home family caregivers. *Aging and Mental Health, 11*, 323–329.

Maniaci, M. J., Heckman, M. G., & Dawson, N. L. (2008). Functional health literacy and understanding of medications at discharge. *Mayo Clinic Proceedings, 83*, 554–558.

Martire, L. M., Lustig, A. P., Schulz, R., Miller, G. E., & Helgeson, V. S. (2004). Is it beneficial to involve a family member? A meta-analysis of psychosocial interventions for chronic illness. *Health Psychology, 23*, 599–611.

McAndrew, S., Warne, T., Fallon, D., & Moran, P. (2012). Young, gifted, and caring: A project narrative of young carers, their mental health, and getting them involved in education, research and practice. *International Journal of Mental Health Nursing, 21*, 12–19.

National Alliance for Caregiving and AARP. (2004). *Caregiving in the U.S.* Retrieved from http://www.caregiving.org/. . ./Caregiving_in_the_US_2009_full_report.pdf

Nielsen-Bohlman, L., Panzer, A. M., & Kindig, D. A. (Eds.). (2004). *Health literacy: A prescription to end confusion*. Institute of Medicine (U.S.) Committee on Health Literacy. Washington, DC: The National Academies Press. Retrieved from http://books.nap.edu/catalog/10883.html

Northouse, L. L., Katapodi, M. C., Song, L., Zhang, L., & Mood, D. W. (2010). Interventions with family caregivers of cancer patients: Meta-analysis of randomized trials. *CA: A Cancer Journal for Clinicians, 60*, 317–339.

Parker, C., Teel, C., Leenerts, M. H., & Macan, A. (2011). A theory-based self-care talk intervention for family caregiver-nurse partnerships. *Journal of Gerontological Nursing, 37*, 30–35.

Pedersen, A. F., Olesen, F., Hansen, R. P., Zachariae, R., & Vedsted, P. (2011). Social support, gender and patient delay. *British Journal of Cancer, 104*, 1249–1255.

Ragan, S., Wittenberg-Lyles, E. M., Goldsmith, J., & Sanchez-Reilly, S. (2008). *Communication as comfort: Multiple voices in palliative care*. New York: Routledge.

Rains, S., & Young, V. (2009). A meta-analysis of research on formal computer-mediated support groups: Examining group characteristics and health outcomes. *Journal of Health Communication, 35*, 309–336.

Reinhard, S. C., Given, B., Petlick, N.H, & Bemis, A. (2008). Supporting family caregivers in providing care. In R. G. Hughes (Ed.), *Patient safety and quality: An evidence-based handbook for nurses* (Chapter 14). Rockville, MD: Agency for Healthcare Research and Quality. Retrieved from http://www.ncbi.nlm.nih.gov/books/NBK2665

Rivera, H. R. (2009). Depression symptoms in cancer caregivers. *Clinical Journal of Oncology Nursing, 13*, 195–202.

Rokach, A., Matalon, R., Safarov, A., & Bercovitch, M. (2007). The loneliness experience of the dying and of those who care for them. *Palliative & Supportive Care, 5*, 153–159.

Rosland, A., Heisler, M., & Piette, J. D. (2012). The impact of family behaviors and communication patterns on chronic illness outcomes: A systematic review. *Journal of Behavioral Medicine, 35*, 221–239.

Roter, D. L. (2011). Oral literacy demand of health care communication: Challenges and solutions. *Nursing Outlook, 59*, 79–84.

Segrin, C., & Passalacqua, S. A. (2010). Functions of loneliness, social support, health behaviors, and stress in association with poor health. *Health Communication, 25*, 312–322.

Sherman, D. W. (1998). Reciprocal suffering: The need to improve family caregivers' quality of life through palliative care. *Journal of Palliative Medicine, 1*, 357–366.

SmithBattle, L. (2009). Pregnant with possibilities: Drawing on hermeneutic thought to reframe home-visiting programs for young mothers. *Nursing Inquiry, 16*, 191–200.

Stoltz, P., Udén, G., & Willman, A. (2004). Support for family carers who care for an elderly person at home—a systematic literature review. *Scandinavian Journal of Caring Sciences, 18*, 111–119.

Swanberg, J. (2006). Making it work: Informal caregiving, cancer, and employment. *Journal of Psychosocial Oncology, 24*, 1–18.

The Joint Commission. (2009). *"What did the doctor say?": Improving health literacy to protect patient safety.* Oakbrook Terrace, IL.

Thoits, P. A. (1995). Stress, coping, and social support processes: Where are we? What next? *Journal of Health and Social Behavior, 35*(Extra Issue), 53–79.

Vangelisti, A. (2006). Foreward: Variations and challenges. In D. Braithwaite & L. Baxter (Eds.), *Engaging theories in family communication: Multiple perspectives* (pp. xi–xviii). Thousand Oaks, CA: Sage.

Waldrop, D., Milch, R., & Skretny, J. (2005). Understanding family responses to life-limiting illness: In-depth interviews with hospice patients and their family members. *Journal of Palliative Care, 21*, 88–96.

Wilder, H., Parker Oliver, D., Demiris, G., & Washington, K. T. (2008). Informal hospice caregiving: The toll on quality of life. *Journal of Social Work in End-of-Life and Palliative Care, 4*, 312–332.

Wittenberg-Lyles, E., Demiris, G., Parker Oliver, D., & Burt, S. (2011). Reciprocal suffering: Caregiver concerns during hospice care. *Journal of Pain and Symptom Management, 41*, 383–393.

Wittenberg-Lyles, E., Goldsmith, J., Parker Oliver, D., Demiris, G., Kruse, R. L., & Van Stee, S. (2013). Exploring oral literacy with hospice family caregivers. *Journal of Pain and Symptom Management, 13*, 111–115.

Wittenberg-Lyles, E., Goldsmith, J., Parker Oliver, D., Demiris, G., & Rankin, A. (2012). Targetting communication interventions to decrease oncology family caregiver burden. *Seminars in Nursing Oncology, 28*, 262–270.

Wittenberg-Lyles, E., Goldsmith, J., & Ragan, S. (2011). The shift to early palliative care: A typology of illness journeys and the role of nursing. *Clinical Journal of Oncology Nursing, 15*, 304–310.

Wittenberg-Lyles, E., Goldsmith, J., Ragan, S., & Sanchez-Reilly, S. (2010). *Dying with comfort: Family illness narratives and early palliative care.* Cresskill, New Jersey: Hampton Press.

Wright, K., & Miller, C. (2010). A measure of weak-tie/strong-tie support network preference. *Communication Monographs, 77*, 500–517.

Zhang, A. Y., & Siminoff, L. A. (2003). Silence and cancer: Why do families and patients fail to communicate? *Health Communication, 15*(4), 415–429.

Zulman, D. M., Schafenacker, A., Barr, K. L., Moore, I. T., Fisher, J., McCurdy, K., . . . & Northouse, L. (2012). Adapting an in-person patient-caregiver communication intervention to a tailored web-based format. *Psycho-Oncology, 21*, 336–341.

4

Providers' Perspectives on Health Communication: Influences, Processes, and Outcomes

Melinda Villagran and
Melinda R. Weathers

Is healthcare a science or an art? Is the job of a healthcare provider to conduct tests and experiments like scientists, or do they also interpret symptoms and feelings and build relationships with patients? If healthcare providers were nothing more than a source of health information, we could skip the human doctor and stick with Dr. Google. If our relationships with providers did not matter, we could visit any doctor, nurse, or pharmacist and have the exact same experience. In reality, our relationships with healthcare providers are some of the most important and productive relationships in our lives. Providers greet us when we are born and care for us until the day we die. Providers engage in the science and art of medicine. They discuss evidence from scientific research to create shared meaning with their patients.

Communication is central to the study of healthcare providers because our relationships with providers create the foundation for our healthcare experience. There is no test, no surgery, and no piece of technology that can be used with maximum effectiveness to heal patients unless it is coupled with effective information sharing, problem solving, coordination, and affiliation among patients, providers, and caregivers (Jones & Stubbe, 2004). A lack of competent communication on the part of providers can lead to medical errors, uninformed patients, and inconsistent patient outcomes (Epstein & Street, 2007).

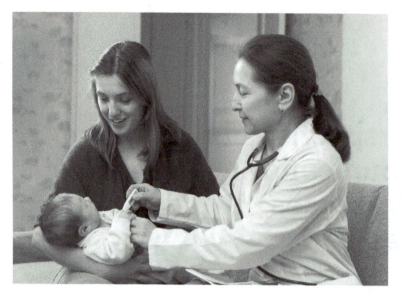

This chapter explores the most significant issues, influences, and challenges of healthcare provider communication. We begin by discussing the term **provider**, used as a way to describe and discuss characteristics of various healthcare professions.

WHAT'S IN A NAME? CLINICIANS, PHYSICIANS, AND PROVIDERS

Much has been written about the use of the term *provider* as a generic way to describe all healthcare professionals. In a blog post on the topic, Ofri (2011) recalled,

> I can't quite remember when the term "provider" slipped into the hospital lexicon. It was perhaps 10 years ago, when our hospital started hiring physician assistants and nurse practitioners to share the clinical load. In contrast to the regular staff nurses, who cared for the patients in conjunction with the doctors, physician assistants and nurse practitioners would see patients independently, the way the rest of the doctors did. So there needed to be a term that would include all three groups—physician assistants, nurse practitioners and doctors—who could have primary responsibility for patients.

WHO ARE HEALTHCARE PROVIDERS?

Providers are nurses, therapists, dentists, pharmacists, clinicians, physicians, technicians, paramedics, and any other person working in the business of caring for patients and family members.

Hartzband and Groopman (2011) denounced describing physicians as providers because of the term's generic and impersonal connotation. Ofri (2011) felt being called a provider, "makes [physicians] feel like a vending machine, pushing out hermetically sealed bags of 'healthcare' after the 'consumer's' dollar bill is slurped eerily in." However, Ofri also conceded the term provider can actually minimize hierarchy among physicians, nurses, and other healthcare professionals by reducing perceptual status judgments on the part of patients regarding the quality of care by different members of their healthcare team. Specifically, Ofri wrote, "Physician assistants, nurse practitioners, and doctors have more similarities than differences in their day-to-day interactions with patients, even as they come from unique backgrounds and bring different strengths to the table."

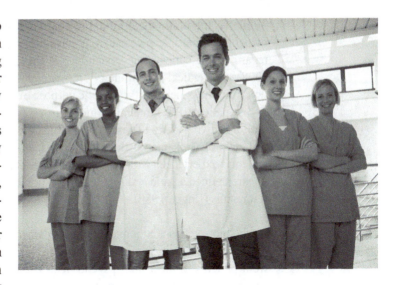

In this chapter we use the term provider, not as a value-laden judgment intended to minimize differences in the education, roles, or relative contributions to patient care among healthcare professionals, but as an all-encompassing term for those whose primary task is to deliver healthcare services to individuals, families, or communities. Providers are nurses, therapists, dentists, pharmacists, clinicians, physicians, technicians, paramedics, and any other person working in the business of caring for patients and family members. From a communication perspective, all providers share a responsibility to interact with patients in ways that promote shared meaning and satisfaction and lead to optimal health outcomes. This chapter begins with a discussion of historical issues of healthcare provider communication, followed by an examination of patient-centered communication, one of the most common approaches to patient and provider interaction today.

HISTORICAL APPROACHES TO PROVIDER COMMUNICATION

When providers make healthcare decisions on behalf of their patients without regard to the patients' wishes, they are taking a paternalistic approach to care (Gafni & Charles, 2009). Although the **paternalistic model** of healthcare is typically provider-directed and hierarchical, patient care often requires open dialogue among patients, providers, and family members (Jones & Stubbe, 2004). Traditional provider roles, however, were developed based on task-oriented and verbally dominant conversations with patients (Graugaard, Holgersen, Eide, & Finset, 2005).

Similarly, the **biomedical model** of communication reflects a scientific approach by focusing on hard sciences such as physiology, biochemistry, and genetics, without regard to the patients' understanding of these issues (Geist-Martin, Sharf, & Jeha, 2008). Biomedical patient interviews used closed-ended questions to gather information from the patient for the specific purpose of providing diagnostic information back to that patient. The biomedical model of care was common in the 1970s and 1980s, until a growing body of research demonstrated how patients' psychological, social, and relational characteristics work in conjunction with biological issues to shape patients' experiences with disease and illness. The resulting **biopsychosocial model** of care defined a patient as whole person, not just as a set of biological symptoms and test results (Engel, 1980).

As the biopsychosocial model of care became more prevalent, providers began using medical interviewing techniques such as open-ended questions to gather evidence from patients to meet their psychosocial needs (Engel, 1980). The biopsychosocial approach relied more on interactions seeking to gather and interpret information from patients and to engage patients in dialogue about potentially relevant attitudes, emotions, and behaviors (McWhinney, 1989). The increased acceptance and popularity of biopsychosocial clinical interviewing in healthcare interactions marked a turn toward a decidedly interpretive approach to care.

The biopsychosocial model is based in part on Delia's (1977) constructivist framework, which stressed "the interplay of shared and individual interpretive processes by

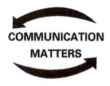

COMMUNICATION MATTERS

John Stewart, MD, FACP, Division of Internal Medicine & Pediatrics, University of Kentucky College of Medicine

As a primary care physician, effective communication is one of the most necessary skills required to perform my job well. I see patients of all ages and educational levels in my practice, so I am constantly assessing the best method to communicate with each individual patient. In our medical training, doctors learn another language that we use to communicate with each other. That language is often confusing and unintelligible to most patients. I have to translate what I think is going on and what the patient needs to do using language they can understand and remember. I also have to communicate well in my written documentation to ensure that other health care professionals understand my care plans for the patient. Most of the frustrations I encounter with patients have to do with miscommunication of expectations for the patient's care, while the primary frustration I encounter with fellow colleagues is lack of communication regarding their thoughts or plans for a patient due to insufficient documentation.

which individuals define situations and construe the perspectives of others within them" (p. 70). This view of provider communication falls clearly within the interpretive paradigm and draws from the distinction introduced by Bernstein (1971) as person-centered and position-centered communication. In other words, when we form a specific impression of a person, we tend to engage in communication that focuses on the unique qualities of that person (Cerposki & Kline, 1982). According to Applegate and Delia (1980), person-centered communication assumes that the "motivation, intentions, and feelings of individuals are unique; consequently, communication messages must rely on the recognition and elaboration of individual differences" (p. 253). Thus, person-centered communication is rooted in the notion that communication is created and interpreted based on individual and situational influences (Applegate & Delia, 1980; Cerposki & Kline, 1982).

While literature directly linking person-centered communication to the healthcare context is fairly sparse, a body of provider and patient communication research employs interpretive, critical, and cultural perspectives (Dutta & Zoller, 2008). These studies emphasize the social construction of interaction between providers and patients (Sharf & Vanderford, 2003) and the nature of power in the relationship (Lupton, 1994).

Patient-centered Communication

In 2001, patient-centered care was endorsed by the Institute of Medicine as one of six domains of quality leading to safer healthcare practices and more effective patient outcomes. As a fundamental part of patient-centered care, patient-centered communication incorporates scientific/biomedical and interpretive/biopsychosocial evidence, and it helps providers understand and build relationships with patients as unique individuals. Patient-centeredness seeks to avoid potential provider dominance in medical interactions by establishing more equal participation in clinical consultations.

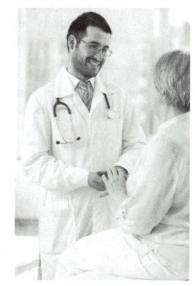

The patient-centered communication approach responds directly to the needs and desires of the patient, and it revolves around three core attributes: (a) consideration of patients' needs, perspectives, and individual experiences; (b) provision of opportunities to patients to participate in their care; and (c) enhancement of the provider–patient relationship (Epstein et al., 2005). For communication to contribute to increased health, providers, patients, and their families must have the capacity to engage in communication behaviors that contribute to the objectives of patient-centered care. For all parties involved, this means having adequate and appropriate **motivation**; having sufficient **knowledge**, understanding, and self-awareness of what is required to communicate effectively; and having suitable perceptual and linguistic **skills** to produce effective communication behaviors and adapt them appropriately (Epstein & Street, 2007).

PATIENT-CENTERED COMMUNICATION AND COMMUNICATION COMPETENCE

The patient-centered communication approach responds directly to the needs and desires of the patient, and it revolves around three core attributes: (1) consideration of patients' needs, perspectives, and individual experiences; (2) provision of opportunities to patients to participate in their care; and (3) enhancement of the provider-patient relationship (Epstein et al., 2005).

Communication competence consists of three components: (1) knowledge: understanding what communication skills are required to interact effectively with patients, (2) skills: the ability to apply communication knowledge in interactions with patients, and (3) motivation: the willingness to engage in the skills during interactions with patients.

Over the last decade, numerous studies on patient-centered communication have been conducted by researchers from both the interpretive and scientific paradigms. Interpretive studies seek to understand patients' experiences with healthcare, while scientific studies tend to seek more generalizable findings about the complexities of patients' and providers' motivations, knowledge, and skills that lead to effective patient-centered care.

Role of motivation. In the past, all too often the shifting structure of patient-centered care may have led providers to be less motivated to engage in dialogue with patients. Why? Because many providers worked under an assumption that patients who came to the clinic with an illness would automatically comply with providers' treatment recommendations and take prescribed medication. Today, however, patients are less likely to automatically comply with "doctor's orders" and more likely to seek treatment options from their doctors, friends, and sources on the Internet. Furthermore, patients are motivated to comply with providers' recommendations when they perceive that the provider made an effort to understand and validate the patient's perspective (both psychologically and socially), come to a shared understanding of the patient's problem and treatment, and empower patients by offering involvement in treatment choices during clinical visits (Epstein & Street, 2007). When providers communicate to find common ground with patients, they create a relationship based on mutual trust, respect, and commitment, all of which contribute to higher levels of patient satisfaction (Epstein & Street, 2007).

An example of interpretive research on patient-centered communication with providers is a study by Ledford and colleagues (2010). Through interviews and focus groups, the researchers sought to better understand how patients decided whether to take medication on the basis of patient-centered communication with a provider. Previous research on this topic found that even when providers were motivated to elicit participation from patients in conversations during a medical visit, patients were often unwilling to interact if they were unsure what to ask, believed their questions would waste the physicians' time, or felt the provider might think they were stupid for asking a question (Sepucha, Belkora, Mutchnick, & Esserman, 2002). On the basis of these findings, Ledford and colleagues gathered narratives from patients in one-on-one interviews and used that initial data to formulate questions in follow-up focus groups. Results revealed that, regardless of their own knowledge and preparedness to interact with a provider, patients were most likely to participate in discussions with providers when they viewed the provider as trustworthy and credible. When providers seemed more motivated to *sell* the patient on a specific medication, or when they failed to give an accurate diagnosis or prescription on a patient's first visit, participants in this study felt the provider was not delivering patient-centered care.

Although you might think that providers should make it a point to always use patient-centered communication, sometimes providers experience fatigue and scheduling conflicts, or they choose to avoid interactions that are uncomfortable or involve emotionally laden topics (Epstein & Street, 2007). When providers approach patient-centered communication as the basis for forming a relationship with their patients, however, clinical visits tend to involve more participation from motivated patients and providers (Beach & Roter, 2000; Zoppi & Epstein, 2002).

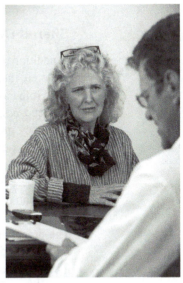

Role of knowledge. Today, effective communication requires providers to consider not only a patient's health condition but also their perspectives and the purpose of the interaction (Epstein & Street, 2007). By having sufficient knowledge, providers are better positioned to personalize treatment recommendations, use language the patient understands, provide clear explanations, and validate or address the patient's emotional state (Marvel, Epstein, Flowers, & Beckman, 1999). Unfortunately, acquiring an accurate understanding of their patients' perspectives, which include their concerns, feelings, preferences, beliefs, and values, is challenging for many providers. Although such knowledge can be learned through direct experience or observation, research indicates that providers often misjudge patients' perspectives, including their preferences, likelihood to follow treatment, satisfaction with care, understandings and beliefs about health, or emotional states (Epstein & Street, 2007).

Role of skills. Providers need both medical skills and communication skills, but communication is not always stressed as part of medical education for all types of healthcare providers (Ledford, Seehusen, Villagran, Cafferty, & Childress, 2013). A nonverbal skills training protocol that has been used in nursing education is SOLER. SOLER has five key elements: Providers should face patients *squarely* (S), sitting at eye level and fairly close to the patient to demonstrate immediacy behaviors; create an *open* (O) body posture by keeping arms uncrossed during patient interactions; *lean* (L) toward the patient when possible to show intimacy and flexibility; in Western cultures, providers are also encouraged to use *eye contact* (E) to demonstrate attention and interest in the patient; finally, providers should maintain a *relaxed* (R) posture to help decrease patient anxiety. Patient-centered skills such as those taught through SOLER help providers demonstrate their interest in what the patient has to say by connecting with patients (Epstein & Street, 2007). This protocol and other approaches to communication skills training must be taught to providers to enhance their ability to engage in patient-centered communication through nonverbal immediacy.

Shared Decision Making

In addition to engaging in specific provider communication behaviors to foster patient-centered interactions, providers must demonstrate **competent communication** in their roles as the links between patients and the larger healthcare system (Bredart, Bouleuc, & Dolbeault, 2005). Providers are stakeholders in their organizations, and as such they must advocate for patients. They must also share in decision making with patients when decisions relate to the health and welfare of the patient (Elwyn, Frosch, & Rollnick, 2009). Providers are most likely to engage in shared decision making when there is **clinical equipoise**, which means there are equivalent pros and cons for more than one treatment option for a patient's condition (Elwyn et al., 2009).

The process of making shared clinical decisions involves two distinct phases: determination and deliberation. Determination occurs when providers and patients choose a particular course of treatment, most often based on the provider's advice or clinical guidelines. Deliberation involves joint and reciprocal consideration of information, discussing options, considering concerns, and addressing preferences, including preference for roles in the decision-making process. **Shared decision making** occurs when providers relinquish total control of healthcare decisions in favor of a more

Teach-back Training

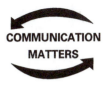

COMMUNICATION MATTERS

The American Medical Association promotes a communication skills technique called "teach-back" to help providers and patients demonstrate a shared understanding of information provided during a medical visit. Using teach-back, providers seek to encourage patient-centered communication with statements such as, "I tend to give a lot of information. May I ask you to tell me what you'll remember most? I want to make sure you have the information you need." Or, "That was a lot of information to absorb. What will you tell your family and friends about what we just discussed?" Patients demonstrate their understanding of what their provider has said by teaching the information back to the provider in response to these types of questions. You can learn more about teach-back training by visiting this website: http://teachbacktraining.com

Table 4.1 Examples of Patient-centered Provider Behaviors

Nonverbal Behaviors

Maintaining eye contact
Forward lean to indicate attentiveness
Nodding to indicate understanding
Absence of distracting movements (e.g., fidgeting)

Verbal Behaviors

Avoiding interruptions
Establishing purpose of the visit
Encouraging patient participation
Soliciting the patient's beliefs, values, and preferences
Eliciting and validating the patient's emotions
Asking about family and social context
Providing sufficient information
Providing clear, jargon-free explanations
Checking for patient understanding
Offering reassurance
Offering encouragement and support

Adapted from Epstein and Street (2007).

collaborative process that aims to help patients and families understand key issues with the diagnosis and treatment options (Makoul & Clayman, 2006). Even though providers typically have more knowledge about the disease and illness, patients have more knowledge about their own symptoms and their readiness to engage in various treatments.

In the healthcare context, **concordance** is defined as a perceived similarity, or shared identity, between physicians and patients (Street, O'Malley, Cooper, & Haidet, 2008). Although the term concordance has been used to examine perceived similarity between patients and providers on the basis of demographic characteristics such as gender (Schmittdiel, Grumbach, Selby, & Quesenberry, 2000) and race/ethnicity

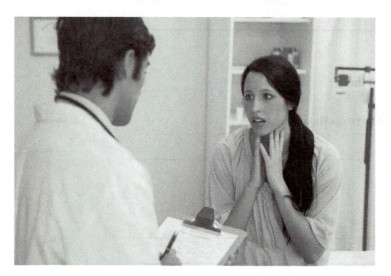

(Stepanikova, 2006), among many scholars concordance is used to describe identification stemming from interpersonal interactions that build interpersonal trust and patient empowerment through patient-centered communication (Banerjee & Sanyal, 2012).

An example of patient-centered communication that led to concordance with a patient was described in an interview conducted just before the death of a 24-year-old woman who was generally fit and healthy until the day her provider told her she had Stage 4 cancer.

I was sitting on the doctor's table, and instead of leaning over, or towering over me to talk to me, he actually leaned back against the cabinet so we were at eye level. I guess that is part of the reason he made me feel comfortable because he looked right at me and I could tell he was assessing the situation as we were talking. I think he was trying to assess my friend and myself to think about our education levels to see how to handle things. It may have only taken him like two minutes, but he paused and spoke directly to my friend and me. He didn't talk *over* me, and he didn't talk *down* to me, he just talked to us like people. He said I'm not going to tell you anything worse than it is, and I'm not going to tell you anything better than it is . . .

(Sparks & Villagran, 2010, p. 110)

Concordance takes effort over the course of the relationship, and providers must continually demonstrate their willingness to adapt to meet the needs of their patients. A lack of support in provider interactions, like in marriage, can lead to a lack of concordance and an unhealthy relationship.

Research has consistently shown that interpersonal skills are crucial to patient–provider interactions, and providers who lack effective communicative skills may jeopardize the medical care process. As Cerposki and Kline (1982) described,

> The physician must perceive the patient as having unique feelings, motivations and beliefs that affect significantly the character of interaction. Moreover, the physician must conceptualize his/her own interactional roles as requiring variations in approach, flexibility in accommodation to emergent circumstances, and the pursuit of interpersonal as well as instrumental objectives.
>
> (p. 10)

Strong interpersonal skills exhibited through a patient-centered orientation will, at the very least, help providers to learn their patient's needs, attitudes, and feelings, thereby producing a more holistic picture of the patient as diagnosis and treatment decisions are made.

Clinical interventions from the scientific perspective have linked shared decision making with a number of improvements in patient outcomes, including greater understanding of the clinical problem, lower decisional conflict, and higher overall satisfaction with care (Joosten et al., 2008). Unfortunately, while shared decision making between providers and patients can reduce patients' anxiety and distress and improve quality of life, many providers are often reluctant to relinquish complete control of patient care because all too often, they are held responsible by patients and loved ones for negative health outcomes (Elwyn et al., 2009).

Health Literacy

Shared decision making often hinges on the ability of providers to present scientific information in ways that are easily understandable for patients and their families. Although health literacy is often portrayed as a problem rooted in patients' lack of knowledge or education (e.g., Does the patient understand diagnosis and treatment information?), much of the health literacy research focuses on teaching providers to adapt language and scientific information to meet the needs of their patients. As defined by the Institute of Medicine (IOM, 2004, p. 32), **health literacy** is "[t]he degree to which individuals have the capacity to obtain, process, and understand basic health information and services needed to make appropriate health decisions that may affect the health of Americans and the ability of the healthcare system to provide effective, high quality care."

As the most common and trusted source of health information (Cutilli, 2010), providers must use competent communication to effectively convey the most relevant and up-to-date health information to patients. Surprisingly, healthcare providers and medical establishments are often equally unprepared to provide patients and care-givers with pertinent health-related information—information that is necessary for informed medical decision making. Providers seeking to present health information based on the tenets of health literacy must consider how to best communicate with patients in a manner that exemplifies the four components of health literacy (IOM, 2001): (a) cultural and conceptual knowledge, (b) listening and speaking (oral literacy), (c) writing and reading (print literacy), and (d) numeracy (knowledge of statistics and other numeric data). Chapter 7 of this text also addresses health literacy.

HEALTH LITERACY

National Library of Medicine (NLM) and the Institute of Medicine (IOM) define health literacy as "[t]he degree to which individuals have the capacity to obtain, process, and understand basic health information and services needed to make appropriate health decisions that may affect the health of Americans and the ability of the healthcare system to provide effective, high quality care." It consists of four components: (a) cultural and conceptual knowledge, (b) oral literacy, (c) print literacy, and (d) numeracy.

Cultural and conceptual knowledge. The first component of health literacy includes cultural and conceptual knowledge—an understanding of health, illness, risk, and benefits (IOM, 2001). Cultural and conceptual knowledge typically deals with a person's ability to navigate the health system in order to obtain health information and information about preventive activities. However, in recent years the definition has been broadened to include healthcare providers and healthcare systems within this process. Providers' roles include using effective communication to present opportunities for patients to participate in healthy lifestyles. By employing patient-centered communication, providers are able to create shared meaning and under-standing of the most important concepts and cultural issues affecting health-related decisions (Epstein & Street, 2007). System-wide interventions build on best practices to optimize healthcare through self-management support, decision support, clinical information systems, delivery system design, and community resources and policies, all of which are aligned to optimize care (Epstein & Street, 2007). Coupled with provider and/or patient training, improved communication with patients is a likely outcome of such a system.

Listening and speaking. Listening and speaking skills, also known as oral literacy, are crucial in the provider–patient interaction. Patients and providers must work toward possessing strong oral communication skills so as to adequately and accurately describe the diagnosis and any health concerns and be able to competently ask for and understand health information. Improving oral communication in the medical encounter begins with the disuse of medical jargon and the assurance of patient understanding. This is important as providers often have a poor grasp of what patients do and do not know about relevant medical concepts and information, making it difficult for patients with limited literacy to understand their diagnosis and treatment options (Schwartzberg, VanGeest, & Wang, 2005).

Furthermore, providers must be able to perceive whether or not a patient understands the message being conveyed in the medical encounter. For instance, when a patient presents symptoms related to asthma, the provider must be able to explain the diagnosis in a way that the patient can comprehend and in a way that then allows the

---

Julie Green, RN/case manager, Crossroads Hospice

COMMUNICATION
MATTERS

Being kindly referred to as a well-seasoned nurse by my co-workers, I've had the opportunity and pleasure of meeting many culturally diverse people over the years. Working the majority of my career in the hospital setting, I've seen the industrialization of the healthcare system. There have been so many high-tech changes with the intention of communicating patient information to members of the healthcare team. Electronic charting is a great convenience, so much information you can get without even meeting the patient! But we must always keep in mind that our patients are often confused with this technology, frightened and anxious about being in the hospital. Many patients are in pain and generally they are not at their best when we meet them. I've learned long ago that the best way to communicate with anyone, no matter what their cultural background, is to take a quiet moment with them and listen to their concerns and answer their questions. By being present in the moment with them and not distracted by other tasks, we convey our respect and concern for their dignity and well-being. This can be calming for them, making a stressful situation more bearable. Though technology is great we must always remember we are dealing with human beings and we must always be wary that the human touch does not give way to the high-tech.

patient to ask follow-up questions to ensure complete understanding. However, providers are often in a hurry and do not take the time needed to ensure that patients understand what they have been told (Schwartzberg et al., 2005). Techniques such as "asking patients to explain or demonstrate what they've been told" and slowing the speed of the communication have been shown to enhance patients' understanding of critical health information (Weiss, 2007, p. 33).

Writing and reading. Also known as print literacy, writing and reading skills are needed for tasks related to the use of the printed word. This could be in health education brochures, on medicine bottles, or in informed consent documents (IOM, 2001). The utilization of effective written materials by providers can reinforce patients' understanding, knowledge, and use of relevant health information. As the most trusted source of health information, providers must arm themselves with as much information as possible and learn to be savvy consumers of that information (Kutner, Greenberg, Jin, & Paulsen, 2006). To ensure the most effective use of written materials, providers can read them aloud, highlight specific passages, or number the key points for a particular patient (Weiss, 2007).

Numeracy. Providers are often highly trained in mathematical and science skills. Translation of these skills through communication requires providers to consider "the patient's ability to understand and act on numerical directions given by a healthcare provider" (IOM, 2001, p. 304). Patients and providers need these skills to understand nutrition labels, compare health insurance benefit packages, and determine the proper dosage and timing of medication (IOM, 2001). A patient's ability to understand health risks may be undermined by poor numeracy skills (Schwartzberg et al., 2005). There-fore, providers must ensure statistical information is both relevant and easily understood by the patient.

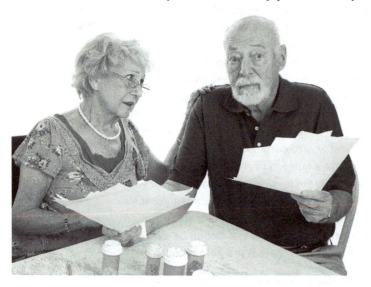

Health literacy fosters shared decision making in patient-centered interactions. Providers are the genesis of shared power, and patients benefit from providers who possess the knowledge and skills to help patients navigate healthcare systems. Most providers gain a tremendous amount of experience with technical skills necessary to do their jobs, but communication skills are all too often learned on the job with patients or through interactions with other providers working as part of the healthcare team. This type of "on the job" training may not lead to the best health outcomes for patients.

Primary care physician Hanan Aboumatar and colleagues (2013) conducted a study from the scientific approach with interesting results regarding the relationships among health literacy, shared decision making, and patient-centered communication. In this experimental study, half of the 275 patient participants and half of the 41 physician participants received intensive communication skills training to improve patient-centered communication and shared decision making in their healthcare interactions. Patients were also divided into groups based on their existing levels of health literacy. Results revealed that despite similar desires to participate in medical decision making with their physicians, patients with low health literacy were significantly less likely than high literacy patients to act on that desire by asking questions during their medical visits. In fact, low literacy patients asked significantly fewer questions of their doctors, even after they received intensive communication skills training. In addition, even among doctors who received intensive patient-centered communication training as part of the experiment, the amount of shared decision making with low literate patients did not differ significantly from physicians who did not receive communication training. This study highlights some of the challenges faced by providers who seek to improve health outcomes for low literate patients through patient-centered communication (Aboumatar, Carson, Beach, Roter, & Cooper, 2013).

Professional Communication Challenges for Healthcare Providers

Although much of the literature on patient-centered communication examines physician communication with patients, a whole host of providers engage in communication that directly impacts health outcomes for their patients. In this section, we focus on three groups: nurses, emergency room providers, and dentists.

Nurses. Research regarding communication challenges experienced by nurses is extensive (Schriner, 2007; Willard & Luker, 2007). Apker (2001) described a "complex array of expectations communicated to nurses regarding how to fulfill their professional roles in an organizational environment that lacks the resources necessary to enact those roles" (p. 132). Nurses have varying educational backgrounds, and the nursing profession is rooted in a hierarchy guided by varied educational requirements. Collaboration among nurses and other providers requires a shared power structure that has traditionally been dominated by physicians. All too often, the shifting structure of patient-centered care puts nurses in the middle of conflict between patients and other providers, and communication conflict involving nurses can become a cyclical pattern when problems are not properly addressed (Duddle & Boughton, 2007).

As the healthcare environment has moved to a more equal and supportive climate of patient-centered communication, increasing complexity of nurses' roles has resulted in increased stress, burnout, and poor physical and mental health among some nurses (Mackintosh, 2007; Patrick & Lavery, 2007). Hospitals now operating in a managed care structure frequently place increased performance demands on nursing staff. These changes often mean that nurses take on more managerial and clinical responsibilities, caring for a larger number of patients, and learning skills once considered outside the scope of nursing practice.

Emergency room providers. Challenging communication for hospital emergency room (ER) providers emerges as a result of time constraints and emotional pressures (Laposa, Alden, & Fullerton, 2003). In fact, healthcare providers working in hospital

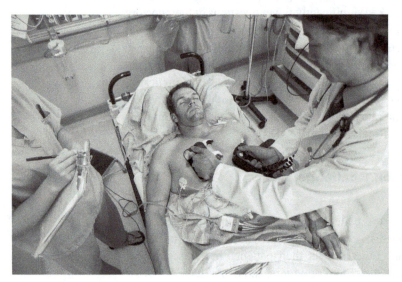

ERs often experience emotional stress, anxiety, depression, and even post-traumatic stress disorder due to the demands of delivering care to critically and terminally ill patients. Although few ER health professionals ever seek medical care for their symptoms, studies have found that 12% of ER nurses and 11.7% of ER medical residents met the full criteria for post-traumatic stress disorder and an additional 30% of ER nurses and 30% of medical residents had severe stress-related illnesses (Laposa et al., 2003; Mills & Mills, 2004).

An ER provider described the stress experienced in a hospital ER:

> I was once in the military, in a war zone. I got what was called "hazardous duty pay". It is extra money because you are in an area of danger. You know what? Nurses in the ER deserve hazardous duty pay . . . The average person is not going to come to ER unless they truly are very sick or have an accident . . . These patients are the dysfunctional, criminal, crazy people among us. They are the people you move to the suburbs to avoid. Every day we deal with [patients] who are verbally abusive, even physically abusive. They threaten us. They sometimes get out of control. We never know what's coming through the door and what they

are going to do next. (*Madness: Tales of an emergency room nurse*. Emergency-room-nurse.blogspot.com)

The nature of ER medicine means providers rarely have the chance to build lasting relationships with their patients before the patient is admitted to the hospital or sent home. Relationships among ER providers are more long-lasting, so perhaps more supportive relationships among ER health-care providers could help alleviate some of the emotional pressures from working in the ER.

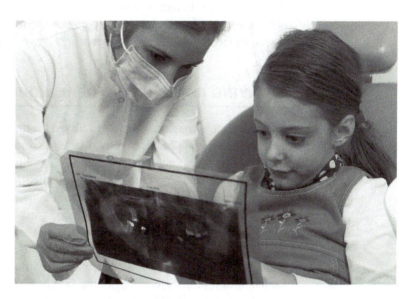

Dentists. Among dentists, stressful interactions often stem from heavy workload and anxious patients (Moore & Brodsgaard, 2001). A 2010 review of existing literature in this area reported that while several studies assessed the

Pam Stein, DMD, MPH, Division of Public Health Dentistry, University of Kentucky College of Dentistry

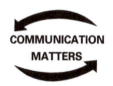

COMMUNICATION MATTERS

As a public health dentist, appropriate communication strategies are a must. I provide dental care and oral health education for a diverse population—expectant mothers, nursing home residents, school children in underserved areas and the homeless. One of the most important aspects of my job is being a good listener. It is essential to find out my patient's concerns, fears, medical history and desires and then to respond appropriately. Experience has taught me that I provide the best care when I am communicating effectively. Whether it's discussing with a new mom how to prevent tooth decay and toothaches in her child, talking a frightened pre-schooler through their first dental visit, or employing threat reduction techniques with a cognitively impaired older adult, I daily utilize my toolbox of communication strategies. The most rewarding part of my job is relieving and preventing suffering and improving self-esteem in my patients. Knowing that I have had even a small role in improving the lives of my patients is very gratifying.

effectiveness of various communication skills training programs for dental students, almost no research examined patients' communicative experiences during dental visits (Carey, Madill, & Manogue, 2010). Moreover, dental schools are required to ensure that undergraduates are adequately trained in communication skills, yet little evidence exists to suggest what constitutes appropriate training and how competency can be assessed. Future research on patient-centered communication in dental inter-actions should focus on how providers can use messages that reduce patients' stress levels, which could in turn improve dentists' overall effectiveness.

APPLYING RESEARCH TO REAL WORLD SETTINGS

Throughout this chapter, we have discussed the importance of active, patient-centered communication that requires providers' conscious attention to patients' psycholog-ical, emotional, and interpersonal needs. To cultivate more effective communication skills among providers, numerous **communication skills training programs** have been designed and delivered (Bylund et al., 2008; Hoffman & Steinberg, 2002; Villa-gran, Baldwin, Goldsmith, & Wittenberg-Lyles, 2010). Upon completion, providers usually report these programs to be satisfying and meaningful, and many programs leave providers feeling more confident to handle difficult communication issues with patients (Bylund et al., 2008). For example, in a study conducted by Hoffman and Steinberg (2002), before beginning a communication skills training program, providers expressed difficulty with a number of communication issues such as giving complex information, obtaining informed consent, and handling cultural differences. Three months after the three-day course, providers reported having greater confidence in handling these matters, a more positive attitude toward patients' psychosocial needs, and a more patient-centered orientation. Communication interventions for providers have also been linked to patients' perceptions of quality of care. In a study conducted by Razavi and colleagues (2003), for example, patients of trained providers reported that they understood their disease better, felt less depressed, and believed they were more in control than did patients whose providers did not have training.

Providers in real world settings also use communication skills training as a tool to help them adapt to an increasingly team-based healthcare environment (Hollenbeck, Beersma, & Schouten, 2012). Chapter 6 of this text addresses interprofessional communication in healthcare teams from a group and organizational perspective. Here, we consider the more interpersonal aspects of interdisciplinary **healthcare team** communication.

Like nurses, ER providers, and dentists, all providers are increasingly being asked to work in interdisciplinary healthcare teams where they experience stressful and often complex roles, structures, regulations, and contexts in their pursuit of optimal health outcomes for patients (Villagran & Baldwin, 2014). Recent healthcare reforms place a strong emphasis on use of interprofessional collaboration among providers. However, a shift away from the traditional model of provider leadership in healthcare can cause fragmentation and turbulence across the continuum of care as patients, nurses, nurse practitioners, and other health professionals become co-equal partners in shared decision making with providers (Kuziemsky et al., 2009).

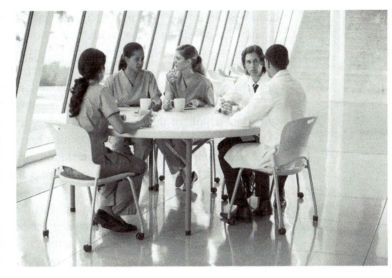

In hospitals and large clinical practices, providers in real world settings increasingly engage in interactions framed by differing levels of knowledge and skills, decision-making authority, and temporal stability in their organizations. Communication training programs often seek to educate providers about the importance of teamwork based on respect and differentiation of skills and authority within the team (Hollenbeck et al., 2012).

Skill differentiation is "the degree to which members have specialized knowledge or functional capacities that make it more or less difficult to substitute members" (Hollenbeck et al., 2012, p. 84) of the healthcare organization. The interdisciplinary composition of healthcare creates differentiation among members on the basis of professional and personal training and experiences. **Authority differentiation** among healthcare providers is a term used to describe how tasks are divided among providers and how decision-making power is viewed in different situations (Hollenbeck et al., 2012). Authority differentiation is a major factor in healthcare because of regulations and professional norms mandating physicians' authority and leadership in managing patients. Providers gain **temporal stability** on the basis of their "history of working together in the past and an expectation of working together in the future" (Hollenbeck et al., 2012, p. 94). Temporal stability is a significant challenge for providers who work simultaneously at multiple healthcare facilities, each with its own staff, set of rules, and processes for patient care. For example, physicians may have their own office where they see patients, but they also have hospital privileges enabling them to admit patients, order labs and treatments, and perform procedures at a hospital. Even though the physician is not actually employed or directly supervised by hospital administrators, there is a professional relationship, supported by nurses and healthcare technicians who work with various providers on the basis of whether or not the provider has patients at the facility. Providers working on different time shifts in the same hospital may not know each other personally, despite working to keep up with important details of their patients' prognoses and treatment plans. Specialists delivering care only to patients with a specific disease, or to a specific patient population, can be isolated within a health organization, making it difficult to collaborate across subspecialties to solve unusual or persistent patient concerns.

The interdisciplinary composition of healthcare creates differentiation among providers on the basis of professional and personal training and experiences. A study of patient communication challenges among healthcare providers offered an illustration of one providers' struggle with authority differentiation:

> It was a no win situation because someone would end up a victim, the doctor or the patient . . . you're damned if you do, damned if you don't . . . you want to make sure the patient knows what is going on, but you're not the doctor. It'd probably be a real sticky situation . . . As a patient advocate . . . it's important to tell them [patients] what their rights are . . . but it would get me into trouble with the surgeons.
>
> (Marin, Sherblom, & Shipps, 1994, p. 205)

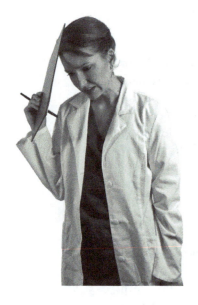

In real world settings, healthcare providers may gain the knowledge and skills to deal with authority differentiation through innovative communication skills curricula. For example, Kneebone, Nestel, Chrzanowska, Barnet, and Darzi (2006) designed an innovative program to maximize learning outcomes among providers on a surgical team by using external evaluators to identify conflicts and issues of role strain. Results from this intervention included a new sense of respect among some participants for differing roles and challenges among team members and new role development in areas of team weakness and conflict.

Cultural communication training. Critical–cultural research on healthcare providers has revealed that even the most well-intentioned provider can face unconscious barriers to effective communication based on unequal power in their patient relationships, unconscious stereotypes, and cultural biases. Recent communication skills training programs also focus on a lack of cultural awareness among providers as a barrier to positive health outcomes for diverse patients. Culture "is conceptualized as both transformative and constitutive, providing an axis for theorizing the discursive processes through which meaning is socially constructed" (Dutta-Bergman, 2004, p. 241). Here, culture represents both an interpretive and critical–cultural approach to health communication. While few providers consciously choose different care options for patients on the basis of the patient's cultural background, considerable evidence suggests that subconscious biases among providers lead to health disparities based on patients' race, education, sex, and ethnicity (Dovidio et al., 2008; Green et al., 2007; Penner et al., 2010). Providers can unconsciously develop biases that influence their views of their own power in making decisions on behalf of patients during clinical interactions.

Unconscious biases can negatively impact patient care by reducing providers' willingness to engage in shared decision making or refer non-White patients to specialists. Recent research conducted from the interpretive perspective involved interviews with physicians and nurses to explore participants' views on racial disparities and the validity of studies reporting health disparities (Clark-Hitt, Malat, Burgess, & Friedemann-Sanchez, 2010). Communication researcher Rose Clark-Hitt and colleagues informed participants that researchers found White patients generally received better healthcare than African American patients, regardless of the patients' insurance/healthcare access, existing health conditions, education, or income. Then the researchers asked participants why they believed these disparities occur. A physician participant responded, "It doesn't seem right to me . . . do the African Americans actually go to the . . . provider? Maybe they wait longer . . . Do they access that healthcare?" (p. 393). Another participant expressed concern about the existence of unconscious biases toward patients: "You wonder if it is because we as humans want people who look like us to get the care that we would want. You know that there's somehow a better identification of, this could be my grandfather, this could be my dad, or this could be me" (p. 393).

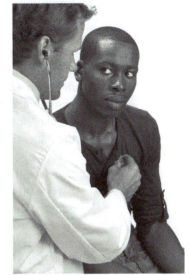

Although explicit racial biases are not shared among all providers, responses to evidence of racial bias and health disparities are typically evaluated based on providers' existing values and beliefs (Frantz, Cuddy, Bernett, Ray, & Hart, 2004). To improve culturally competent communication between diverse patients and providers, an intervention was recently conducted among oncologists to teach skills for delivering controversial diagnoses in a culturally appropriate manner (Quinn et al., 2011). Providers who participated in the training reported feeling more confident about their own cultural sensitivity and a greater willingness to adapt communication to meet diverse patients' needs.

CONFLICTING RESULTS IN RESEARCH ON HEALTHCARE PROVIDER PERSPECTIVES

Despite a growing body of evidence about the positive impact of patient-centered care, there are conflicting views regarding how the assumption of patient-centered communication on the part of patients might impact providers in an increasingly dynamic healthcare environment. Specifically, providers have expressed concerns for how to maintain optimal health outcomes and patient safety in a system of shared decision making and patient-centered care. Some providers remain leery of threats to patient confidentiality despite improvements in available communication technology used to interact with patients between clinical visits (Wu et al., 2012). After all, it was not too long ago that physicians relied on pagers to stay connected with patients and their healthcare team. Today, new technologies may help providers interact in real time with patients and their families, but little research exists to examine the logistics and impact of patient-centered communication across geographically separated patient care environments (Wu et al., 2012).

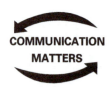

COMMUNICATION MATTERS

Patricia A. Donohoue, MD, Department of Pediatrics, Endocrinology & Diabetes, Medical College of Wisconsin

As I reflected on writing about physician–patient communication, I realized its immense complexity, particularly since the vast majority of physicians lack any formal training in communication skills. The stakes are usually high, and the stress levels of the patient and family are often equally high. This puts the decision-makers in a place where they are least equipped to understand new material or make important decisions. The physician must ask the right questions and understand the answers in order to obtain the information needed to guide an evaluation and treatment regimen. Facts and recommendations must be communicated by the physician in a clear and understandable manner for listeners of all ages and backgrounds. The communication style must be flexible enough to reach listeners of all ages—the parents (for the youngest patients), the parents and patient (for older children), and the patients themselves (for teens and older). There is often an educational process that must occur for the family to understand the situation and the recommendations, and face-to-face time is nearly always limited. There are many, many potential barriers to successful communication in these settings. The most significant include spoken language, cultural background, emotional state, and knowledge base of both the physician and the family. Physicians must be skilled at delivering very bad news, and no one is comfortable in those situations. The rewards are huge, though, when there is a solid and trusting relationship between the physician and the family.

Even though research tends to suggest that the process of patient-centered communication has a generally positive impact on patient satisfaction, this process relies on the ability of providers and patients to access each other on a regular and timely basis. Providers who work around the clock, in various locations, and on time-sensitive issues may feel conflicted by the increasing need to engage in face-to-face interactions with patients and other providers in today's healthcare environment (Wu et al., 2012). As patients and providers grow increasingly accustomed to shared decision making in clinical interactions, new challenges may focus on making sure providers are ready and available to spend the time needed to achieve this goal.

FUTURE RESEARCH ON HEALTHCARE PROVIDER PERSPECTIVES

Future research in the area of healthcare providers and their perspectives is needed to

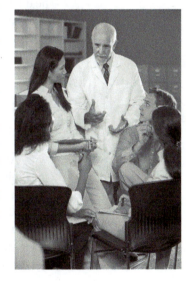

(a) better understand how to overcome unconscious biases among providers that negatively impact patient care, (b) improve providers' communication training to help them more effectively use plain language to overcome health literacy challenges, (c) improve interprofessional healthcare team communication, and (d) more fully explore interventions that improve cultural challenges in the patient–provider interaction. Medical interventions and technology help us live longer lives than ever before, and as our world becomes more diverse, providers will spend more time caring for diverse patient populations. This means providers will need effective tools to identify and overcome personal and systemic barriers to effective care. Increased expectations for effective communication with patients and healthcare team members will require new research on how to educate and train all providers to work together through coordinated communication.

CONCLUSION

This chapter examined issues and opportunities for healthcare providers who deliver care to patients and their families. The evolution of the provider and patient relationship has led to increased interaction and shared decision making through patient-centered communication. Providers of all kinds, trained not just as clinicians but also as communicators, engage with other humans in psychologically challenging, scientifically complex, and emotionally turbulent interactions that seek to improve health outcomes for patients. Patient-centered communication provides a framework for shared decision making and collaboration based on knowledge, skills, and motivation needed to solve healthcare challenges for patients.

DISCUSSION QUESTIONS

1. What challenges do you have when you communicate with your healthcare provider?
2. It's often easy to become confused when faced with health information. For example, you may have heard or read that a certain group has a certain percentage chance of getting a disease. What do those numbers really mean? Have you ever actually read the information pharmacists insert into your prescription bottles? Talk about complicated! What is your experience with receiving health information? Have you ever experienced a sense of confusion? Why was that?
3. How could better communication and coordination of care among members of a healthcare team reduce medical errors for patients?
4. What are some of the unique communication challenges for dentists? Nurses? Pharmacists? Emergency room providers? How could these providers improve patient-centered communication?

IN-CLASS ACTIVITIES

1. Watch the Institute for Healthcare Improvement open school video interview with Anthony M. DiGioia, MD, on patient-centered care: www.IHI.org/offerings/ihiopenschool/resources/Pages/TonyDiGioiaOnShadowing.aspx
    Have a discussion about the points that Dr. DiGioia makes.
2. The American Medical Association provides a series of interactive learning modules on their website: www.teachbacktraining.com
    Select some of the learning modules and use them as an in-class role play activity in which pairs of students practice teach-back in various healthcare settings.

RECOMMENDED READINGS

Epstein, R. M., & Street, R. L. (2007). *Patient-centered communication in cancer care: Promoting healing and reducing suffering.* NIH Publication No. 07-6225. Bethesda, MD: National Cancer Institute.

This is a comprehensive monograph on all aspects of patient-centered communication in the cancer context.

Ledford, C., Villagran, M., Kreps, G., Zhao, X., & Weathers, M. (2010). Practicing medicine: Patient activation and perceptions of physician communication in the process of medication prescription. *Patient Education and Counseling, 80*, 384–392.

This article examines how patients perceive providers who use trial and error to decide on appropriate treatment for their patients.

McCormack, L., Treimanb, K., Rupert, D. Williams-Piehota, P., Nadler, E., Arora, N., . . . Street, R. (2011). Measuring patient-centered communication in cancer care: A literature review and the development of a systematic approach. *Social Science & Medicine, 72*, 1085–1095.

This article offers a review of patient-centered communication in the context of cancer care.

REFERENCES

Aboumatar, H. A., Carson, K., Beach, M. C., Roter, D. & Cooper, L. (2013). The impact of health literacy on desire for participation in healthcare, medical visit communication, and patient reported outcomes among patients with hypertension. *Journal of General Internal Medicine, 28*, 1469–1476.

Apker, J. (2001). Role development in the managed care era: A case of hospital-based nursing. *Journal of Applied Communication Research, 29*, 117–136.

Applegate, J. L., & Delia, J. G. (1980). Person-centered speech, psychological development, and the contexts of language usage. In R. St. Clair (Ed.), *The social and psychological contexts of language* (pp. 245–282). Hillsdale, NJ: Lawrence Erlbaum.

Banerjee, A., & Sanyal, D. (2012). Dynamics of doctor–patient relationship: A cross-sectional study on concordance, trust, and patient enablement. *Journal of Family & Community Medicine, 19*, 12–19.

Beach, M. C., & Roter, D. L. (2000). Interpersonal expectations in the patient-physician relationship. *Journal of General Internal Medicine, 15*, 825–827.

Bernstein, B. (1971). *Class, codes and control: Theoretical studies towards a sociology of language*. London: Routledge & Kegan Paul.

Bredart, A., Bouleuc, C., & Dolbeault, S. (2005). Doctor-patient communication and satisfaction with care in oncology. *Current Opinion in Oncology, 17*, 351–354.

Bylund, C., Brown, R., Lubrano di Ciccone, B., Levin, T.T., Gueguen, J.A., Hill, C., & Kissane, D. W. (2008). Training faculty to facilitate communication skills training: Development and evaluation of a workshop. *Patient Education and Counseling, 70*, 430–436.

Carey, J. A., Madill, A., & Manogue, M. (2010). Communications skills in dental education: A systematic research review. *European Journal of Dental Education, 14*, 69–78.

Cerposki, J. M., & Kline, S. L. (1982). *Social perception processes and person-centered communication in the medical setting: Research findings and implications for medical education*. Paper presented at the annual meeting of the Speech Communication Association, Louisville, KY.

Clark-Hitt, R., Malat, J., Burgess, D., & Friedemann-Sanchez, G. (2010). Doctors' and nurses' explanations for racial disparities in medical treatment. *Journal of Health Care for Poor and Underserved, 21*, 386–400.

Cutilli, C. C. (2010). Seeking health information: What sources do your patients use? *Orthopaedic Nursing, 29*, 214–219.

Delia, J. G. (1977). Constructivism and the study of human communication. *Quarterly Journal of Speech, 63*, 66–83.

Duddle, M., & Boughton, M. (2007). Intraprofessional relations in nursing. *Journal of Advanced Nursing, 59*, 29–37.

Dutta, M., & Zoller, H., (2008). Theoretical foundations: Interpretive, critical, and cultural approaches to healthcare. In M. Dutta & H. Zoller (Eds.), *Emerging perspectives in health communication: Meaning, culture, power* (pp. 1–28). London: Routledge.

Dutta-Bergman, M. (2004). The unheard voices of Santalis: Communicating about health from the margins of India. *Communication Theory, 14*, 237–263.

Dovidio, J. F., Penner, L. A., Albrecht, T. L., Norton, W. E., Gaertner, S. L., & Shelton, J. N. (2008). Disparities and distrust: The implications of psychological processes for understanding racial disparities in health and health care. *Social Science & Medicine, 67*, 478–486.

Elwyn, G., Frosch, D., & Rollnick, S. (2009). Dual equipoise shared decision making: Definitions for decision and behavior support interventions. *Implementation Science, 4*, 75.

Engel, G. L. (1980). The clinical application of the biopsychosocial model. *American Journal of Psychiatry, 137*, 535–544.

Epstein, R. M., & Street, R. L. (2007). *Patient-centered communication in cancer care: Promoting healing and reducing suffering*. NIH Publication No. 07-6225. Bethesda, MD: National Cancer Institute.

Epstein, R. M., Franks, P., Fiscella, K., Shields, C. G., Meldrum, S. C., Kravitz, R. L., & Duberstein, P. R. (2005). Measuring patient-centered communication in patient-physician consultations: Theoretical and practical issues. *Social Science & Medicine, 61*, 1516–1528.

Frantz, C. M., Cuddy, A. J., Burnett, M., Ray, H., & Hart, A. (2004). A threat in the computer: The race implicit association test as a stereotype threat experience. *Personality and Social Psychology Bulletin, 30*, 1611–1624.

Gafni, A. & Charles, C. (2009). The physician-patient encounter: An agency relationship? In A. Edwards & G. Elwyn (Eds.), *Shared decision making: Achieving evidence-based patient choice* (pp. 73–78). New York, NY: Oxford University Press.

Geist-Martin, P., Sharf, B., & Jeha, N. (2008) Communicating healing holistically. In M. Dutta & H. Zoller (Eds.), *Emerging perspectives in health communication: Meaning, culture, power* (pp. 85–112). London: Routledge.

Graugaard, P. K., Holgersen, K., Eide, H., & Finset, A. (2005). Changes in physician–patient communication from initial to return visits: A prospective study in a haematology outpatient clinic. *Patient Education and Counseling, 57*, 22–29.

Green, A. R., Carney, D. R., Pallin, D. J, Ngo, L. H., Raymond, K. L., Lezzoni, L. I. & Banaji, M. R. (2007). Implicit bias among physicians and its prediction of thrombolysis decisions for black and white patients. *Journal of General Internal Medicine, 22*, 1231–1238.

Hartzband, P., & Groopman, J. (2011). The new language of medicine. *New England Journal of Medicine, 365*, 1372–1373.

Hoffman, M. & Steinberg, M. (2002). Development and implementation of a curriculum in communication skills and psycho-oncology for medical oncology fellows. *Journal of Cancer Education, 17*, 196–200.

Hollenbeck, J. R., Beersma, B., & Schouten, M. E. (2012). Beyond team types and taxonomies: A dimensional scaling conceptualization for team description. *Academy of Management Review, 37*, 82–106.

Institute of Medicine. (2001). *Crossing the quality chasm: A new health system for the 21st century.* Washington, DC: National Academy of Sciences Press.

Institute of Medicine. (2004). *Health literacy: A prescription to end confusion.* Washington, DC: The National Academies Press.

Jones, D., & Stubbe, M. (2004). Communication and the reflective practitioner: A shared perspective from sociolinguistics and organizational communication. *International Journal of Applied Linguistics, 14*, 185–211.

Joosten, E. A. G., DeFuentes-Merillas, L., de Weert, G. H., Sensky, T., van der Staak, C. P. F., de Jong, C. A. J. (2008). Systematic review of the effects of shared decision-making on patient satisfaction, treatment adherence and health status. *Psychotherapy and Psychosomatics, 77*, 219–226.

Kneebone, R., Nestel, D., Chrzanowska, J., Barnet, A., & Darzi, A. (2006). Innovative training for new surgical roles — the place of evaluation. *Medical Education, 40*, 987–994

Kutner, M., Greenberg, E., Jin, Y., & Paulsen, C. (2006). *The health literacy of America's adults: Results from the 2003 National Assessment of Adult Literacy.* US Department of Education. National Center for Education Statistics (NCES). Publication No. 2006-483.

Kuziemsky, C. E., Borycki, E. M., Purkis, M. E., Black, F., Boyle, M., Cloutier-Fisher, D., . . . & Wong, H. (2009). An interdisciplinary team communication framework and its application to healthcare "e-teams" systems design. *BMC Medical Informatics and Decision Making, 9*, 43–55.

Laposa, J. M., Alden, L. E., & Fullerton, M. (2003). Work stress and posttraumatic stress disorder in ED nurses/personnel. *Journal of Emergency Nursing, 29*, 23–28.

Ledford, C., Seehusen, D., Villagran, M., Cafferty, L., & Childress, M. (2013). Resident scholarship expectations and experiences: Sources of uncertainty as barriers to success. *Journal of Graduate Medical Education, 5*, 564–569.

Ledford, C. J, Villagran, M. M., Kreps, G. L., Zhao, X., McHorney, C., Weathers, M., & Keefe, B. (2010). "Practicing medicine": Patient perceptions of physician communication and the process of prescription. *Patient Education and Counseling, 80*, 384–392.

Lupton, D. (1994). Toward the development of critical health communication praxis. *Health Communication, 6*, 55–67.

Mackintosh, C. (2007). Protecting the self: A descriptive qualitative exploration of how registered nurses cope with working in surgical areas. *International Journal of Nursing Studies, 44*, 982–990.

Makoul, G., & Clayman, M. L. (2006). An integrative model of shared decision making in medical encounters. *Patient Education and Counseling, 60*, 301–312.

Marin, M. J., Sherblom, J. C., & Shipps, T. B. (1994). Contextual influences on nurses' conflict management strategies. *Western Journal of Communication, 58*, 201–228.

Marvel, M. K., Epstein, R. M., Flowers, K., & Beckman, H. B. (1999). Soliciting the patient's agenda: Have we improved? *Journal of the American Medical Association, 281*, 283–287.

McWhinney, I. (1989). The need for a transformed clinical method. In M. Stewart & D. Roter (Eds.), *Communicating with medical patients* (pp. 25–42). London: Sage Publications.

Mills, L. D., & Mills, T. D. (2004). Symptoms of post-traumatic stress disorder among emergency medical residents, *Journal of Emergency Medicine, 28*, 1–4.

Moore, R. & Brodsgaard, I. (2001). Dentists' perceived stress and its relation to perceptions about anxious patients. *Community Dental Oral Epidemiology, 29*, 73–80.

Ofri, D. (2011, December 29). The provider will see you now. *Well.* Retrieved from http://well.blogs.nytimes.com/2011/12/29/the-provider-will-see-you-now/?ref=health

Patrick, K., & Lavery, J. F. (2007). Burnout in nursing. *Australian Journal of Advanced Nursing, 24*, 43–48.

Penner, L. A., Dovidio, J. F, West, T. V., Gaertner, S. L., Albrecht, T. L., Dailey, R. K., & Markova, T. (2010). Aversive racism and medical interactions with black patients: A field study. *Journal of Experimental Social Psychology, 46*, 436–440.

Quinn, G. P., Jimenez, J., Meade, C. D., Muñoz-Antonia, T., Gwede, C. K., Castro, E., . . . Brandon, T. H. (2011). Enhancing oncology health care provider's sensitivity to cultural communication to reduce cancer disparities: A pilot study. *Journal of Cancer Education, 26*(2), 322–325.

Razavi, D., Merckaert, I., Marchal, S., Libert, Y., Conradt, S., Boniver, J., . . . Delvaux, N. (2003). How to optimize physicians' communication skills in cancer care: Results of a randomized study assessing the usefulness of post-training consolidation workshops. *Journal of Clinical Oncology, 21*, 3141–3149.

Schmittdiel, J., Grumbach, K., Selby, J. V., Quesenberry, C. P., Jr. (2000). Effect of physician and patient gender concordance on patient satisfaction and preventive care practices. *Journal of General Internal Medicine, 15*, 761–769.

Schriner, C. L. (2007). The influence of culture on clinical nurses transitioning into the faculty role. *Nursing Education Perspectives, 28*, 145–149.

Schwartzberg, J. G., VanGeest, J. B., & Wang, C. C. (Eds.). (2005). *Understanding health literacy: Implications for medicine and public health*. United States: American Medical Association.

Sepucha, K., R., Belkora, J., K., Mutchnick, S., & Esserman, L. J. (2002). Consultation planning to help breast cancer patients prepare for medical consultations: Effect on communication and satisfaction for patients and physicians. *Journal of Clinical Oncology, 20*(11), 2695–2700.

Sharf, B., & Vanderford, M. L. (2003). Illness narratives and the social construction of health. In T. Thompson, A. Dorsey, K. Miller, & R. Parrot (Eds.), *Handbook of health communication* (pp. 9–34). Mahwah, NJ: Lawrence Erlbaum.

Sparks, L., & Villagran, M. M. (2010). *Provider-patient communication: Global perspectives.* London: Polity Press.

Stepanikova, I. (2006). Patient-physician racial and ethnic concordance and perceived medical errors. *Social Science & Medicine, 63,* 3060–3066.

Street, R. L., Jr., O'Malley, K. J., Cooper, L.A., & Haidet, P. (2008). Understanding concordance in patient-physician relationships: personal and ethnic dimensions of shared identity. *Annals of Family Medicine, 6,* 198–205.

Villagran, M. M., & Baldwin, P. (2014). Health care team communication. In S. Chou & H. Hamilton (Eds.) *The Routledge handbook on language and health communication* (pp. 339–354). New York, NY: Routledge.

Villagran, M. M., Baldwin, P., Goldsmith, J., & Wittenberg-Lyles, E. (2010). Communicating comfort: Audience-centered communication in the medical encounter. *Communication Education, 59,* 220–235.

Weiss, B. D. (2007). *Health literacy and patient safety: Help patients understand* (2nd ed.) United States: American Medical Association.

Willard, C., & Luker, K. (2007). Working with the team: Strategies employed by hospital cancer nurse specialists to implement their role. *Journal of Clinical Nursing, 16,* 716–724.

Wu, R., Lo, V., Rossos, P., Kuziemsky, C., O'Leary, K., Cafazzo, J., & . . . Morra, D. (2012). Improving hospital care and collaborative communications for the 21st century: Key recommendations for general internal medicine. *Interactive Journal of Medical Research, 1,* e9.

Zoppi K, & Epstein RM. (2002). Is communication a skill? Communication behaviors and being in relation. *Family Medicine, 34,* 319–324.

5

Approaches to Studying Provider–Patient Communication

Carma L. Bylund and
Christopher J. Koenig

Imagine that you are a parent and you take your one-year-old baby to the pediatrician for a check-up. During the short visit, the pediatrician quickly checks the child over and asks you a series of closed-ended questions. At the end of the visit, the physician recommends a prescription for oral vitamin drops and tells you to get it filled. Recently, you had read on a parenting website that oral vitamins are not necessary, and you had a similar discussion about this issue with a colleague. As the physician is on her way out the door, you realize you have no intention of filling the prescription, but you don't tell the pediatrician this. You wouldn't want her to think you are a bad parent or that you are questioning her authority.

Healthcare interactions like this are not uncommon. Healthcare providers have little time and often feel rushed. Patients and family members do not always bring up treatment preferences or concerns they might have. These and a multitude of other issues often lead to poor provider–patient communication, which can lead to poor health outcomes.

The study of **provider–patient communication** has spanned several decades. From early work by Barbara Korsch in the late 1960s (Korsch, Gozzi, & Francis, 1968), research on provider–patient communication today is multidisciplinary and multi-methodological. In this chapter, we provide a broad overview of the knowledge gained from these studies, followed by a more critical analysis of some of this work.

METATHEORETICAL APPROACHES TO STUDYING PROVIDER–PATIENT COMMUNICATION

What we know about provider–patient communication has come primarily from two different metatheoretical approaches: the scientific and the interpretive.[1] We will explain in more detail in the next section about the methods of these approaches, starting with an overview of findings.

The Scientific Approach: Communication is Measurable

From a scientific approach, we know that provider–patient communication matters in many ways. We also know that processes of communication that occur

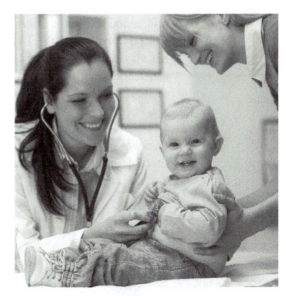

during a healthcare encounter are affected by many factors and that good healthcare communication leads to positive outcomes. The definition of *good* depends on how the researchers have defined the conceptual framework of their study, but ultimately most ways of conceptualizing good healthcare communication can be categorized as being *patient-centered*.

Communication and outcomes. Many factors of patient-centered provider–patient communication have been shown to be related to the outcome of **patient satisfaction**. A sizeable body of studies using the **Roter Interaction Analysis System** (RIAS; Roter & Larson, 2002), which analyzes each utterance of communication in the clinical consultation, has provided a great deal of information about how clinical communication affects patient satisfaction. This research shows that satisfaction is affected positively by physician question asking and counseling about psychosocial topics and affected negatively by physician dominance (Bertakis, Roter, & Putnam, 1991), that physician informal talk is related to patient satisfaction during the history taking phase (Eide, Graugaard, Holgersen, & Finset, 2003), and that patients are most satisfied when the majority of the talk is psychosocial (Roter et al., 1997) and when certain types of humor are used (Sala, Krupat, & Roter, 2002).

An Australian study showed that involving a patient in the decision-making process about cancer treatment during a consultation to the extent they want to be involved led to more satisfaction (Gattellari, Butow, & Tattersall, 2001). Study participants have also reported that when they have talked with their healthcare providers about Internet information they have read about their health issue, that provider's validation of their efforts and taking the information seriously was related to their satisfaction with the visit (Bylund et al., 2007; Bylund, Gueguen, D'Agostino, Li, & Sonet, 2010). Research has also shown that patient characteristics such as age, race, and literacy may affect satisfaction (Jensen, King, Guntzviller, & Davis, 2010), but even when many patient factors are accounted for, providers' communication still makes a difference (Clever, Jin, Levinson, & Meltzer, 2008).

Good provider–patient communication also can have a significant impact on the outcome of patient **adherence** to treatments and recommendations. A recent meta-

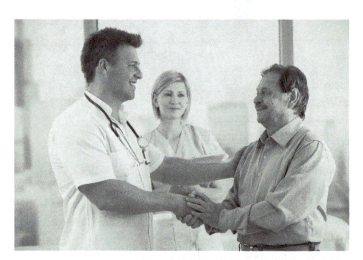

analysis found a 19% higher risk of **nonadherence** for patients with physicians who communicated poorly than for those with physicians who communicated well (Zonierek & DiMatteo, 2009). One recent study from the Netherlands suggested that the positive or negative words used when the provider delivers bad news about a diagnosis to the patient may impact adherence (Burgers, Beukeboom, & Sparks, 2012). As an example of adherence, provider–patient communication can play an important role in whether or not individuals adhere to regular screening recommendations, such as for breast and colon cancers (Fox & Stein, 1991). Factors associated with screening intent or adherence include a physician's simply recommending the screening test (Brenes & Paskett, 2000), the enthusiasm of the physician about the screening test (Fox et al., 2009), and the extent to which the patient feels the doctor communicates in a trusting way (Liang, Kasman, Wang, Yuan, & Madelblatt, 2006). Similarly, Schoenthaler and colleagues found that African-Americans being treated for hypertension were more likely to be adherent to their medications when their providers used collaborative communication (Schoenthaler et al., 2009).

Other research has demonstrated that patients report less anxiety after a consultation when provider communication is compassionate (Fogarty, Curbow, Wingard, McDonnell, & Somerfield, 1999) and when patients' preferences for decision making are matched (Gattellari et al., 2001). Often cited as well are studies that show that good patient communication is related to lower malpractice risk (Levinson, Roter, Maullooly, Dull, & Frankel, 1997). Whether and how communication affects actual patient health outcomes is not well understood. Patient health may be operationalized in several ways, including pain, disease markers such as blood sugar or blood pressure, or functional capacity (Street, Makoul, Arora, & Epstein, 2008). A review of randomized controlled trials testing the effect of communication interventions on patient outcomes found that although the interventions helped to improve communication, less than half of the studies found a significant impact on the outcomes of interest (Griffin et al., 2004).

Impacts on provider–patient communication. Provider–patient communication doesn't happen in a vacuum, as there are many factors that affect that communication. First, **patient characteristics** can affect the interaction. Many studies have shown that patients differ on how much information they want (e.g., Nagler et al., 2010) and how involved they want to be in decision making (Chewning et al., 2012). Second, **provider characteristics** can also affect the interaction. For example, female physicians tend to use more patient-centered communication (Roter, Hall, & Aoki, 2002). Finally, physician and patient demographic characteristics, such as race and gender **concordance**, can also affect provider–patient communication (Schmittdiel, Grumbach, Selby, & Quesenberry, 2000; Schoenthaler, Allegrante, Chaplin, & Ogedegbe, 2012). Street (2003) offers an ecological model that summarizes the many factors that can impact provider–patient communication. Chapter 2 of this text describes Street's model in more detail.

SCIENTIFIC AND INTERPRETIVE APPROACHES TO RESEARCH

Scientific approaches to research on provider-patient communication start from the premise that communication is measurable. High quality scientific research studies can measure behaviors to show how the communication process influences various aspects of healthcare delivery, including quality, safety, and other phenomena. Tightly fitted measurements can show both direct and indirect effects on health and health outcomes. Interpretive approaches to research, on the other hand, start from the premise that communication is a process. High quality interpretive research documents the techniques and practices for documenting the relationship between communication and how we live our lives socially. In-depth analysis of the communication process can document social practices according to different granularity.

The Interpretive Approach: Communication is a Social Process

An interpretive approach to the study of provider–patient interaction is one that acknowledges the intertwined nature of communication and social life. Interpretive approaches tend to take the position that communication occurs in social interaction as a part of larger social processes. Interpretive approaches document the communication process in varying levels of detail by describing recurrent interactional and linguistic patterns that lead to different interactional outcomes (Hodges, Kuper, & Reeves, 2008; Roberts & Sarangi, 2005).

One fundamental premise of an interpretive approach to provider–patient interaction is that communication is a form of **social action**. This means that *saying* something is also *doing* something. Consider the case of a person going to a primary care physician for a sore throat. When asked about her symptoms, the patient can describe the type of pain she has when she swallows hot tea, when the soreness started and how long it has persisted, and the other associated symptoms. When she describes these symptoms to a physician in the context of a primary care visit, she starts a communication process in which describing her problem is also doing something, namely, engaging with the physician about a medical problem. After hearing the symptoms, the physician examines her before deciding if the patient's symptoms merit treatment, such as antibiotics, or some other course of action, such as lab tests or referral to a specialist.

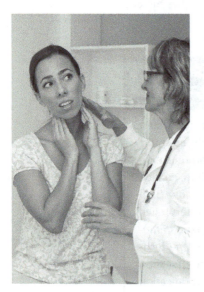

Two things are significant about this example. First, the patient's description started a communication process, namely, requesting medical help for an acute medical problem. Second, the patient's request leads to a variety of interactional outcomes. Depending on what the physician finds in her independent exploration of the problem, the physician may recommend antibiotics or two days' bed rest with an over-the-counter remedy.

While interpretive approaches often focus on communication as social action, previous research has shown that social action can occur at different levels of detail, or **granularity**. Some actions occur at a very fine granularity, while others occur at very gross granularity (Schegloff, 2000, 2006). For example, a social action that occurs at a fine level of granularity might be discovered from close examination of how a speaker constructs the individual words she uses in a speaking turn at talk. Alternatively, a social action that occurs at a gross level of granularity might be discovered by examining how different activities, such as patient history taking and the physical examination, are ordered and distributed across a whole medical visit. In the next two sections, we will describe each of these points along the continuum.

Fine granularity: Turn design and lexical choice. At the fine level of granularity, previous research has shown how physicians and patients enact social actions through how they construct their turns at talk. This form of analysis is known as **turn design** (Schegloff, 2007). Theoretically, the idea behind turn design is the notion that speakers have some control over not only *what* they say but also *how* they say it. One basic research technique is to examine lexical choices, that is, the individual words a speaker uses to make up an individual turn at talk (Heritage, Robinson, Elliot, Beckett, & Wilkes, 2007; Koenig, 2008). Paying close attention to a physician's or patient's lexical choice can result in powerful observations about how language is used in the communication process.

For example, when primary care providers recommend treatment in an acute medical visit, they have many choices to refer to the treatment itself (Koenig, 2008). When recommending treatment for a sore throat, a physician might use a very general term, like "I'm going to recommend *some medicine* to help your throat." Another choice the physician has is to refer to the treatment in slightly more specific terms, "I'm going to recommend *antibiotics* to help your throat." Yet another alternative is to refer to the treatment according to its trade or marketing name, "I'm going to recommend *Zithromax* to help your throat." Finally, the physician could refer to the treatment in technical terms, "I'm going to recommend *azithromycin* to help your throat." The lexical choices physicians make when recommending treatment lead to different interactional outcomes. Specifically, very general and technical terms appear to lead to immediate patient acceptance, whereas more specific and trade names can lead to delayed patient acceptance. Overall, this research shows that small differences in turn design can lead to large differences in interactional outcomes.

Gross granularity: Overall sequence organization. At the gross level of granularity, within a single medical visit, multiple activities can and do occur. Considering a medical visit for a new medical problem, researchers using actual audio-recorded medical visits identified recurrent activities to construct a theoretical model showing how specific activities relate to one another (Byrne & Long, 1976). Figure 5.1 illustrates the recurrent activities for a single acute medical visit.

Medical visits begin with physicians and patients opening the visit with general social greetings, like "hello" and "how are you?" Soon, the visit

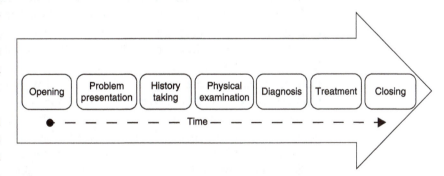

Figure 5.1 Overall Structural Organization of the Acute Medical Visit As an Episode of Social Interaction

moves into the main order of business in which physicians solicit patients' reason(s) for the visit, to which patients respond with symptom descriptions. Next, physicians conduct verbal and physical examinations in which they observe and document the presence or absence of a legitimate medical problem. Once physicians have identified the problem, they announce a diagnosis and recommend possible treatments for the problem. Finally, visits end with talk of future contact and a farewell. This recurrent organization defines tacit roles and responsibilities for both physician and patient where each activity has a distinct organization with unique norms for how it is conducted.

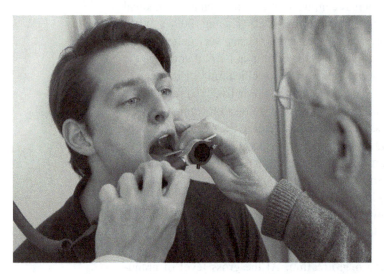

The form of analysis that identifies these gross activities to determine how each one is ordered relative to one another is called **overall structural organization** (Robinson, 2012; Schegloff, 2006). This form of analysis is significant because how a patient presents a new medical problem may indicate what kind of diagnosis or treatment the patient may want, such as antibiotics (Stivers, 2005a, 2005b). Similarly, physicians may orient to patient questions about complementary and alternative treatment in different ways depending on *where* the question is asked in the visit (Koenig, Ho, Yadegar, Tarn, & Yaedgar, 2012). Further, overall structural organization may help explain apparently contradictory differences in patient satisfaction, a common outcome measure discussed above. For example, some research recognizes that when physicians ask questions during the activity of history taking, patients indicate being satisfied overall with the relationship with their physician (Robinson & Heritage, 2006). Contradictorily, other research indicates that when physicians ask questions during the activity of the physical examination, patients indicate being unsatisfied overall with their relationship with their physician (Eide et al., 2003). Overall structural organization can explain this apparent discrepancy because this form of analysis recognizes that each activity has unique norms and expectations that have an overall effect on communication during the medical visit. Whereas asking questions may be perceived as normative during the verbal examination, patients may perceive question asking during a physical exam to be challenging the legitimacy of their illness.

Overall, characterizing talk as a form of social action, interpretive approaches acknowledge the intertwined nature of communication and social life. Whereas some actions are transparent and have everyday labels to help recognize them, like apologizing or thanking, other actions require more technical analysis to understand the social action accomplished. For example, a patient can make a declarative statement to make a request, such as, "I am almost out of refills for my prescription." Interpretive approaches draw attention to the diversity of ways in which talk constructs our daily lives by recognizing that small differences in what or how something is said can have large social consequences.

RESEARCH DESIGNS AND ANALYTIC STRATEGIES

When considering how we know about provider–patient communication, both research design and analytic strategy are important considerations. Research design includes epistemological, theoretical, and practical aspects of how a research project is to be carried out, which all influence what kinds of analytic strategies are possible for a given study.

Research Design

From both the scientific and interpretive approaches, a common component of research design in provider–patient communication research is the recording of actual healthcare encounters. Below, we explain how recording healthcare encounters can be used in both naturalistic and interventional research designs.

Naturalistic. One form of research design is naturalistic (Lincoln & Guba, 1985). **Naturalism** is an epistemological orientation that values investigating the total environment within which communication and other factors interact holistically. Naturalism seeks to investigate settings, episodes, and interactions to include not only *what* is said (e.g., the content) but also *how* something is said (e.g., the manner), *where* something is said (e.g., the context, environment), and *to whom* it is said (e.g., the participants). Because these components are inter-related, naturalism recognizes that communication occurring between participants is more than the sum of its individual parts. For example, in studies of physician–patient interaction, while physician and patient age, sex, and ethnicity/race may all influence aspects of the communication between participants, many other factors may also influence what actions are enacted, including the structure of the examination room, the process through which the patient arrived at the medical visit, and even how long participants have known one another.

Methodologically, naturalism mandates documenting social situations in as much detail as possible and practical to minimize disruption of the interaction as it unfolds. Modes of data collection associated with naturalism include both participant observation, such as sitting in the exam room writing notes about what happens during the medical visit, and non-participant observation, such as audiovisual recording. Audiovisual recording is a common method to naturalistically document communication between provider and patient during a healthcare visit because it is relatively unobtrusive and portable, which encourages participants to forget about the fact they are being recorded.

Recordings are a rich form of data because they document various aspects of the communicative situation, including the rate of speech, pauses, interruptions, and emphasis, and they are easily used for both qualitative and quantitative analysis and from various epistemological and theoretical perspectives. Using a single video recorded interaction between a physician and patient, Gill, Halkowski, and Roberts (2001) analyzed the complex dynamics that occur when patients initiate requests of their providers in subtle ways. In this case, they used the video to show that patients sometimes request medical procedures, such as an HIV diagnostic test, in indirect ways. The researchers used audiovisual recording naturalistically to capture the actual details of how the patient issued the request over the course of the visit and how the physician understood and ultimately responded to the patient's request. Overall, naturalism approaches communication as a social process that emphasizes non-interference with the activity at hand in order to capture the details of how people actually interact with one another in real time.

RESEARCH DESIGN: NATURALISTIC AND INTERVENTION RESEARCH

A naturalistic research design seeks to document the communication process in its natural environment. An intervention research design seeks to manipulate the communication process in order to determine if changing one variable can lead to a change in another variable.

Intervention. Another type of research design in studying physician–patient communication is an experimental research design. The most common type is an **intervention** design, which typically manipulates some aspect of the communication between provider and patient to see how much of an effect the manipulated variable may have on the resulting communication (i.e., interactional outcome) as measured by audiovisual recordings, surveys, interviews, or other self-report methods. For example, Richard Brown and colleagues developed a Question Prompt List (QPL), a patient-focused intervention to help cancer patients plan which questions they wanted to ask their doctors (Brown, Butow, Boyer, & Tattersall, 1999). A QPL is a list of common questions that patients can read in order to choose which ones they will ask. To test the intervention, the researchers randomized patients waiting to see a medical oncologist into one of three groups: control, QPL, and QPL plus an interactive coaching session. Brown and colleagues analyzed the subsequent visits between the medical oncologists and the patients and found that receiving the QPL increased total question asking in the encounter but that the coaching did not make a difference. The work on physician communication training also takes an intervention approach, and we will be discussing that work more later in the chapter.

A creative method for experimental studies about provider–patient encounters is the use of the **"unannounced" standardized patient**, referred to as a USP (Siminoff et al., 2011). An actor, playing the role of a patient, is scheduled for a regular visit with a clinician who has previously consented ahead of time to have a USP visit him or her sometime in the future (e.g., 12 months; Epstein et al., 2006). The USP has an audio recorder hidden that captures the conversation. The physician and his or her office are reimbursed for a comparable amount of money that a real patient would have paid. This approach allows the researcher to manipulate variables that can't be manipulated in a naturalistic setting, such as patient gender and race or what the patient says. For instance, Epstein and colleagues (2007) had primary care physicians meet with two USPs. The USPs were trained to say that they were worried about "something serious" and were randomized to present either straightforward gastroesophageal reflux or chest pain with medically unexplained symptoms.

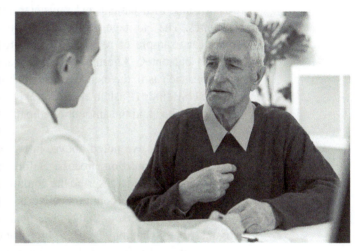

The researchers found that physician empathy was associated with overall USP ratings of interpersonal care in the scenario of medically unexplained symptoms.

As described above, naturalistic and experimental research designs use recordings as primary data. However, analytic strategies of the recordings differ significantly depending on whether one is using a scientific or interpretive approach.

Analytic Strategies

Scientific. From the scientific approach, the most common analysis of provider–patient communication applies interaction analysis systems to the recorded consultations. Coding may be done on a transcript or directly from a recording. The most frequently used system is the RIAS (Roter & Larson, 2002), which codes every utterance of patient or provider speech into a predetermined category. Researchers then use descriptive statistics to describe quantitatively how interactions happen.

Other studies may code only a piece or pieces of the interaction depending on their research interests. For instance, Bylund and Makoul (2002) developed the Empathic Communication Coding System wherein patient-initiated empathic opportunities are first identified and coded, and then doctors' responses are coded. Other researchers have looked specifically at talk about clinical trials (Brown, Butow, Ellis, Boyle, & Tattersall, 2004).

Analyses of recordings from the scientific approach may be used in different ways. Researchers may look for statistical associations between the quantitative descriptions of talk with patient and physician characteristics and/or patient or physician outcomes. The Heritage et al. (2007) study described in the introductory chapter is a clear example of research looking for a statistical association between word use and outcomes. Alternatively, the quantitative descriptions of talk may be the outcome, such as in the examples given above of the QPL study (Brown et al., 1999) and the USP study (Epstein et al., 2007) in which researchers examined the number of questions asked and the amount of empathic statements, respectively.

Interpretive. As we noted above, interpretive approaches are typically concerned with the communication process. Before the process can be effectively analyzed, researchers typically transcribe the communication. **Transcription** is the conversion of spoken and visible communicative behavior into a represented text (Hepburn & Bolden, 2012; Jefferson, 2004). The goal of transcription is to capture as much as possible about what may be heard by participants, including what is said (the words) and how it is said (the intonation, emphasis, speaking pauses, laughter), although gestures, patterns of head position and eye gaze, and the built environment in which the interaction takes place can also be included.

Transcription frequently uses standard written English orthography to represent participants' speech using punctuation and other symbols to represent key features of vocal delivery (Roberts & Robinson, 2004). Rather than a mechanical exercise, transcription is an active and creative part of the researchers' process. Many researchers consider transcription the first *analytic* pass of conversational data because analysts must focus on the details of both the content and form of what is said during transcription. Transcripts are always used in combination with recordings because even the best transcripts only textually represent oral and interactive features of the recorded data.

Example Transcription Symbols Commonly Used to Represent Speech Textually

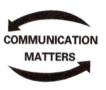

COMMUNICATION
MATTERS

DOC:/PAT:	Speaker designations identify who is speaking, such as physician (DOC) or patient (PAT).
[overlap]	Square brackets indicate onset and offset of overlapping talk.
=	Equal signs indicate utterances are run together with no gap of silence.
-	Hyphens indicate a preceding sound is cut off or self-interrupted.
°word°	Degree signs indicate decreased volume relative to surrounding talk.
(0.8)	Numbers in parentheses measure silences in seconds, tenths of a second.
(.)	Parenthesis with period indicates a "micropause" less than 2/10s of a second.
wo:rd	Colons represent prolongation or stretching of the preceding sound.
word.	Periods represent falling or turn-final intonation contours.
word,	Commas represent continuing or turn-continuative intonation contours.
word¿	Inverted question marks represent intonation rising higher than comma.
word?	Question marks represent rising intonation contours.
word	Underlining represents emphasis relative to surrounding talk.
<slow>	Less than-greater than symbols indicate decreased pace relative to surrounding talk.
>fast<	Greater than-less than symbols indicate increased pace relative to surrounding talk.
.hh	Period followed by h's indicate in-breaths; the more h's, the longer.
hh	H's alone indicate out-breaths or laughter; the more h's, the longer.
wo(h)rd	Single parenthesis filled with h's indicate breathy delivery of talk.
(word)	Single parenthesis filled indicates transcriptionist doubt.
((word))	Double parenthesis filled indicates transcriber's description or characterization of some event.

Once data are transcribed, interpretive approaches typically employ one of three general analytic strategies (Have, 2000). **Single case analyses** can be compared to a significant case study, which is common across qualitative research traditions. Single case analyses typically reveal important points of connection that only a sustained in-depth analysis can provide. Single cases analyses provide a robust analysis of specific social actions through in-depth analysis for how participants enact those actions in context. The strength of single case analysis is that individual interactions can be explored in-depth to raise key questions and demonstrate key moments to problematize taken-for-granted notions about communication or interactional conduct during medical visits. For example, Gill et al. (2001) used a single case analysis to

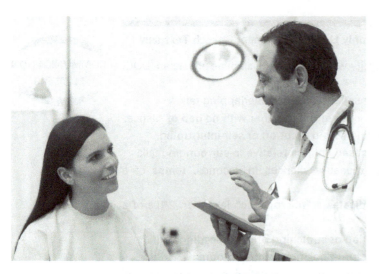

show that sometimes when patients make declarative statements about medical tests or procedures, they may also be indirectly requesting the physician to order the test or subtly eliciting the physician's opinion about a procedure. Because the unit of analysis is the single case, these analyses can present in-depth discussions of contingencies and local outcomes that may not otherwise be noticeable. In the case analyzed in Gill et al.'s study, the declarative sentence subtly does the social action of doing a request.

A second analytic strategy is based on collecting multiple cases or instances of some social action. A **multiple case collection** is an assembled group of instances of a candidate social action to demonstrate the regularity of its occurrence. These collections can be variously assembled but typically include different participants, situations, and, potentially, settings to ensure a generalizable finding. Collections building can demonstrate the regular distribution and the variability of a social action across settings and episodes. In contrast to the single case analysis, multiple case collections identify one or more key interactional features in order to systematically characterize how small differences can make big differences in action trajectories and interactional outcomes. For example, Koenig (2011) found that after physicians recommended treatment for a new medical problem, patients normatively accepted the recommendation immediately and verbally with *okay*. However, when patients did not immediately accept the recommendation or produced other talk other than *okay*, the delay was related to unarticulated treatment preferences or concerns. Rather than enacting a brief treatment recommendation sequence lasting seconds, the delay resulted in an expanded sequence that could last several minutes.

Finally, **deviant case analysis** is a general analytic strategy used across interpretive research. Through the process of building a collection, the analyst establishes inclusion and exclusion criteria for that practice. A "deviant" case is typically an instance that resembles a practice within the collection but, due to the gradually evolving inclusion/exclusion criteria established through assembly of the collection, that instance is disconfirmed as a case for inclusion. Deviant cases are good for a collection because they can show how variation is systematic and how absence of a feature can alter an interactional trajectory and, potentially, its outcome.

INTERPRETIVE ANALYTIC APPROACH

Interpretive approaches often employ single case, multiple case, or deviant case analyses. Single case analysis examines one interaction or a part of an interaction in-depth in order to understand the fine details of how the interaction works or how the component parts fit together. Multiple case analyses examine a phenomenon across many interactions to show the variation and variety of trajectories or social actions. Deviant case analyses examine cases that are unusual in some way. While each of these analytic strategies can be used individually, high quality research employs all three strategies recursively to refine a practice and its variation both within and across cases.

PATIENT PARTICIPATION IN THE HEALTHCARE ENCOUNTER

One construct of interest in provider–patient communication research is **patient participation**. We will use this construct as a context for our review of exemplar studies.

Scientific Research on Patient Participation

From a scientific perspective, patient participation is operationalized broadly as the extent to which patients communicate actively during their encounters with their providers. Two studies by Don Cegala and colleagues provide a contrast of how patient participation in the clinical encounter can be conceptualized as either the independent or dependent variable.

The first study used patients' participation as the independent variable and examined its association with physician behaviors (Cegala, Street, & Clinch, 2007). The researchers audio-recorded and transcribed physician and patient interactions, which they subsequently coded for components of patient participation, operationalized as information seeking, assertive utterances, information provision, and expression of concern. They also coded transcriptions for elements of physicians' information provision, including total information given, information elicited by a question, and information that was unprompted by the patient. Consistent with study hypotheses, results showed that patient participation in a medical visit impacted the physicians' communication. When communicating with patients with high participation, physicians provided more total information, question-elicited information, and unprompted information.

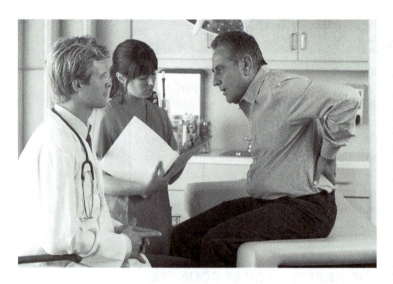

The second study was an intervention that examined how a patient communication training intervention impacted patients' participation during their consultations with their providers (Cegala, McClure, Marinelli, & Post, 2000). The researchers randomly assigned patients to receive no intervention, an instructional communication training booklet in the mail two to three days before their appointment, or a brief written summary of the major points in the booklet while patients were in the waiting room waiting to see the doctors. Twenty-five family practice physicians participated, each with six patients randomly assigned to the three interventions. The study team coded audio recordings of the consultations for varying communication behaviors that the researchers defined as patient participation, including information seeking and receiving, providing detailed information, and using information-verifying communication. Patients who received the training book asked more direct, verifying, and assertive questions, provided more information, and summarized information from the physician more frequently than those who received nothing and those who received the summary only.

Interpretive Research on Patient Participation

From an interpretive perspective, patient participation is studied as part of the communication process by examining how patients do (or do not) actively contribute to the various activities throughout the medical visit. The literature on prescribing medication is one area in which interpretive studies have been able to highlight patient participation. For example, studies involving prescriptions for antibiotics have been particularly important because primary care providers in the United States restrict access to antibiotics due to increasing concerns about increasing antibiotic resistance across the U.S. (and global) population. While the evidence-based literature shows that antibiotics do not help viral infections and therefore should only be used to treat bacterial infections, several studies show that when primary care providers perceive patients to expect antibiotics, providers are more likely to prescribe antibiotics, regardless of whether they are medically indicated (e.g., Cockburn & Pit, 1997). Interpretive research has provided evidence for how and why physicians inappropriately prescribe these medications.

Examining interactions between physicians and parents during pediatric visits, Stivers (2005b) demonstrated that parents advocate for antibiotics for children who have upper respiratory infections. She found that in interaction, parents use both direct and indirect communication techniques to exert pressure on physicians for antibiotics prescriptions. For example, parents can directly request antibiotics for their child's illness by asking the physician to write the prescription that the parent can fill at a later time only if the child's illness persists. However, this request puts physicians in a position to deny a parent's request because it does not actually propose treating the child's symptoms. Instead, it defers treatment until a later time in which it is the parent, rather than the physician, who decides whether the child will use the antibiotic. In other words, parents' direct requests orient to physicians' recommendations not as final but as negotiable.

Similarly, Stivers (2005a) showed that parents can indirectly request antibiotics for their children as well by asking if the physician will recommend antibiotics. For example, after presenting the child's problem, parents may directly ask, "Do you think we need antibiotics for this?" While it may seem counter-intuitive, asking questions is an effective technique to raise the possibility of antibiotics as an item for discussion, rather than as a request for treatment. Stivers suggests that by simply raising the possibility of antibiotics, parents position themselves in favor of antibiotics as a treatment for their child's illness, which can challenge the physician's diagnosis and projected non-antibiotic treatment plan. Asking about antibiotics therefore displays parents' preferences toward antibiotics, potentially influencing physicians' prescribing decisions.

Interpretive approaches also show that patients can actively participate in medical visits in ways that physicians sometimes do not readily recognize. For example, Koenig (2011) argues that in interactions between adult patients and their primary care providers, patients sometimes withhold acceptance of physicians' treatment recommendations as a way to advocate for their treatment preferences and concerns. When patients withhold acceptance, they subtly demonstrate being active participants in the medical visit by preventing physicians from moving

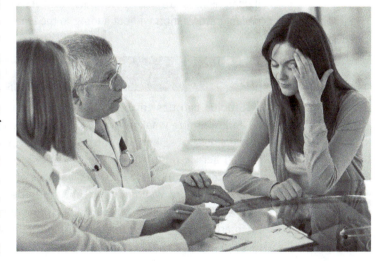

on to a next activity, which prolongs the treatment recommendation sequence. While this behavior can be subtle, physicians overtly orient to patient non-acceptance by recycling the treatment recommendation, providing additional explanation or justification for the treatment, and even changing the original recommendation to something potentially more acceptable to the patient's preferences.

Blended Scientific and Interpretive Approaches

Mixed methods are an increasingly important trend in research about physician–patient communication (Creswell, Klassen, Plano Clark, & Smith, 2011). Mixed methods is an umbrella term for research that combines multiple paradigms, such as scientific and interpretive, or multiple approaches to analysis, such as quantitative or qualitative. While mixed methods promise a more balanced picture of social phenomena, few studies are successful in combining different approaches. Heritage et al. (2007), however, successfully blended scientific and interpretive approaches to show the difference one word can make during a medical visit on patient participation. Building on the qualitative and interpretive tradition of conversation analysis, the authors hypothesized that at the end of the visit when physicians ask patients, "Do you have *any* other questions?" the use of the word *any* curtails further patient participation. Conversely, if physicians ask patients, "Do you have *some* other questions?" the use of the word *some* elicits further patient participation. The results showed a statistically significant result in which the qualitatively generated hypothesis was quantitatively confirmed. Moreover, patients presented more of their problems without significantly altering the length of the visit. The significance of this study shows that small differences in how something is said, typically an interpretive concern, can alter an outcome of the visit, typically a scientific concern. This study has important implications for communication skills training for providers because it demonstrates how the appropriate word at a crucial point in the visit leads to increased patient participation without adding to the length of the visit overall.

MIXING METHODS

Studies can use mixed-methods research designs to capitalize on strengths and minimize weaknesses of different research approaches. For example, one weakness of scientific approaches is that while results can be widely generalized across populations, processes that lead to results may be poorly documented and understood. One weakness of interpretive approaches is that while processes are well-documented, the in-depth study of a process often sacrifices generalizability. Mixed methods research designs can combine approaches to answer a research question. This methodology is relatively new, and standard practices are currently under development.

CONFLICTING RESULTS IN RESEARCH

As we introduced earlier in the chapter, patient satisfaction is a commonly examined outcome of provider–patient communication. Although components of provider–patient communication are often shown to be associated with patient satisfaction, scientific research has questioned the utility of patient satisfaction as a construct (Gil & Whilte, 2009). First, there is concern about the "ceiling effects" of patient satisfaction; patients generally give quite high ratings of satisfaction about their care (O'Connor & Shewchuk, 2003). Second, there is some conflict about how communication is associated with satisfaction and which components of communication are associated (Oliveira et al., 2012). A third conflict surrounds the construct of patient satisfaction and whether or not "patient satisfaction" measures really measure satisfaction, or if "satisfaction" is even the right construct at all. One study found that although patients reported high satisfaction scores on a self-report measure, they also gave negative evaluations of the healthcare service they received when asked in a face-to-face interview (Williams, Weinman, & Dale, 1998). Furthermore, others have suggested that instead of thinking of patient satisfaction and patient dissatisfaction as opposite ends of the same continuum, we should consider them to be two different constructs, requiring different measurement and definitions (Biering, Becker, Calvin, & Grobe, 2006).

From an interpretive perspective, the notion of patient satisfaction is problematic. Patient satisfaction is typically assessed using measures (or coding schemes) that treat "satisfaction" without specificity to the context in which it is situated, that is, in a context-free manner. For example, while in general, provider information giving is typically associated with patient satisfaction, one study of oncologist information giving (Eide et al., 2003) showed that provider information giving is paradoxically associated with negative patient satisfaction during the physical examination phase of the post-surgical cancer visit. From an interpretive perspective, this finding makes sense because the context of giving information matters: Different phases of the medical visit have unique norms and values that govern what may and may not be said. While in general, patients may value being given information, the physical examination is a unique phase of the medical visit in which particular types of information may be more or less difficult to hear. Here's an example to show you what we mean.

Imagine that you are a cancer patient seeing your oncologist during a post-surgical medical visit. While the physician has her hands on your body, she tells you that while the surgery seems to be successful, there is a high percentage of recurrence. That information, in addition to being vulnerable and at the mercy of the physician, may be too much for people who are struggling with the medical uncertainty of a cancer prog-

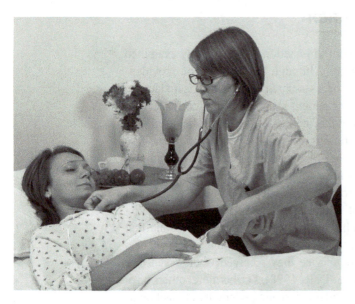

nosis, the physical challenge in recovering from surgery, and the emotional nature of being vulnerable. These findings imply that the communication behavior "information giving" has different values depending on the context in which it is presented, in this case during a particular phase of the visit.

HOW THE RESEARCH HAS BEEN APPLIED IN REAL WORLD SETTINGS

Provider–patient communication as it has been discussed in this chapter so far is very applied and real world. The body of research describing provider–patient communication from both the scientific and interpretive perspectives is best served when it is put into practice by providers and patients. There have been some research studies focusing on training patients to communicate better, as noted above. Here we will briefly overview how healthcare providers are trained in communication skills.

The teaching and assessment of communication in medical schools across the country has increased over the past few decades (Novack, Volk, Grossman, & Lipkin, 1993). The notion that communication is a core clinical skill that must be taught and evaluated during medical school (Makoul, 1999, 2001) is well accepted. In many medical schools communication skills instruction occurs across multiple years of training. On the next page we present a typical example of a role play scenario from a physician communication training class. How would you handle this situation if you were the medical student?

Changes in **communication skills education** in residency and fellowship programs has been driven by accreditation. In 1999, the Accreditation Council for Graduate Medical Education (ACGME) introduced a set of six general competencies, three of which have communication skills as a critical component: Interpersonal & Communication Skills, Patient Care, and Professionalism (Swing, 2007; also see www.acgme.org). Post-graduate training programs must demonstrate that they are teaching and assessing these skills in their trainees. Some scholars suggest that graduate medical trainees are ideal to be engaged in

Example Role Play Scenerio for Physician Communication Education

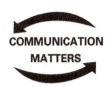

COMMUNICATION
MATTERS

Maribel McAllister, 44, lives with her husband, Peter, and four kids ages 9–17. Peter is an executive vice president at a Madison Avenue advertising agency. Maribel works part-time as a special events coordinator for the Mayor's Office in her local town. Maribel has always been quite athletic. She's run in three marathons and goes to the gym several times each week.

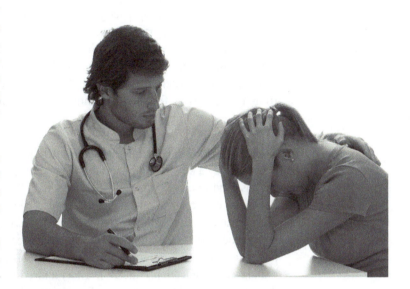

Maribel discovered a lump in her breast after showering. She has had cysts in her breasts previously, so she delayed visiting her doctor as she expected it would subside. After a month, it seemed to be getting larger, so she finally visited her doctor.

Maribel's doctor sent her for a mammogram, which revealed a cluster of three irregular dense masses with a few small calcifications in her left breast. The dominant mass measured approximately 2.0 cm. Axillary lymph nodes were suspicious for evidence of macro metastasis. Her biopsy demonstrated a poorly differentiated infiltrating ductal carcinoma. Maribel's doctor has not given her this news yet but has referred her to you, the surgeon, for advice and management of the findings. This is your first time meeting with Maribel.

Your task today is to give Maribel the bad news about her cancer.

advanced communication skills training, as they have enough experience to feel comfortable with the clinical content but have not yet established engrained communication patterns that are difficult to change (Back, Arnold, Tulsky, Baile, & Fryer-Edwards, 2003).

Practicing providers do not generally receive communication skills training. Providers at academic medical centers may have the opportunity to participate in communication skills training projects; however, these are not usually ongoing programs but instead are research studies that are only offered for a limited amount of time. Some scholars advocate that hospitals and medical centers should offer communication skills training as part of an overall strategy of quality of care (Bylund et al., 2011).

The critical importance of both patient communication and interprofessional communication to the ability of nurses and other allied health professionals to do their jobs is widely acknowledged (American Association of Colleges of Nursing, 2008). Despite its importance, nursing educators have also criticized the lack of attention to communication skills training in nursing education (Rosenzweig et al., 2008). Nurse communication is conceptualized by some educators as something that is learned through experience (Kotecki, 2002), while others have called for a move away from a behaviorally focused curriculum, focusing more on the relationship (Hartrick, 1999).

Communication skills training is an important piece of pharmacy education, as pharmacists can play a key role in interviewing patients, providing counseling regarding medications, and educating patients (McDonough & Bennett, 2006). As with medicine, pharmacy communication education has also been guided by standards set by accrediting agencies. In 2006, the Accreditation Council for Pharmacy Education (2007) listed communication skills as one of its emphasis areas in its standards and guidelines for pharmacy education programs. Pharmacy schools teach communication skills by integrating communication education into required courses, as well as offering training through specific elective courses (Beardsley, 2001). Communication training in pharmacy includes topics such as basic communication theory, basic skills such as interviewing, and assertiveness. Some schools teach more advanced skills such as risk management, leadership development, and crisis management (Beardsley, 2001). Other programs have focused on assertive communication in talking with physicians (Hasan, 2008).

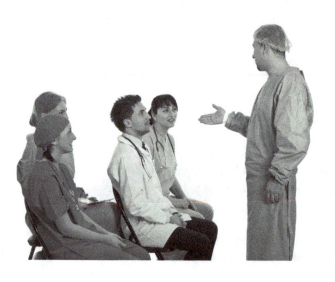

WHAT WE DO NOT KNOW

Of course, there is much we still do not know about provider–patient communication. Here we focus on two particular areas: longitudinal communication and patient-centered communication.

Longitudinal Communication

Because most studies of communication are cross-sectional, a research design that captures communication at a point in time, one of the things we do not know about is how patient–provider communication might change over time.

However, communication helps build a relationship between provider and patient through and across time (Epstein et al., 2005). Conventional notions about relationships presuppose that the longer you know someone, the stronger the relationship might be along various measurable dimensions, such as intimacy, trust, and disclosure of psychosocial information, and along various processes, such as important life course events (marriage, birth, graduations, divorce, serious illness, etc.). Yet very few studies of patient–provider communication have considered communication in its relationship to time and temporality.

This is a significant lack because longitudinal studies can empirically document how some topic or concern gets raised at one point and is (or is not) followed up at a later point. For example, a primary care provider managing a person with diabetes may hold off discussions about moving from oral medication to injectable insulin until she feels enough rapport to raise that sensitive topic in a way that will not be immediately perceived as (face) threatening. Conversely, providers who know their patients for a long period of time may routinely use extremely direct communication strategies, thereby disregarding potentially (face) threatening communication because they have a stable relationship achieved over time (Koenig et al., 2012). Longitudinal studies of provider–patient communication would help to fill this gap and begin to answer questions about how communication is embedded in the flow of time, as well as how communication between healthcare providers and patients contributes more generally to continuity of care within and across practice settings.

Patient-centered Communication

Amid the current debates about healthcare reform in the United States, patient-centeredness has become one of the main concepts guiding transformation. The Institute of Medicine characterizes patient centeredness as encompassing "qualities of compassion, empathy, and responsiveness to the needs, values, and expressed preferences of the individual patient" (2001, pp. 48–51). While the concept has been productive in re-examining the role of safety and treatment within the healthcare system, it has had both ethical and empirical setbacks. Conceptually, Berwick (2009) asserts that patient-centeredness is a unique dimension of healthcare in its own right, regardless of its relationship to other desirable aims. Empirically, though, little research has identified what observable activities might actually be considered "patient-centered." For example, shared decision making is universally included under the umbrella of patient-centeredness. However, substantive questions still persist about both the process and outcomes of what a "shared decision" actually looks like in practice.

On the one hand, scientific research suggests that patients' views of shared decision making may be different from researchers' definitions of shared decision making. In a study examining communication about colorectal cancer screening, Wunderlich and colleagues (2010) asked patients to report if they felt that the cancer screening decision had been shared between them and their doctor. In addition, outside raters coded the decision-making process to see if it met the published, academic criteria for shared decision making (Charles, Gafni, & Whelan, 1997). The researchers found no association between the patients' reports and the outside raters' codings.

On the other hand, interpretive research criticizes shared decision making because "a decision" is typically thought of as a discrete event that happens at a discrete point in time during a medical visit. However, when actual recordings are examined, decisions between providers and patients as discrete events are more rare than "decisions as a process" that occur diffusely throughout an interaction across more than one

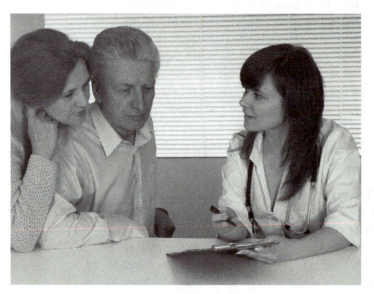

activity within a medical visit. For example, a decision about whether to adjust blood sugar medication will depend not only on the patient's report of blood sugar control but also the medical test that determines average blood sugar level over a six-month period, the amount of physical activity, dietary monitoring, and other medical, psychological, and idiosyncratic aspects of the person's life.

While shared decision making does not encompass the totality of patient-centeredness, it is a key construct that raises questions about what is measured and how those measures are clinically and social relevant to the organization of medical care and, ultimately, health outcomes. If patient-centeredness is a useful construct, more empirical work must be done to carefully operationalize specific components of patient-centeredness.

CONCLUSION

Communication between patients and providers occupies a central role for understanding health communication. In their interactions, patients explain the experience of health-related problems, and providers help to diagnose, treat, and educate patients about those problems. This healthcare delivery process depends on effective communication to build a strong therapeutic alliance and to improve health outcomes. To reach these goals, research into communication has adopted scientific and interpretive approaches to answer questions that treat communication in different ways, such as an ingredient of the healthcare process and as a variable that influences healthcare outcomes. One key area of application of the results of these studies is communication education in which a range of healthcare providers, from medical and nursing students to professional clinicians and specialists, can learn to improve their communication skills in order to strengthen the patient–provider therapeutic alliance. This alliance is an essential ingredient for patient-centered communication and healthcare delivery. Communication is both complex and multifaceted. How we study communication in healthcare settings must reflect the techniques and practices used in everyday communication to better understand how communication works and the outcomes different forms of communication have to positively influence health.

DISCUSSION QUESTIONS

1. What are some of the key differences and key assumptions between scientific and interpretive approaches to conducting research in health communication? Give two examples for how each approach can be applied to the study of health communication.
2. What is naturalism? Is naturalism associated exclusively with an interpretive approach to research? Explain why or why not.
3. Give an original example to study some aspect of healthcare delivery using a *naturalistic* approach.
4. What is an intervention? Are interventions associated exclusively with a scientific approach to research? Explain why or why not.

5. Scientific and interpretive approaches use transcription in different ways. What are some typical uses for transcription according to each approach?

IN-CLASS ACTIVITIES

1. View a television program or movie that is focused on healthcare. Find instances of provider–patient communication and consider whether you think this was effective or ineffective communication and discuss why or why not.
2. Role play a provider–patient interaction using the scenario about Maribel. Have one student play the doctor and one student play the patient. Afterwards have each participant report on challenges faced in that particular setting.
3. Devise an original communication intervention to change some aspect of health-care delivery. Be specific about the setting, participants, and measurement.

RECOMMENDED READINGS

Cegala, D. J., McClure, L., Marinelli, T. M., & Post, D. M. (2000). The effects of communication skills training on patients' participation during medical interviews. *Patient Education and Counseling, 41*(2), 209–222.

This article reports the impact of a patient-directed communication intervention study on patients' communication behavior during consultations with their physicians.

Heritage, J., Robinson, J. D., Elliot, M. N., Beckett, M., & Wilkes, M. (2007). Reducing patients' unmet concerns in primary care: The difference one word can make. *Journal of General Internal Medicine, 22*, 1429–1433.

This article reports a communication intervention that combines interpretive research findings with scientific methods to show that the words physicians use can have a large impact on local communication outcomes within a medical visit.

Street, R. L., Makoul, G., Arora, N. K., & Epstein, R. M. (2008). How does communication heal? Pathways linking clinician-patient communication to health outcomes. *Patient Education and Counseling, 74*(3), 295–301.

This article reviews the research literature on provider-patient communication and outlines several pathways through which communication can affect proximal, intermediate, and distal health outcomes.

NOTES

1 Throughout this chapter, we use the terms "scientific" and "interpretive" to refer to two distinct approaches to the study of communication. However, these terms are somewhat imprecise. As we discuss throughout the chapter, the name something is called matters for communication. When we refer to "scientific" research throughout the text, we actually mean post-positivist science. The reader should guard against the implication that one approach is systematic and the other results from "an interpretation." We affirm that both approaches are different and equally systematic ways of doing social science to study how communication affects the delivery and reception of healthcare encounters. Readers interested in learning more about theoretical approaches to the study of human communication should refer to Craig (1999); those who wish to learn more about the metatheoretical perspectives that inform methodology in human communication research should refer to Polkinghorne (1983).

REFERENCES

Accreditation Council for Pharmacy Education. (2007). *Accreditation standards and guidelines for the professional program in pharmacy leading to the doctor of pharmacy degree*. Chicago, IL: Author.

American Association of Colleges of Nursing. (2008). *The essentials of baccalaureate education for professional nursing practice*. Washington, DC: Author.

Back, A. L., Arnold, R. M., Tulsky, J. A., Baile, W. F., & Fryer-Edwards, K. A. (2003). Teaching communication skills to medical oncology fellows. *Journal of Clinical Oncology*, *21*(12), 2433–2436.

Beardsley, R. S. (2001). Communication skills development in colleges of pharmacy. *American Journal of Pharmaceutical Education*, *65*, 307–314.

Bertakis, K. D., Roter, D., & Putnam, S. M. (1991). The relationship of physician medical interview styles to patient satisfaction. *The Journal of Family Practice*, *32*(2), 175–181.

Berwick, D. M. (2009). What "patient-centered" should mean: Confessions of an extremist. *Health Affairs*, *28*(4), w555–w565.

Biering, P., Becker, H., Calvin, A., & Grobe, S. J. (2006). Casting light on the concept of patient satisfaction by studying the construct validity and the sensitivity of a questionnaire. *International Journal of Health Care Quality Assurance*, *19*, 246–258.

Brenes, G. A., & Paskett, E. D. (2000). Predictors of stage of adoption for colorectal cancer screening. *Preventive Medicine*, *31*(4), 410–416.

Brown, R. F., Butow, P. N., Boyer, M. J., & Tattersall, M. H. N. (1999). Promoting patient participation in the cancer consultation; evaluation of a prompt sheet and coaching in question asking. *British Journal of Cancer*, *80*(1/2), 242–248.

Brown, R. F., Butow, P. N., Ellis, P., Boyle, F., & Tattersall, M. H. N. (2004). Seeking informed consent to cancer clinical trials: describing current practice. *Social Science & Medicine*, *58*, 2445–2457.

Burgers, C., Beukeboom, C. J., & Sparks, L. (2012). How the doc should (not) talk: When breaking bad news with negations influences patients' immediate responses and medical adherence intentions. *Patient Education and Counseling, 89*, 267–273.

Bylund, C. L., Brown, R. F., Bialer, P. A., Levin, T. T., Lubrano di Ciccone, B., & Kissane, D. W. (2011). Developing and implementing an advanced communication training program in oncology at a comprehensive cancer center. *Journal of Cancer Education, 26*, 604–611.

Bylund, C. L., Gueguen, J. A., D'Agostino, T. A., Li, Y., & Sonet, E. (2010). Doctor-patient communication about cancer-related internet information. *Journal of Psychosocial Oncology, 28*(2), 127–142.

Bylund, C. L., Gueguen, J. A., Sabee, C., Imes, R., Li, Y., & Sanford, A. (2007). Provider-patient dialogue about internet information: An exploration of strategies to improve the provider-patient relationship. *Patient Education and Counseling, 66*, 346–352.

Bylund, C. L., & Makoul, G. (2002). Empathic communication and gender in the physician-patient encounter. *Patient Education and Counseling, 48*, 207–216.

Byrne, P. S., & Long, B. E. L. (1976). *Doctors talking to patients*. London: Her Majesty's Stationary Office.

Cegala, D. J., McClure, L., Marinelli, T. M., & Post, D. M. (2000). The effects of communication skills training on patients' participation during medical interviews. *Patient Education and Counseling, 41*(2), 209–222.

Cegala, D. J., Street, R. L., & Clinch, C. R. (2007). The impact of patient participation on physicians' information provision during a primary care medical interview. *Health Communication, 21*(2), 177–185.

Charles, C., Gafni, A., & Whelan, T. (1997). Shared decision-making in the medical encounter: What does it mean? (or it takes at least two to tango). *Social Science & Medicine, 44*(5), 681–692.

Chewning, B., Bylund, C. L., Shah, B., Arora, N. K., Gueguen, J. A., & Makoul, G. (2012). Patient preferences for shared decisions: A systematic review. *Patient Education and Counseling, 86*, 9–18.

Clever, S. L., Jin, L., Levinson, W., & Meltzer, D. O. (2008). Does doctor-patient communication affect patient satisfaction wtih hospital care? Results of an analysis with a novel instrumental variable. *HSR: Health Services Research, 43*(5), 1505–1519.

Cockburn, J., & Pit, S. (1997). Prescribing behaviour in clinical practice: patients' expectations and doctors' perceptions of patients' expectations—A questionnaire study. *BMJ, 315*(7107), 520–523.

Craig, R. T. (1999). Communication theory as a field. *Communication Theory, 9*(2), 119–161.

Creswell, J. W., Klassen, A. C., Plano Clark, V. L., & Smith, K. C. (2011). *Best practices for mixed methods research in the health sciences*. Rockville, MD: National Institutes of Health. Retrieved from http://obssr.od.nih.gov/mixed_methods_research

Eide, H., Graugaard, P., Holgersen, K., & Finset, A. (2003). Physician communication in different phases of a consultation at an oncology outpatient clinic related to patient satisfaction. *Patient Education and Counseling, 51*(3), 259–266.

Epstein, R. M., Franks, P., Shields, C. G., Meldrum, S. C., Miller, K. N., Campbell, T. L., & Fiscella, K. (2005). Patient-centered communication and diagnostic testing. *Annals of Family Medicine, 3*(5), 415–421.

Epstein, R. M., Hadee, T., Carroll, J., Meldrum, S. C., Larndner, J., & Shields, C. G. (2007). "Could this be something serious?" Reassurance, uncertainty, and empathy in response to patients' expressions of worry. *Journal of General Internal Medicine, 22,* 1731–1739.

Epstein, R. M., Shields, C. G., Meldrum, S. C., Fiscella, K., Carroll, J., Carney, P. A., & Duberstein, P. R. (2006). Physicians' responses to patients' medically unexplained symptoms. *Psychosomatic Medicine, 68,* 269–276.

Fogarty, L. A., Curbow, B. A., Wingard, J. R., McDonnell, K., & Somerfield, M. R. (1999). Can 40 seconds of compassion reduce patient anxiety? *Journal of Clinical Oncology, 17,* 371–379.

Fox, S. A., Heritage, J., Stockdale, S. E., Asch, S. M., Duan, N., & Reise, S. P. (2009). Cancer screening adherence: Does physician-patient communication matter? *Patient Education and Counseling, 75,* 178–184.

Fox, S. A., & Stein, J. A. (1991). The effect of physician-patient communicaiton on mammography utilization by different ethnic groups. *Medical Care, 29*(11), 1065–1082.

Gattellari, M., Butow, P. N., & Tattersall, M. H. (2001). Sharing decisions in cancer care. *Social Science & Medicine, 52*(12), 1865–1878.

Gil, L., & Whilte, L. (2009). A critical review of patient satisfaction. *Leadership in Health Services, 22,* 8–19.

Gill, V. T., Halkowski, T., & Roberts, F. (2001). Accomplishing a request without making one: A single case analysis of a primary care visit. *Text – Interdisciplinary Journal for the Study of Discourse, 21*(1/2), 55–81.

Griffin, S. J., Kinmonth, A. L., Veltman, M. W. M., Gillard, S., Grant, J., & Stewart, M. (2004). Effect on health-related outcomes of interventions to alter the interaction between patients and practitioners: A systematic review of trials. *Annals of Family Medicine, 2*(6), 595–608.

Hartrick, G. (1999). Transcening behaviorism in communication education. *Journal of Nursing Education, 38*(1), 17–68.

Hasan, S. (2008). A tool to teach communication skills to pharmacy students. *American Journal of Pharmaceutical Education, 72*(3), 1–6.

Have, P. T. (2000). *Doing conversation analysis: A practical guide.* London: Sage.

Hepburn, A., & Bolden, G. (2012). The conversation analytic approach to transcription. In T. Stivers & J. Sidnell (Eds.), *The handbook of conversation analysis* (pp. 57–76). Cambridge, England: Cambridge University Press.

Heritage, J., Robinson, J. D., Elliot, M. N., Beckett, M., & Wilkes, M. (2007). Reducing patients' unmet concerns in primary care: The difference one word can make. *Journal of General Internal Medicine, 22,* 1429–1433.

Hodges, B. D., Kuper, A., & Reeves, S. (2008). Qualitative research — Discourse analysis. *BMJ, 337*(7669), 570–72.

Institute of Medicine. (2001). *Crossing the quality chasm: A new health system for the 21st century.* Washington, DC: Institute of Medicine.

Jefferson, G. (2004). Glossary of transcript symbols with an introduction. In G. Lerner (Ed.), *Conversation analysis: Studies from the first generation* (pp. 14–31). Amsterdam/Philadelphia: John Benjamins Publishing Co.

Jensen, J. D., King, A. J., Guntzviller, L. M., & Davis, L. A. (2010). Patient-provider communication and low-income adults: Age, race, literacy, and optimism predict communication satisfaction. *Patient Education and Counseling, 79,* 30–35.

Koenig, C. J. (2008). *The structure and dynamics of negotiation treatment between physician and patient in the acute medical care visit.* Doctoral Dissertation. Department of Applied Lingusitics. Los Angeles: University of California.

Koenig, C. J. (2011). Patient resistance as agency in treatment decisions. *Social Science & Medicine, 72*(7), 1105–1114.

Koenig, C. J., Ho, E. Y., Yadegar, V., Tarn, D. M., & Yaedgar, V. (2012). Negotiating complementary and alternative medicine use in primary care visits with older patients. *Patient Education and Counseling, 89*(3), 368–373.

Korsch, B. M., Gozzi, E. K., & Francis, V. (1968). Gaps in doctor-patient communication: Doctor-patient interaction and patient satisfaction. *Pediatrics, 42*(5), 855–870.

Kotecki, C. N. (2002). Baccalaureate nursing students' communication process in the clinical setting. *Journal of Nursing Education, 41*(2), 61–68.

Levinson, W., Roter, D. L., Maullooly, J. P., Dull, V. T., & Frankel, R. M. (1997). Physician – patient communication: The relationship with malpractice claims among primary care physicians and surgeons. *JAMA, 277*(7), 553–559.

Liang, W., Kasman, D., Wang, J. H., Yuan, E. H., & Madelblatt, J. S. (2006). Communication between older women and physicians: Preliminary implications for satisfaction and intention to have mammography. *Patient Education and Counseling, 64*, 387–392.

Lincoln, E. S., & Guba, Y. S. (1985). *Naturalistic inquiry*: Beverly Hills, CA: Sage Publications, Inc.

Makoul, G. (1999). *Contemporary issues in medicine: Communication in medicine (report III)*. Washington, DC: Association of American Medical Colleges.

Makoul, G. (2001). The SEGUE framework for teaching and assessing communication skills. *Patient Education and Counseling, 45*, 23–34.

McDonough, R. P., & Bennett, M. S. (2006). Improving communicaton skills of pharmacy students through effective precepting. *American Journal of Pharmaceutical Education, 70*(3), article no. 58, 1–9.

Nagler, R. H., Gray, S. W., Romantan, A., Kelly, B. J., DeMichele, A., Armstrong, K., ... Hornik, R. C. (2010). Differences in informaiton seeking among breast, prostate, and colorectal cancer patients: results from a population-based survey. *Patient Education and Counseling, 81*, S54–62.

Novack, D. H., Volk, G., Grossman, D. A., & Lipkin, M. (1993). Medical interviewing and interpersonal skills teaching in U.S. medical schools: Progress, problems, and promise. *JAMA, 269*(16), 2101–2105.

O'Connor, S. J., & Shewchuk, R. (2003). Patient satisfaction: What is the point? *Health Care Management Review, 28*, 21–24.

Oliveira, V. C., Refshauge, K. M., Ferreira, M. L., Pinto, R. Z., Beckencamp, P. R., Negrao Filho, R. F., & Ferreira, P. H. (2012). Communication that values patient automomy is associated with satisfaction with care: a systematic review. *Journal of Physiotherapy, 58*, 215–229.

Polkinghorne, D. (1983). *Methodology for the human sciences: Systems of inquiry*. Albany, NY: State University of New York Press.

Roberts, C., & Sarangi, S. (2005). Theme-oriented discourse analysis of medical encounters. *Medical Education, 39*(6), 632–640.

Roberts, F., & Robinson, J. D. (2004). Interobserver agreement on first-stage conversation analytic transcription. *Human Communication Research, 30*(3), 376–410.

Robinson, J. D. (2012). Overall structural organization. In T. Stivers & J. Sidnell (Eds.). *The handbook of conversation analysis* (pp. 257–280). Cambridge, England: Cambridge University Press.

Robinson, J. D., & Heritage, J. (2006). Physicians' opening questions and patients' satisfaction. *Patient Education and Counseling, 60*(3), 279–285.

Rosenzweig, M., Hravnak, M., Magdic, K., Beach, M. C., Clifton, M., & Arnold, R. (2008). Patient communication simulation laboratory for students in an acute care nurse practitioner program. *American Journal of Critical Care, 17*(4), 364–372.

Roter, D. L., Hall, J. A., & Aoki, Y. (2002). Physician gender effects in medical communication: A meta-analytic review. *JAMA, 288*(6), 756–764.

Roter, D. L., & Larson, S. (2002). The Roter Interaction Analysis System (RIAS): Utility and flexibility for analysis of medical interactions. *Patient Education and Counseling, 46*(4), 243–251.

Roter, D. L., Stewart, M., Putnam, S. M., Lipkin, M. J., Stiles, W., & Inui, T. S. (1997). Communication patterns of primary care physicians. *JAMA, 277*(4), 350–356.

Sala, F., Krupat, E., & Roter, D. (2002). Satisfaction and the use of humor by physicians and patients. *Psychology and Health, 17*(3), 269–280.

Schegloff, E. A. (2000). On granularity. *Annual Review of Sociology, 26*, 715–720.

Schegloff, E. A. (2006). Interaction: The infrastructure for social institutions, the natural ecological niche for language, and the arena in which culture is enacted. In N. J. Enfield & S. C. Levinson (Eds.), *Roots of human sociality: Culture, cognition, and interaction* (pp. 70–96). Oxford, UK: Berg Publishers.

Schegloff, E. A. (2007). *A primer for conversation analysis: Sequence organization.* Cambridge, England: Cambridge University Press.

Schmittdiel, J., Grumbach, K., Selby, J. V., & Quesenberry, C. P. (2000). Effect of physician and patient gender concordance on patient satisfaction and preventive care practices. *Journal of General Internal Medicine, 15*, 761–769.

Schoenthaler, A., Allegrante, J. P., Chaplin, W., & Ogedegbe, G. (2012). The effect of patient-provider communication on medication adherence in hypertensive black patients: Does race concordance matter? *Annals of Behavioral Medicine, 43*, 372–382.

Schoenthaler, A., Chaplin, W. F., Allegrante, J. P., Fernandez, S., Diaz-Gloster, M., Tobin, J. N., & Ogedegbe, G. (2009). Provider communication effects medication adherence in hyptertensive African Americans. *Patient Education and Counseling, 75*, 185–191.

Siminoff, L. A., Rogers, H. L., Waller, A. C., Harris-Haywood, S., Esptein, R. M., Carrio, F. B., . . . Longo, D. R. (2011). The advantages and challenges of unannounced standardized patient methodology to assess healthcare communication. *Patient Education and Counseling, 82*, 318–324.

Stivers, T. (2005a). Non-antibiotic treatment recommendations: Delivery formats and implications for parent resistance. *Social Science & Medicine, 60*(5), 949–964.

Stivers, T. (2005b). Parent resistance to physicians' treatment recommendations: One resource for initiating a negotiation of the treatment decision. *Health Communication, 18*(1), 41–74.

Street, R. L. (2003). Communication in medical encounters: An ecological perspective. In T. Thompson, A. M. Dorsey, K. I. Miller, & R. Parrott (Eds.), *Handbook of health communication* (pp. 63–89). Mahwah, NJ: Lawrence Erlbaum Associates.

Street, R. L., Makoul, G., Arora, N. K., & Epstein, R. M. (2008). How does communication heal? Pathways linking clinician-patient communication to health outcomes. *Patient Education and Counseling, 74*(3), 295–301.

Swing, S. R. (2007). The ACGME outcome project: Retrospective and prospective. *Medical Teacher, 29*, 648–654.

Williams, S., Weinman, J., & Dale, J. (1998). Doctor-patient communication and patient satisfaction: A review. *Family Practice, 15*(5), 480–492.

Wunderlich, T., Cooper, G., Divine, G., Flocke, S., Oja-Tebbe, N., Stange, K., & Elston Lafata, J. (2010). Inconsistencies in patient perceptiosn and obser ratings of shared decision making: The case of colorectal cancer screening. *Patient Education and Counseling, 80*, 358–363.

Zonierek, K. B. H., & DiMatteo, M. R. (2009). Physician communication and patient adherence to treatment: A meta-analysis. *Medical Care, 47*(8), 826–834.

6

Interprofessional Communication

Health Care Teams and Medical Interpreters[1]

Kevin Real and
Marjorie M. Buckner

Communication between medical professions—**interprofessional communication**—is required for the complex care provided by most hospitals and healthcare organizations. Few, if any, individual providers can care for patients in the 21st century without some form of collaboration and assistance from other healthcare professions. Communication across professions is not easy, and there are barriers to simple and effective communication between different medical professionals. For example, physicians have their own specialties (family medicine, cardiology, surgery, radiology, etc.), as do nurses (operating room, hospital floor, medical records), and these specialties create the need for specialized vocabularies and different clinical functions. Healthcare itself has a traditional medical hierarchy that presents a number of problems to effective interprofessional communication. In addition, there are a number of other medical professions beyond nurses and doctors, such as therapists, technicians, and specialists, that add to the complexity of interprofessional communication.

We all know that a major problem in the U.S. healthcare system is ineffective communication and that it has an impact on both quality of patient care and patient safety. As the Institute of Medicine reported in its landmark study, *To Err is Human* (Kohn, Corrigan, & Donaldson, 2000), preventable medical errors account for as many as

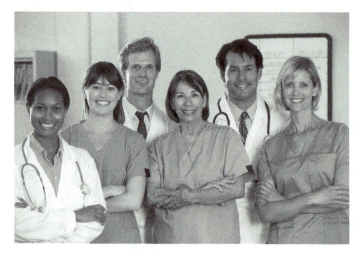

98,000 deaths in U.S. healthcare organizations each year. This finding led to a number of changes, including an emphasis on team training and recognition of the importance of communication in health care teams and organizations. Furthermore, the Joint Commission, which is the primary accrediting body for healthcare organizations, has found that more than 66% of the root causes of patient sentinel events are related to ineffective or poor communication (The Joint Commission, 2006). A **sentinel event** is an unexpected occurrence (or risk thereof) involving death of a patient or serious physical or psychological injury that signals the need for an immediate response or investigation (The Joint Commission, 2012). When people suggest that communication is not that important to the process of what people do in healthcare, they obviously are not as well informed as the readers of this book. As you can see, there is a need for clear, effective communication in healthcare. The lives of patients depend on good communication.

In this chapter, we focus on two specific areas of interprofessional communication: health care teams and medical interpreters. Within each section, we examine how leading research from multiple perspectives has informed our knowledge. We describe theories and methods, present exemplar studies, and show how the research has been applied in real world settings.

HEALTH CARE TEAMS

Medical care is complex, and the increasing need for team care is a result of a number of factors: greater specialization of care, use of healthcare professionals from different specialties, influence of the Joint Commission, and newer forms of healthcare financing and delivery. **Health care teams** are an important context where interprofessional communication occurs, and they have been examined from many different perspectives. In addition to communication scholarship, research in health care teams has been conducted in medicine, gerontology, geriatrics, nursing, surgery, group dynamics, social work, and more. For example, as you can see in Table 6.1, communication in surgical teams has been studied from a number of different perspectives, including surgery, communication, public health, medical education, and more.

Table 6.1 Examination of Surgical Team Communication from Multiple Perspectives

Authors	Discipline	Focus and Purpose	Findings
Awad et al. (2005)	Surgery	Surgical Teams Pre-post intervention at four points in time	Preoperative team briefings developed through interactive training increased communication scores of surgeons and anesthesiologists but not nurses; implementation of patient safety procedures also increased as a result of briefings.
Haynes et al. (2009)	Public Health	Surgical Teams Use of communication checklist in surgical teams for nearly 4,000 patients across globe	Patients' post-surgical rate of complications, in-hospital morbidity, surgical-site infections, and unplanned re-operations all decreased after introduction of a 19-item communication checklist in surgical teams.
Williams et al. (2007)	Medical Education/ Assessment	Surgical Teams Information transfer and communication errors assessed using focus groups	Information transfer and communication errors (boundaries of responsibility, decreased surgeon familiarity with patients, diversion of surgeon attention and distorted or inhibited communication) led to delays in patient care, wasted time, and serious adverse patient consequences.
Mills et al. (2008)	Psychiatry	Surgical Teams Survey of 384 surgical staff members in six facilities	There were perceptual differences among healthcare providers: Surgeons perceived stronger organizational culture, better communication, and better teamwork than either nurses or anesthesiologists.
Lingard et al. (2008)	Communication	Surgical Teams Introduced a communication intervention to 86 surgical teams	Average number of communication failures per procedure declined from 3.95 before the intervention to 1.31 after the intervention.

(*Continued*)

Table 6.1 Continued

Authors	Discipline	Focus and Purpose	Findings
Gardezi et al. (2009)	Critical Ethnography	Surgical Teams Observed over 700 procedures to examine whether a preoperative briefing was effective	Identified three forms of recurring "silences": absence of communication, not responding to queries or requests, and speaking quietly; these silences may be defensive or strategic and may be influenced by institutional, structural, and situational power dynamics.
Reddy & Jansen (2008)	Information Sciences	Surgical Teams Ethnography: interviews, observations of two teams	Information seeking in health care teams is a collaborative, not individual, enterprise that shapes how individuals interact with each other, the complexity of the information need, and the role of information technology.

What is interesting about these studies is that they engage the topic from different perspectives, but each points out how valuable effective team communication is to patient care.

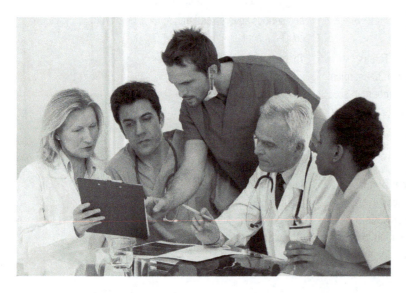

Communication in health care teams has played a significant role in patient care and has become more important over time (Poole & Real, 2003). From a communication perspective, a health care team can be defined as "an intact group of health care providers motivated to communicate with each other regarding the care of specific patients" (Real & Poole, 2011, p. 101). In the following section, we discuss what we know about communication in health care teams from different perspectives.

COMMUNICATION IN HEALTH CARE TEAMS FROM DIFFERENT PERSPECTIVES

As we mentioned, communication in health care teams has been studied from a number of perspectives. Poole and Real (2003) examined the subject from a **group dynamics perspective**, suggesting that teams can be understood on the basis of their varying degrees of **interaction, interdependence, boundedness** (the extent that members report to a supervisor within the team), **commonality** (shared knowledge, experiences, values, and norms), and **motivation** to work together.

HEALTH CARE TEAMS AS GROUPS

By examining health care teams from a group perspective, we are able to understand how and why healthcare professionals interact in certain ways. Members of each type of group (ad hoc, nominal, unidisciplinary, multidisciplinary, interdisciplinary, or transdisciplinary) may interact with each other differently depending on:

- how much group members rely on others in the group (interdependence)
- how frequently group members communicate (interaction)
- how much group members inform the group supervisor (boundedness)
- what is shared among the members (commonality)
- how invested members feel to work as a group (motivation)

Why do health care teams vary? Healthcare professionals often serve on multiple teams at the same time. A pediatrician could be part of a pediatric care team that sees patients but also could serve on a quality improvement team aimed at reducing wait time for patients. A nurse could belong to that same pediatric care team and serve on two other teams: a quality improvement team designed to improve flu care and a team devoted to reducing hospital-acquired infections. For this reason, health care teams can have high levels of interaction and commonality but low levels of interdependence and boundedness. Healthcare professionals may see each other and communicate often about some patients (interaction), but they may not need to depend on each other (interdependence) to get their work done, nor may they report to the same supervisor or work together on a regular basis (boundedness). (Chapter 4 of this text considers interpersonal aspects of interdisciplinary teams in the healthcare setting.)

Poole and Real (2003) developed a typology of health care teams, highlighting the specific purpose of particular teams and how they fulfill their functions. Table 6.2 provides an example of each type of team across various healthcare contexts.

Table 6.2 Types of Health Care Teams

Type of Team	Description	Example: Multiple Perspectives
Ad hoc	Formed for a limited period of time to address a problem and disbands when they achieve their goals	Design: Advisory group established to work with architects in the redesign of a hospital floor
Nominal Care	Provides care through independent consultation of professionals directed by a primary care physician	Patient: Individual patient is referred to specialists because of need identified by primary care MD, who stays involved with both the patient and specialists
Uni-disciplinary	Organized around a single discipline or healthcare profession such as nursing or surgery	Surgery: Surgeons develop new communication protocol for use in the operating room
Multi-disciplinary	Composed of practitioners from multiple disciplines who work in conjunction with each other but function independently	Cancer: Team composed of nurses, oncologists, surgeons, social workers, nutritionists, pharmacists, and more can provide a continuum of care
Inter-disciplinary	Practitioners from two or more disciplines working interdependently in the same setting, communicating to share information from various disciplines and to integrate care	Geriatrics: Geriatric MD, nurses, physical therapists, dentists, social workers, pharmacists, clergy, and more collaborate to address elderly patient problems
Trans-disciplinary	Team members are proficient in their own specialty and, through cross-training and working together on the team, develop overlapping skills	Chronic Disease: Shared responsibilities and blurred professional boundaries of the team allow for treatment of diseases like diabetes through improving health literacy and overcoming disparities

Adapted from Poole and Real (2003).

Ad hoc teams work together on an issue until it has been addressed. For example, a healthcare facility undergoing a redesign of a hospital floor would use an ad hoc team to work on the project. In **nominal care teams**, the physician refers patients to different specialists who provide care independently, with the "big picture" being coordinated by the physician. Communication in this type of team has a classic "wheel" structure (Leavitt, 1951) in which the primary care physician is at the center and other care providers interact with and deliver services as requested. **Unidisciplinary teams** are organized around a single discipline (e.g., surgery, anesthesiology). A unidisciplinary team could work on the development of a new communication protocol or instrument, such as a checklist that requires surgeons to verbally communicate the specifics of an operation or procedure (e.g., "removing cartilage from left knee," or "patient has no known allergies") before performing surgery on a patient.

Multidisciplinary teams are composed of practitioners from multiple disciplines who work in conjunction, but their actual patient care is often sequential. In Table 6.2, we used cancer care as an example because patients will first see an oncologist, who may or may not refer the patient to a surgeon. If the patient needs surgery, he or she would return to the care of the oncologist after the surgery and would also likely be treated by nurses, social workers, nutritionists, and more. But the health professionals would work separately on the patient's case. In contrast, **interdisciplinary teams** consist of practitioners from multiple disciplines who work interdependently in the same setting. In geriatrics, a number of healthcare professionals work together and communicate at the same time and in the same setting to address patient concerns. For example, a combi-

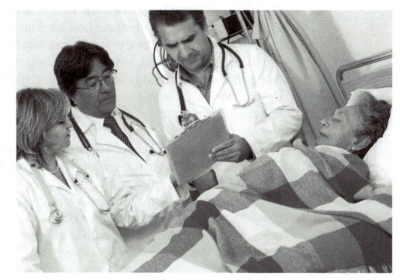

nation of physicians, nurses, physical therapists, dentists, social workers, pharmacists, and clergy could be in a patient room together, treating the patient and talking about their work with each other and their patient and families.

The final type of team is the **transdisciplinary team**, where healthcare professionals not only are proficient in their own specialty but also develop overlapping skills through cross-training and working together on the team. This is a type of interdisciplinary team in which "members have developed sufficient trust and mutual confidence to engage in teaching and learning across disciplinary boundaries" (Weiland, Kramer, Waite, & Rubenstein, 1996, p. 656). Effective transdisciplinary teams require interprofessional communication that enhances the context for both teaching and learning among care professionals. A number of studies have noted the positive impact of interdisciplinary and transdisciplinary forms of interprofessional communication in end-of-life care (Connor, Egan, Kwilosz, Larson, & Reese, 2002; Wittenberg-Lyles, Parker Oliver, Demiris, Regehr, 2010).

Each and every one of the typologies described above can be used in a variety of healthcare settings, and all have distinctive types of communication. For healthcare professionals, understanding the type of team they are working in can help clarify the kind of communication that can be effective within that context. For example, communication in ad-hoc teams tends to be task focused and characterized by information exchange. On the other hand, interprofessional communication in inter- and transdisciplinary teams is highlighted by both relational and task interaction. Reflecting the scientific and interpretive paradigms, communication in these teams involves both information exchange (scientific) and the social construction of meaning (interpretive). We will discuss this research in greater depth later in the chapter.

Real and Poole (2011) extended our understanding of communication in health care teams by drawing on the **input-process-output (IPO) model** (McGrath, 1984) derived from the group dynamics perspective. This classic framework continues to provide a useful model for understanding how groups and teams operate. Real and Poole's contribution was to develop an IPO model focused on communication (see Figure 6.1). Their model illustrates how communication structures shape communication processes and how these processes can then influence health care team outcomes. While the IPO framework originated in group dynamics, much of the research that Real and Poole examined is situated within clinical (e.g., surgical, geriatric, primary care), team (e.g., multidisciplinary, interdisciplinary), and organizational (e.g., hospital, nursing homes) contexts.

The IPO framework is helpful because it asserts that the process of communication that occurs in many health care teams is shaped by the communication structures of the team. An example comes from a large-scale study by Haynes et al. (2009) that evaluated the World Health Organization's surgical checklist. In the study, they tested a 19-item communication checklist intervention in eight hospitals across the globe. The checklist required teams to perform a number of communication activities before and during operations, such as orally confirming the patient's identity, noting that the surgical site was marked (if applicable), and confirming that members of the team were aware of the patient's allergies. The checklist also required, before incision, that all members of the team orally review any concerns they had related to the procedure. Haynes et al. found that use of the communication checklist significantly decreased negative outcomes for patients. Specifically, post-surgical rate of complications, in-hospital death rate, rates of surgical-site infection, and unplanned reopera-tions were all significantly reduced after introduction of the checklist.

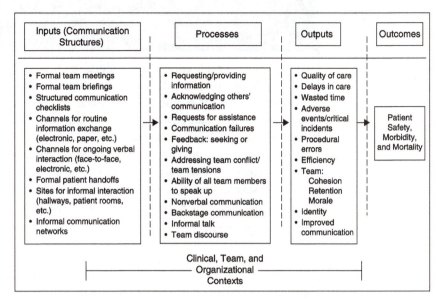

Figure 6.1 Input-Output-Process Model of Communication in Health Care Teams.

Source: From Real and Poole (2011).

In the following section we take a look at how research in interprofessional health care teams has been conducted. We also examine two differing perspectives on how interprofessional communication operates in health care teams.

HOW WE KNOW WHAT WE KNOW

A key question for those of us interested in health care teams is how and under what theoretical assumptions the research is conducted. The communication discipline is a useful arena in which to explore distinct theoretical and methodological approaches because it demonstrates a variety of contexts, methods, and primary assumptions. Communication researchers have conducted studies in a variety of applied contexts, including nursing (Apker, Propp, & Ford, 2005), oncology (Ellingson, 2003), chil-dren's mental health (Davis, 2008), emergency medicine (Eisenberg et al., 2005), patient satisfaction (Paulsel, McCroskey, & Richmond, 2006), and end-of-life hospice care (Wittenberg-Lyles et al., 2010).

Research on health care teams reflects both scientific and interpretive paradigms. On one hand, health care teams have to exchange a lot of technical and sometimes sensitive information. Scholars operating under the scientific perspective may study what hinders or improves sharing this information that then impacts patient outcomes. On the other hand, scholars may be interested in how health care team members achieve understanding and investigate how team members interact with each other. The inclusion of both paradigms in this body of scholarship is evident in the variety of methods used to study health care teams, including surveys, interviews, experiments, and observations.

Methodologically, communication research in teams is well-rounded, as there are both qualitative approaches, such as interviews, ethnography, and observations, and quantitative approaches, including surveys, field experiments using interventions, and behavioral observations. There are also elements of rhetorical analysis in some of the qualitative studies, particularly those conducted by Lingard and her colleagues (2005, 2006, 2008).

In terms of metatheoretical assumptions about interprofessional communication, there are two primary ways in which communication is assumed to operate in teams: as information exchange and as the construction of meaning. An **information exchange**

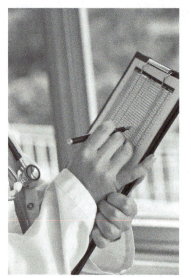

perspective, which reflects the scientific paradigm, operates on the assumption that communication is a means through which to address day-to-day issues facing health care teams. In this view, information is exchanged between members of a team so that all members are clear about their role, the patient's diagnosis, the care that will be delivered, and more. Research in this area examines the role of briefings, checklists, communication errors or information sharing in reducing adverse events, delays in patient care, and patient safety. For example, the Haynes et al. (2009) study we described earlier, which examined the impact of a communication checklist in surgical teams across eight hospitals, is a good example of communication as information exchange.

Further examples of communication as information exchange include work by Lingard and her colleagues from public health, who have conducted a series of studies assessing a preoperative checklist designed to improve communication in team briefings in the operating room

(Lingard et al., 2005, 2006, 2008). These researchers found that using a preoperative checklist provided an opportunity to talk about the details of the surgery, express any concerns, and build teamwork. Additionally, communication failures—communication that happened too late, had inaccurate content, failed to achieve its purpose, or excluded relevant team members—declined significantly after the checklist/briefing intervention. This series of studies provides empirical evidence that formal communication structures (e.g., briefings, checklists) can improve the exchange of information and increase clinical team effectiveness.

A second perspective on how communication operates in interprofessional health care teams emphasizes the socially constructed nature of interactions. In this view, which reflects the interpretive paradigm, much of what occurs in the work of teams is a result of the team's communication, which enables the **construction of meaning**. A good example of this interpretive perspective comes from Sutcliffe and colleagues (2004), who examined how communication failures contributed to medical mishaps in a teaching hospital (where future doctors, known as medical residents, are trained). Medical mishaps were defined as patient-care related incidents ranging from close calls to major incidents.

Sutcliffe and her colleagues (2004) found that communication problems often stemmed from misinterpretation of what individual providers were telling each other as they worked together. First, existing medical hierarchies and social structures led residents to be hesitant to communicate information to their supervising ("attending") physicians for fear of appearing incompetent or offending someone in power. Second, there was often a lack of information about specific patients for the residents. This tended to happen when a resident would be caring for a new patient who had been handed off to them by another doctor who did not take the time to explain the patient's situation to the resident. Third, incorrect use of communication modes or channels resulted in misinterpretation in many instances, when communication links would be so convoluted that any messages that were conveyed would be miscommunicated as they moved through the various links (similar to the telephone game many of us played in elementary school classrooms). Sutcliffe et al. provided evidence for what many in healthcare believe to be true: Miscommunication and misinterpretation lead to problems in patient care.

AN EXEMPLAR STUDY OF HEALTH CARE TEAMS

There are a number of excellent studies examining the impact of communication in health care teams. Apker's, Lindgard's, and Haynes' work are all great examples of good research, and we have discussed them elsewhere in this chapter. Here we call your attention to one additional study that has stood the test of time in terms of its unique and important contributions.

Eisenberg et al. (2005) studied communication in health care teams in two emergency departments (EDs). A number of different approaches, from sociology to health administration to emergency medicine, have sought to understand the issues facing emergency medicine, which include overcrowding, staff shortages, an increasing number of people without health insurance who use the ED to meet their primary care needs, the crisis factor (accidents, injuries, etc.), unplanned arrivals by ambulances diverted to their location, and much more. Directing our attention to competing interpretive frameworks that exist in emergency medicine, Eisenberg et al. argue that past efforts to address these problems have failed because "they have not sufficiently taken into account the real-life communicative dynamics of emergency departments" (p. 197).

The method of the study involved action research. **Action research** promotes a more in-depth collaboration between researchers and practitioners, which enables the researchers to get close to the various actors in the ED in order to conduct a close analysis of their communication. The approach also aims to bring about action in the form of change while developing an understanding of local context, which can then lead to practical improvements. As such, it reflects the critical–cultural paradigm's focus on social change. Eisenberg et al. (2005) conducted a year-long study of communication and used a qualitative, narrative analytical approach to identify the competing frameworks operating within the hospital ED. The researchers believed that unrecognized

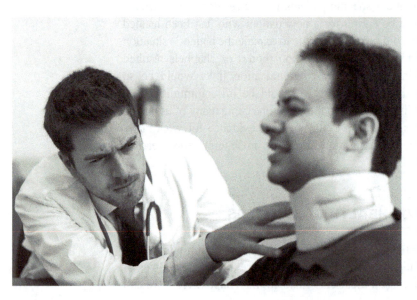

competing frameworks were an underlying factor contributing to persistent problems in the ED. As researchers and ED staff worked together, the process encouraged the staff to recognize and understand the various ways of viewing the world (frames) that operated in the ED.

The findings of this study highlighted the communicative tensions involving how meaning was constructed through communication in two distinct ways, or "rationalities."

Patients typically described their situations in story form, which Eisenberg and colleagues (2005) called "narrative rationality." For example, a driver of a car who was injured in an auto accident could relate the following: "I was crossing the intersection and the next thing I knew I was seeing stars. I figured out later that the airbag deployed when the other car ran the stop sign and hit me. Now my neck and jaw are killing me." Medical professionals, however, are trained to work in clinical contexts that rely on short, detailed information that Eisenberg et al. called "technical rationality." Patients' stories are reconstituted into constructions that work best for emergency teams, such as lists and medical jargon. In keeping with the auto accident example, the patient's story would have to be interpreted as to whether there was temperomandibular joint injury, upper cervical spine fractures, soft tissue damage, bony neck injuries, damage to the vasculature, and the like. All of these descriptors are medical terminology and are important for the diagnosis and treatment of patients.

As you can imagine, there are times when things simply get lost in translation. The construction/translation of patient stories into technical lists failed to capture the full and proper interpretation of patients' descriptions. As patients were processed, Eisenberg et al. (2005) observed miscommunication in evaluations, handoffs, and admissions. This study provides a good example nullifying the idea that communication is simply information exchange. In the ED context, any understanding of communication must fully address interpretation issues. It also highlights the difficulty and complexity in team interaction in healthcare settings.

CONFLICTING RESULTS IN THE LITERATURE

There are not many conflicting results in the literature on health care team communication. This is probably due to the fact that this line of research is in its "first generation" (Lingard, 2012). To the extent that there are differences in research findings, these distinctions are likely due more to metatheoretical perspectives than any directly conflicting results.

For example, the Haynes et al. (2009) study described earlier found that the surgical checklist was an important tool in improving patient safety. This study was based on the scientific paradigm; it used a carefully derived sample from a number of different hospitals across the globe, accounting for socio-demographic and other factors as it tried to eliminate any confounding factors that could have skewed its results. On the other hand, Lingard et al. (2006) conducted an ethnographic study and observation of a phased implementation of a preoperative team briefing. This analysis of observation-based field notes from 302 briefings yielded a model of communicative "utility," suggesting that surgical team members' performance improved as a result of communication, specifically in the areas of team awareness and individual behavior.

Lingard's interpretive approach went beyond the impact of whether or not a particular tool or activity was being utilized successfully to examine *how* teams interacted as they worked together when engaged in the briefing itself. This is not to say that Lingard et al.'s approach was superior to Haynes et al.'s approach, but merely to point out that different perspectives yield different (although not necessarily conflicting) results. Each is limited as it looks at different aspects of health care team communication, but when brought together, the studies can provide a more holistic view.

HOW THE RESEARCH HAS BEEN APPLIED IN THE REAL WORLD

We want to highlight two interesting ways in which research in interprofessional communication has been applied to actual healthcare settings. The first involves a communication protocol called **SBAR**, which stands for Situation, Background, Assessment, and Recommendation (Haig, Sutton, & Whittington, 2006). This practical approach, which was developed in the medical field, provides a structured method for healthcare professionals to communicate about patient care. This approach

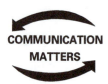

COMMUNICATION MATTERS

SBAR is Effective Communication

Here is a hypothetical example we developed to demonstrate SBAR. It presents a phone call from a nurse, Janet, to a physician, Dr. Smith, about a patient, John Doe. (We are remarkably creative.) We ran the script by a trauma surgeon and ICU nurse at the University of Kentucky Hospital to check its authenticity.

Situation: Hello, Dr. Smith, this is Janet in the 7th floor ICU at UK Hospital. Here is the situation: I am calling about your patient, John Doe, who is having trouble breathing and is complaining of chest pain.

Background: Mr. Doe had hip surgery yesterday and has been complaining of chest pains for about five minutes.

Assessment: I assessed him, and he is short of breath and his pulse is 133 and BP [blood pressure] is 141/63. I believe he is at risk for a cardiac or pulmonary-related event.

Recommendation: I recommend that you see him immediately and that we start him on the chest pain protocol stat. What do you think?

has been used in healthcare organizations to prevent the communication failures mentioned at the beginning of this chapter that have been found to be a root cause of the majority of sentinel patient events. When used regularly, SBAR can become part of a healthcare organization's culture in which healthcare professionals voluntarily use this structure to clearly and effectively communicate information about patients. This approach is particularly useful because it provides a structure that enables clear communication within the context of a busy and complex environment.

SBAR has been implemented successfully in a wide variety of healthcare settings, including intensive care, emergency departments, and operating rooms. Improvements have been seen in team communication, clinical outcomes, and patient and staff satisfaction. As you can see from the scenario presented on the previous page, SBAR is an excellent example of how a structured approach to communication can promote the exchange of critical information in a clear and effective manner. The nurse has a clear idea of what she is going to say and is much less likely to leave out or forget to convey important information. The physician is brought up to speed quickly on the patient and then is asked for input.

A second way in which interprofessional communication research has been applied in the real world is the **COMFORT communication model** developed by communication researcher Elaine Wittenberg-Lyles and her colleagues (Wittenberg-Lyles, Goldsmith, & Ragan, 2010). COMFORT is an acronym designed to assist healthcare professionals who work in end-of-life or palliative care. It stands for seven principles effective for palliative care contexts: Communication (from a narrative approach), Orienting (to health literacy and cultural diversity of patients/families), Mindful (presence), Family (caregiver communication), Openings (that allow for patient/family transition), Relating (and building trust), and Team (effectiveness).

TOOLS TO IMPROVE HEALTHCARE QUALITY

Health care team scholarship has helped develop practices and procedures that improve the quality of healthcare patients receive. Advancements such as the World Health Organization's surgical checklist and SBAR help healthcare providers effectively and expediently communicate with one another. Other communication tools such as COMFORT help healthcare providers communicate with patients and their caregivers. Studying how healthcare professionals interact with each other and with those they serve leads to innovations that can positively impact the care we receive.

As you can see in Figure 6.2, these principles are not a formula for talking to patients, as many physician-based communication protocols are, nor are they aimed at information exchange. Instead, the principles can be used concurrently and reflectively as clinicians care for patients/families with life-limiting illnesses. This approach is more in keeping with communication from the interpretive paradigm, emphasizing communication as the construction of meaning among all participants involved in a patient's care. As with any skill, healthcare professionals can learn these principles in order to facilitate a patient-centered communication perspective.

There are elements from the classic group dynamics perspective in the COMFORT model, with its emphasis on **task** and **relational communication**. As Bales (1950) noted well over 60 years ago, one of the problems facing groups (and teams) is that of **equilibrium** in terms of balancing the group's task and relational interaction. Bales thought groups that failed to attend to their relational needs would not be successful over time. Although the equilibrium problem is not specified in the COMFORT model, the model is designed to teach healthcare professionals that communication is both task and relational. Wittenberg-Lyles and her colleagues imply that failure to attend to both task and relational communication reduces provider effectiveness in communication with patients and families in end-of-life care. For example, providers could pretend to be listening by providing the standard verbal "uh huhs" during interaction

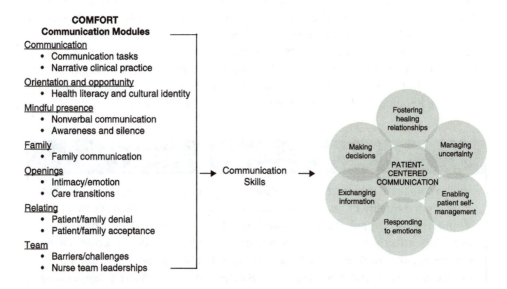

Figure 6.2 COMFORT Communication Model.

Source: From http://www.clinicalcc.com, Elaine Wittenberg-Lyles (2013).

while doing something else. Or they could ask how someone is feeling while looking at the medical chart. Although patients sometimes might overlook these behaviors, these kinds of ineffective communication encounters certainly are not good at fostering productive interactions with patients and families.

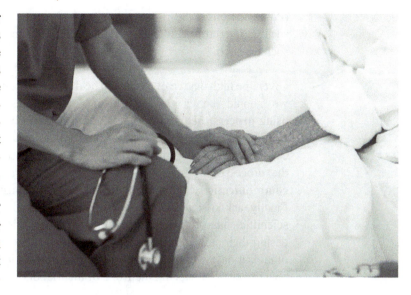

In application, the COMFORT curriculum aims to prevent (or at least reduce) these often vacuous acknowledgments that can occur in everyday interaction within end-of-life care. Instead, clinicians are trained to (a) recognize individuality by listening to the patient, (b) understand the patient's life before illness through reflection, and (c) go beyond medical information by focusing on the patient's story and using that information to re-tell the story. Research has shown that using person-centered approaches can increase perceived communication competence, improve coping skills for patients, increase liking of the clinician, and increase relational satisfaction (Wittenberg-Lyles, Goldsmith, Ferrell, & Ragan, in press). By extension, we believe that clinicians who follow the COMFORT approach and engage in person-centered communication with patients and their families will be more likely to do the same with their professional colleagues. As such, they would tend to be more relationship-centered in their interprofessional communication. This is certainly an area ripe with potential for future research.

FUTURE RESEARCH IN HEALTH CARE TEAMS: WHAT WE STILL NEED TO KNOW

One area in which we still need to know more is why and how health care teams change over time. This line of research, known as group development (Fisher, 1970; McGrath & Tschan, 2004), looks at recurring patterns within groups and teams that can enlighten us as to what goes on in real world settings. A number of interesting possibilities exist in this arena, including whether teams go through a series of stages of regular movement such as forming, storming, norming, and performing (Tuckman, 1965) or whether they go through phases that occur and recur as a group does its work

(Poole & Roth, 1989). The extent to which communication has an impact on factors such as interprofessional coordination and collaboration can be ascertained through such research.

Given the high degree of change in healthcare overall and in healthcare organizations, we should better understand how interprofessional communication operates using **process theories** (Poole & Van de Ven, 2004). This approach would allow us to understand how the process of interprofessional communication unfolds in health care teams, as well as the factors that influence these processes. We can also examine the processes of informal talk that make teams effective. Examining **informal communication** highlights the practices that constitute much of what teams do. Finally, acknowledging the particular perspective from which a study is derived (i.e., scientific, interpretive, critical–cultural) will be important. Researchers can better design their studies, and consumers of this research, including healthcare providers, organizations, and teams, as well as communication scholars and students, will be able to better understand the fruits of their labors.

MEDICAL INTERPRETERS

Imagine not being able to fully explain your symptoms or understand your physician's instructions because you speak a non-native language. You may ask a family

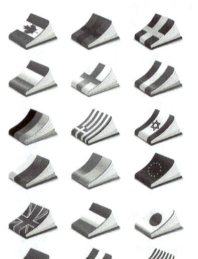

member or friend who speaks the native language to accompany you on your medical visit. However, if they can't come with you, you are left to the mercy of the healthcare system. According to the 2010 U.S. census, 25.2 million people have **limited English language proficiency (LEP)**, and 20.5% speak a language other than English at home. This means that seeking medical assistance may be particularly challenging for a significant number of people living in the United States. To help alleviate the stress of seeking medical attention and facilitate quality healthcare for LEP patients, health systems have employed bilingual speakers, known as medical interpreters, to enhance patient and medical staff communication (Dysart-Gale, 2005, 2007).

Communication View of Medical Interpreters

Theories, models, and frameworks. Traditionally, medical interpreters are viewed as conduits of information, serving only as translators between healthcare providers and patients (Dysart-Gale, 2005, 2007; Hsieh, 2006). The metaphor of the conduit reflects Shannon and Weaver's (1949) **transmission model of communication**. This model is situated within the scientific paradigm and is privileged in the medical field (Dysart-Gale, 2007). The healthcare provider sends a message; the interpreter translates the message to the patient. If the patient sends an explicit verbal message, then the interpreter translates the message for the healthcare provider. Through interviews with medical interpreters, interpreters report frustration with the conduit metaphor, yet they acknowledge the significance of the transmission model in both their training and role (Dysart-Gale, 2005). By limiting interpreters to only translating and relaying messages sent by the healthcare provider or patient, instances of malpractice or spreading faulty information are presumably limited. Thus, medical interpreters' professional codes of ethics generally reflect the transmission model or conduit metaphor of communication.

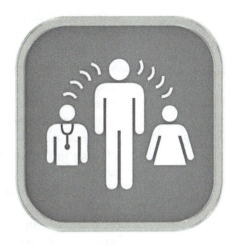

PARADIGMATIC PERSPECTIVES ON MEDICAL INTERPRETER RESEARCH

Medical interpreter research includes scientific, interpretive, and critical scholarship. Although the scientific view of medical interpreting (the interpreter as a translator for the healthcare provider and patient) is often favored because of ethics and regulations, medical interpreters may actually perform multiple roles during a healthcare interaction. Thus, the interpretive paradigm allows researchers to capture how medical interpreters help healthcare providers and patients shape and negotiate meaning. The critical perspective illuminates the tensions between medical interpreter roles and how the tensions relate to patients' care.

However, Beltran Avery (2001) identified three additional roles the medical interpreter serves. First, medical interpreters can serve as **clarifiers**. That is, medical interpreters may have to stray from the direct translation and add information in order to convey the correct meaning. Words and phrases do not always directly translate to the same meaning, so medical interpreters must adjust to make sure the receiver comprehends the message. Second, medical interpreters may also act as **culture brokers**. In other words, medical interpreters may draw on unique knowledge of the patient's culture in order to situate the healthcare provider's message within the cultural context of the patient. For example, some topics may be considered taboo in certain cultures. Although a provider may need information about a culturally taboo topic (e.g., suicide), addressing the topic directly may lead to negative consequences, such as the patient feeling insulted and perhaps refusing medical attention. As a culture broker, the medical interpreter may educate the healthcare provider about the patient's culture and create another way to address the issue that would facilitate the provider's goal of attaining the information without risking negative consequences. Finally, medical interpreters can also function as **patient advocates**. As a patient advocate, the interpreter considers the quality of the patient experience, including care and communication (Dysart-Gale, 2005). Accordingly, the interpreter may do more than translate between the healthcare provider and patient. As Dysart-Gale (2005) noted, an interpreter may chat with the patient about his or her concerns before the doctor arrives or call the patient to remind him or her about a check-up. Advocacy behavior like this is meant to facilitate better care for the patient.

Hsieh (2007) proposed a fourth role of medical interpreters, **co-diagnostician**. In this role, medical interpreters may seek to improve the healthcare interaction through five strategies: "assuming the provider's communicative goals; editorializing information for medical emphasis; initiating information-seeking behaviors; participating in diagnostic tasks; and volunteering medical information to patients" (Hsieh, 2007, p. 924). That is, medical interpreters may ask the patient questions without prompting from the provider, asking follow up questions, editing patient responses, and even examining the patient; they also may give the patient medical advice without direction from a medical provider. All four roles (i.e., clarifier, cultural broker, patient advocate, and co-diagnostician) extend the responsibilities and duties of a medical interpreter beyond providing translations.

Because these roles do not fit within the conduit metaphor, Dysart-Gale (2005, 2007) considered two additional communication models, the **ritual view** and **semiotic model**, that provide medical interpreters with guides for negotiating and switching between all four of the described roles. Both the ritual view and semiotic model describe communication as a process through which symbols are used to negotiate meaning; thus, both approaches are situated within the interpretive paradigm. These frameworks benefit interpreters by guiding their transitions between roles (e.g., conduit to patient advocate), as well as assessing performance within each role (Dysart-Gale, 2007). Despite recommendations for using these communication models to frame the medical interpreter role, researchers and practitioners still commonly rely on the transmission model.

COMMUNICATION MATTERS

Medical Interpreters: More than Translators

Sophia, a 19-year-old woman, lay comatose in the hospital for several weeks. Dr. Adams, her physician, updated the family on Sophia's clinical condition and prognosis through Miguel, a medical interpreter. To the family, Dr. Adams seemed cold and distant. Despite the emotionally charged context, Miguel's main role was to translate Dr. Adams' words to the family and vice versa. As weeks went by and discussions of terminating Sophia's life support began, Miguel noticed an increased tenseness in Sophia's friends and family as they interacted with Dr. Adams. Miguel decided to talk to Dr. Adams and explained to him that the discussion of Sophia's death as inevitable violated the family's cultural values and perspective. With this information about Sophia's family's culture, Dr. Adams chose to try a different way of explaining Sophia's situation. Dr. Adams first explained that Sophia had no brain activity. Sophia's mother, Juanita, protested that God may want to use Sophia to perform a miracle. Dr. Adams acknowledged Juanita's concerns and suggested that God was the only one who could choose to perform a miracle. Dr. Adams asserted that it was important for everyone to follow their journey. Following Dr. Adams' explanation, Sophia's family felt more comfortable with the idea of stopping Sophia's treatment, and finally, Juanita and the rest of the family agreed to stop treatment.

This case study is based on Dysart-Gale (2007).

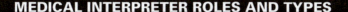

MEDICAL INTERPRETER ROLES AND TYPES

Each of the five medical interpreter roles (translator, clarifier, patient advocate, cultural broker, or co-diagnostician) reflects the way a medical interpreter interacts with a healthcare provider and patient. Whereas the translator role is more distant, some of the other roles reflect concern for the patient and the patient's culture. As the co-diagnostician, the medical interpreter privileges the healthcare provider and strives to perform duties that will help the provider in some way. All five types of interpreters (chance, untrained, bilingual health care providers, on-site, and telephone) may vacillate between roles, although medical interpreter codes of ethics generally reflect the translator role.

Types of interpreters. In addition to identifying the underlying assumptions guiding the multiple roles medical interpreters negotiate, Hsieh (2006, 2007) proposes five different types of medical interpreters: chance interpreters, untrained interpreters, bilingual healthcare providers, on-site interpreters, and telephone interpreters.

Before the widespread use of medical interpreters, chance and untrained interpreters commonly facilitated patient–provider communication (Dysart-Gale, 2005). **Chance interpreters** include family, friends, or bilingual persons who happen to be nearby during an exchange between a patient and healthcare provider. These interpreters have not undergone medical interpreter training and are generally called on because they know the patient well or they are nearby at the time. Although family or friends may be very helpful because they know the patient well and the patient may feel particularly comfortable with them, a chance interpreter may negatively impact the patient's care. For example, chance interpreters may not know the medical terminology, may provide inaccurate interpretations, or may behave inappropriately for the role (e.g., answer for the patient, not maintain confidentiality; Hsieh, 2006).

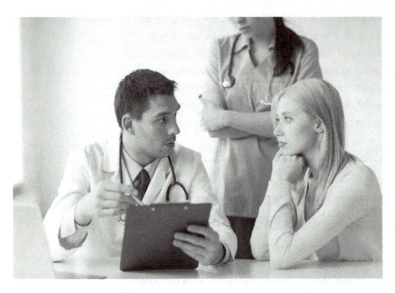

Untrained interpreters refer to untrained bilingual support staff in the healthcare organization, such as a nurse or technician. These people may know organizational policies and medical terminology, but untrained interpreters may only be able to spend limited time with a patient. For example, a nurse serving as an untrained interpreter may be able to sit in during the diagnosis but not have time to accompany the patient to the receptionist or pharmacist following the discussion with the physician. Similar to chance interpreters, untrained interpreters may also interpret information incorrectly or behave inappropriately for the role since they have not received training. Although using chance and untrained interpreters has some benefits, such as knowing the patient well or being easy to contact, these benefits do not outweigh the potential mistakes these interpreters might make, which may ultimately worsen the experience and care for the patient. Consequently, bilingual healthcare providers, on-site medical interpreters, and telephone interpreters are preferred.

Medical providers who learn additional languages are **bilingual healthcare providers**. Although this type of interpreter may seem like the best option, they have their issues. First, they may not know cultural information that can influence language choices or behaviors (i.e., they may fail as culture brokers). Second, they may also perceive themselves as more competent at interpreting and communicating medical information in sensitive situations than they actually are. However, bilingual healthcare providers are able to communicate directly with the patient, thus building rapport between the patient and provider (Baker, Hayes, & Fortier, 1998).

On-site interpreters are professional, bilingual persons who have received training as medical interpreters. In addition to the benefit of being specially trained, on-site interpreters bring with them cultural and medical experiences pertinent to the healthcare environment and "are more likely to play an active role in health communication" (Hsieh, 2006, p. 180). However, on-site interpreters also have their drawbacks: They are expensive, they may not know all the languages various patients speak, and they may not have adequate time to meet with all of the patients who need translation services.

One way to overcome some of the challenges associated with on-site interpreters is to use **telephone interpreters**. Like on-site interpreters, telephone interpreters are professional interpreters. Because the interpreters are part of a telephone service, they may work outside of traditional office hours. Additional benefits include the ability to cater to a variety of languages, including rare languages, and confidentiality. However, telephone interpreters are not able to consider nonverbal cues during an interaction. In light of the conduit model, though, this may be a benefit rather than a disadvantage. Moreover, telephone interpreters are often a more accessible and affordable option for healthcare organizations.

All five types of medical interpreters described here are common in practice; however, on-site interpreters and telephone interpreters are preferred. Although medical interpreters are usually divided into dichotomous groupings as professional or formal interpreters versus untrained, informal, or ad hoc interpreters, the five medical interpreter types provide researchers greater opportunities to understand the dynamic situations and unique role requirements and expectations of different interpreters (Hsieh, 2006).

Other Perspectives on Medical Interpreters

Outside of the communication discipline, a diverse array of scholars representing fields such as socio-linguistics, psychology, and medicine have contributed to the body of knowledge on medical interpreters. Within medicine, doctors have explored specific disease contexts, including cancer (e.g., Butow et al., 2011), diabetes (e.g., McCabe, Gohdes, Morgan, Eakin, & Schmitt, 2006), and end-of-life (e.g., Norris et al., 2005), as well as specific practice settings, such as family practice (e.g., Leanza,

Boivin, & Rosenberg, 2010) and general practice (e.g., Meeuwesen, Twilt, ten Thije, & Harmsen, 2010). In addition to garnering multiple perspectives through diverse fields of study, medical interpreter research reflects the multiple perspectives of those who come into contact with medical interpreters (Davidson, 2000; Hsieh, 2006). Examining multiple perspectives by studying medical interpreters across disciplines and capturing reflections from those who interact with medical interpreters is important to furthering our understanding of medical interpreters.

CONFLICTING RESULTS AND PERSPECTIVES ON MEDICAL INTERPRETERS

Several conflicts emerge across the medical interpreter literature. Perhaps the primary contention is the incongruence in definitions regarding medical interpreters' responsibilities. As mentioned previously, medical interpreters are expected to be neutral conduits of information (Dysart-Gale, 2005), in which the medical interpreter only provides translations of what the healthcare provider says to the patient and vice versa. Medical interpreters' professional ethics reflect this model of communication. Yet, interpreters also respond in socially and culturally appropriate ways, which sometimes require the medical interpreter to communicate with the patient outside of directly translating what the healthcare provider has said (Angelelli, 2006). Although problems may arise when medical interpreters perform duties other than translation, such as offering medical information to patients (Hsieh, 2007), research demonstrates that medical interpreters do perform multiple functions.

A second area of conflicting findings concerns the effectiveness of professional medical interpreters versus other types of interpreters. For example, Bauer and Alegria (2010) assert that the use of professional medical interpreters improves the quality of psychiatric care. Similarly, Karliner, Jacobs, Chen, and Mutha (2007) conducted a literature review that supported professional interpreters as providing improved clinical care for LEP patients. One of the key reasons professional interpreters are seen as more effective is that they commit fewer mistakes in interpretation than non-professional interpreters (Butow et al., 2011). However, Butow et al. (2011) found that not all errors in translations lead to a negative effect. Some errors such as omitting insignificant information may not lead to a change at all. Further, correcting or clarifying information, simplifying the message, or reducing the impact of the message may be considered a positive message change. Thus, scholars recognize the potential benefits of including family members or friends in patient consultations even though professional medical interpreters may provide more accurate translations.

Additionally, patients and healthcare providers report inconsistent preferences regarding types of medical interpreters. Some patients report negative experiences with medical interpreters and prefer family and friends to serve as medical interpreters (Edwards, Temple, & Alexander, 2005). However, nurses report preferring professional interpreters (Fatahi, Mattsson, Lundgren, & Hellstrom, 2010). Differences in patient and provider perspectives may result from encounters with multiple types of medical interpreters. Further investigations assessing interpreter effectiveness and patient or physician preference should distinguish the type of medical interpreter and account for patient and healthcare provider past experience with interpreters. Additionally, healthcare organizations should consider the effectiveness of collaboration not only between physicians and medical interpreters (Butow et al., 2011; Hsieh, 2007) but also among different types of interpreters.

A third area of conflict regarding medical interpreters is the use of face-to-face versus remote interpreters. Remote interpreters are professional interpreters who are not present during a consultation but are at the same facility where the patient is receiving care. An early investigation of remote medical interpreters included an experimental trial in which patients were assigned to a control group consisting of proximate-consecutive (face-to-face) interpreter services or an experimental condition using remote-simultaneous interpretations (Hornberger et al., 1996). Proximate-consecutive interpretation describes a traditional interpreter experience. Interpreters sit in the consultation room during the health appointment and speak after the healthcare provider or patient. When providing remote-simultaneous interpretation, however, the interpreter sits in a separate room, and both the healthcare provider and patient wear headsets. As the healthcare provider speaks, the interpreter translates the messages and the patient receives the translation through the headset and vice versa. Although interpreters indicated preferring proximate-consecutive interpretation, results indicated greater satisfaction for patients and providers using the remote-simultaneous interpretation technology. Further, the remote-simultaneous interpretation technology resulted in physicians' and patients' messages being translated with greater accuracy. Perhaps the interpreters' physical distance from the interaction prevented them

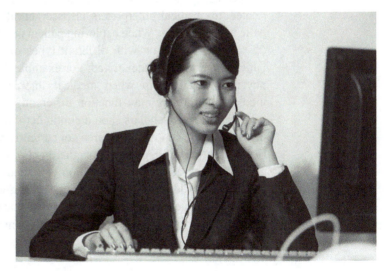

from using context and nonverbal cues to enhance (but possibly complicate) their interpretations. On the other hand, patients and healthcare providers may have had an easier time establishing rapport because others were not present in the consultation and influencing the interaction. Moreover, healthcare providers may also feel able to provide more information to the patient, as the interaction occurred more as a conversation.

Since Hornberger and colleagues' (1996) study, scholars have continued to assess effectiveness of the use of technology and satisfaction for patient, provider, and interpreter. Butow et al. (2011) reported no significant differences between equivocal messages produced by professional on-site medical interpreters versus professional telephone interpreters. However, in a comparison of video conferencing, telephone, and face-to-face medical interpreter experiences, Locatis et al. (2012) found that both providers and interpreters preferred in-person encounters. The research appears to indicate advantages and disadvantages to using each type of medical interpreter. Thus, other factors such as cost and need may dictate a healthcare organization's decision. However, scholars continue to recommend professional on-site medical interpreters when possible (Locatis et al., 2012).

FUTURE RESEARCH ON MEDICAL INTERPRETERS

Scholars continue to study medical interpreters in order to understand the unique characteristics and demands of this role, as well as to make recommendations to healthcare organizations. Future research should particularly consider the patients' perspective (Brisset, Leanza, & Laforest, 2012). In a literature review of 61 articles related to medical interpreters, Brisset et al. found only 12 articles capturing patient perspectives. When exploring patient perspectives, researchers primarily focus on patient satisfaction with different types of interpreters. However, much of the patient experience is unexplored. For example, how do patients perceive the patient–physician relationship when medical interpreters facilitate healthcare? Because medical interpreters may function differently depending on the type of healthcare service provided, scholars should continue to investigate medical interpreters within different health contexts. One area not currently represented in the literature is pediatrics. Interpreting for parent(s) or guardian(s), as well as the child seeking medical attention, may add a new dimension to a medical interpreter's role not previously considered. Additionally, conducting international research can help determine aspects of the medical interpreter experience that are socio-culturally bound and those aspects of performing or interacting with a medical interpreter that are universal (Brisset et al., 2012).

CONCLUSION

Providing care requires communicating effectively with a diverse array of people and across medical professions. Developing team contexts that enable effective communication, including the productive incorporation of medical interpreters in health care teams, will improve healthcare for patients and help meet the diverse needs of healthcare organizations.

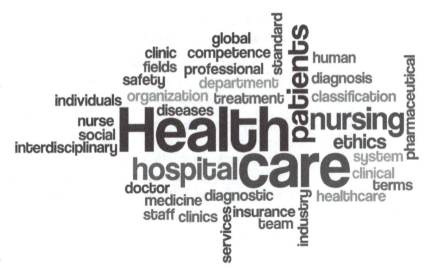

DISCUSSION QUESTIONS

1. How can communication barriers in health care teams, such as hierarchy, status, and other factors, be addressed in hospitals and other healthcare organizations? How can communication experts persuade healthcare providers to better communicate when working together?
2. As a patient, what would be your biggest concerns about including a medical interpreter in your appointment? How might your concerns differ due to the type of medical interpreter included in your appointment? What might the medical interpreter say or do to help you feel more comfortable?
3. Review the International Medical Interpreters Association Code of Ethics (www. imiaweb.org). Which communication paradigm does this code most closely reflect? How would you revise this code to include other communication paradigms? How might the inclusion of other paradigms change the role of medical interpreters?

IN-CLASS ACTIVITIES

1. Non-native speakers seeking medical attention may find the experience particularly daunting. They may be limited to nonverbal communication to describe their symptoms, receive their diagnosis, and understand next care steps.

Directions: Ask students to choose a partner. In each pair, designate one person as the doctor and one person as the patient. Present the class with the following scenario:

> Pretend that you are visiting Italy and have begun to experience an illness. You go to the nearest medical facility and try to explain your symptoms to the doctor. Your teacher will provide you with a list of your symptoms.

Teachers, please refer to the textbook's companion website to see a list of symptoms and share them with the students designated as patients. The patients should explain their symptoms to the students designated as doctors without using English. Instruct the doctors to diagnose and present their patients with instructions for getting better without using English. After five minutes, facilitate a conversation about the experience.

Questions:

- Describe the experience.
- What frustrations did you encounter?
- What communication strategies did you use to try to communicate with each other?
- As the doctor in this scenario, what concerns did you have?
- As the patient in this scenario, how did you feel?
- How could this scenario change for the better?

2. Get in small groups and review the case of Sophia presented earlier in the chapter. Answer the following questions and then share your answers with the class.

- What communication theory informs Miguel's initial role in the interactions between Sophia's family and Dr. Adams?
- What role does Miguel switch to when he recognizes the cultural differences between Sophia's family and Dr. Adams?
- What communication theories or perspectives describe Miguel's role switch?
- What type of medical interpreter is Miguel?
- How would this interaction have been different if Miguel had been a different type of medical interpreter?

RECOMMENDED READINGS

Eisenberg, E., Murphy, A., Sutcliffe, K., Wears, R., Schenkel, S., Perry, S., & Vanderhoef, M. (2005). Communication in emergency medicine: Implications for patient safety. *Communication Monographs, 72*, 390–413.

Eisenberg and colleagues provide fresh insight into how communication plays an important role in emergency medicine.

Lingard, L., Whyte, S., Espin, S., Baker, G. R, Orser, B., & Doran, D. (2006). Towards safer interprofessional communication: Constructing a model of "utility" from preoperative team briefings. *Journal of Interprofessional Care, 20,* 471–483.

Lingard et al. suggest that communication has multiple functions when operating in healthcare.

Seidelman, R. D., & Bachner, Y. G. (2010). That I won't translate! Experiences of a family medical interpreter in a multicultural environment. *Mount Sinai Journal of Medicine, 77,* 389–393.

Seidelman and Bachner illuminate the challenges and benefits associated with different types of medical interpreters by sharing a personal narrative of serving as a chance interpreter, supporting the importance of using professional medical interpreters.

NOTE

1   The distinction between "health care teams" and "healthcare teams" is a fine one. Dr. Real has co-authored chapters in both editions of the *Handbook of Health Communication* on "health care teams." The use of "health care teams," therefore, is maintained with the aim of being consistent with his prior communication research. Beyond reference to teams, however, the term "healthcare" is used to be consistent with the term's usage in this textbook.

REFERENCES

* References marked with an asterisk indicate studies included only in Table 6.1.

Angelelli, C. V. (2006). Validating professional standards and codes: Challenges and opportunities. *Interpreting, 8,* 175–193.

Apker, J., Propp, K. M., & Ford, W. Z. (2005). Negotiating status and identity tensions in health care team interactions: An exploration of nurse role dialectics. *Journal of Applied Communication Research, 33,* 93–115.

*Awad, S. S., Fegan, S. P., Bellows, C., Albo, D., Green-Rashed, B., De La Garza, M. & Berger, D. H. (2005). Bridging the communication gap in the operating room with medical team training. *American Journal of Surgery, 190,* 770–774.

Baker, D. W., Hayes, R., & Fortier, J. P. (1998). Interpreter use and satisfaction with interpersonal aspects of care for Spanish-speaking patients. *Medical Care, 36,* 1461–1470.

Bales, R. F. (1950). *Interaction process analysis: A method for the study of small groups.* Cambridge, MA: Addison-Wesley.

Bauer, A. M., & Alegria, M. (2010). The impact of patient language proficiency and interpreter service use on the quality of psychiatric care: A systematic review. *Psychiatric Service, 61,* 765–773.

Beltran Avery, M. (2001). *The role of the health care interpreter: An evolving dialogue* (Department of Health and Human Services Office of Minority Health). Retrieved from http://www.ncihc.org/workingpapers.htm

Brisset, C., Leanza, Y., & Laforest, K. (2012). Working with interpreters in health care: A systematic review and meta-ethnography of qualitative studies. *Patient Education and Counseling, 91*(2), 131–140.

Butow, P. N., Goldstein, D., Bell, M. L., Sze, M., Alrdidge, L. J., Abdo, S., & Eisenbruch, M. (2011). Interpretation in consultations with immigrant patients with cancer: How accurate is it? *Journal of Clinical Oncology, 29*, 2801–2807.

Connor, S. R., Egan, K. A., Kwilosz, D. M., Larson, D. G., & Reese, D. J. (2002). Inter-disciplinary approaches to assisting with end-of-life care and decision making. *American Behavioral Scientist, 46*, 340–356.

Davis, C. S. (2008). Dueling narratives: How peer leaders use narrative to frame meaning in community mental health care teams. *Small Group Research, 39*, 706–727.

Davidson, B. (2000). The interpreter as institutional gatekeeper: The social-linguistic role of inter-preters in Spanish-English medical discourse. *Journal of Sociolinguistics, 4*, 379–405.

Dysart-Gale, D. (2005). Communication models, professionalization, and the work of medical interpreters. *Health Communication, 17*, 91–103.

Dysart-Gale, D. (2007). Clinicians and medical interpreters: Negotiating culturally appropriate care for patients with limited English ability. *Family & Community Health, 30*, 237–246.

Edwards, R., Temple, B., & Alexander, C. (2005). Users' experiences of interpreters: The critical role of trust. *Interpreting, 7*, 77–95.

Eisenberg, E., Murphy, A., Sutcliffe, K., Wears, R., Schenkel, S., Perry, S., & Vanderhoef, M. (2005). Communication in emergency medicine: Implications for patient safety. *Communication Monographs, 72*, 390–413.

Ellingson, L. L. (2003). Interdisciplinary health care teamwork in the clinic backstage. *Journal of Applied Communication Research, 31*, 93–117.

Fatahi, N., Mattsson, B., Lundgren, S. M., & Hellstrom, M. (2010). Nurse radiographers' expe-riences of communication with patients who do not speak the native language. *Journal of Advanced Nursing, 66*, 774–783.

Fisher, B. A. (1970). Decision emergence: Phases in group decision making. *Speech Mono-graphs, 37*, 53–66.

*Gardezi, F., Lingard, L., Espin, S., Whyte, S., Orser, B., & Baker, G. R.. (2009). Silence, power and communication in the operating room. *Journal of Advanced Nursing, 65*, 1390–1399.

Haig, K. M., Sutton, S., & Whittington, J. (2006). SBAR: A shared mental model for improving communication between clinicians. *Joint Commission Journal on Quality and Patient Safety, 32*, 167–175.

Haynes, A. B., Weiser, T. G., Berry, W. R., Lipsitz, S. R., Breizat, A. S., Dellinger, E. P., & Gawande, A. A. (2009). A surgical safety checklist to reduce morbidity and mortality in a global population. *New England Journal of Medicine, 360*(5), 491–499.

Hornberger, J. C., Gibson, Jr., C. D., Wood, W., Dequeldre, C., Corso, I., Palla, B., & Bloch, D. A. (1996). Eliminating language barriers for non-English-speaking patients. *Medical Care, 34*, 845–856.

Hsieh, E. (2006). Understanding medical interpreters: Reconceptualizing bilingual health communication. *Health Communication, 20*, 177–186.

Hsieh, E. (2007). Interpreters as co-diagnosticians: Overlapping roles and services between providers and interpreters. *Social Science & Medicine, 64*, 924–937.

Karliner, L. S., Jacobs, E. A., Chen, A. H., & Mutha, S. (2007). Do professional interpreters improve clinical care for patients with limited English proficiency? A systematic review of the literature. *Health Service Research, 42*, 727–754.

Kohn, L. T., Corrigan, J. M., & Donaldson, M. S. (Eds.). (2000). *To err is human: Building a safer health system* (Vol. 627). Washington, DC: National Academies Press

Leanza, Y., Boivin, I., & Rosenberg, E. (2010). Interruptions and resistance: A comparison of medical consultations with family and trained interpreters. *Social Science & Medicine, 70*, 1888–1895.

Leavitt, H. J. (1951). Some effects of certain communication patterns on group performance. *Journal of Abnormal and Social Psychology, 46*, 38–50.

Lingard, L. (2012). Productive complications: Emergent ideas in team communication and patient safety. *Healthcare Quarterly, 15*, 18–23.

Lingard, L., Espin, S., Rubin, B., Whyte, S., Colmenares, M., Baker, G. R., & Reznick, R. (2005). Getting teams to talk: Development and pilot implementation of a checklist to promote safer operating room communication. *Quality and Safety in Health Care, 14*(5), 340–346.

Lingard, L., Regehr, G., Orser, B., Reznick, R., Baker, G.R., Doran, D., & Whyte, S. (2008). Evaluation of a preoperative checklist and team briefing among surgeons, nurses, and anesthesiologists to reduce failures in communication. *Archives of Surgery, 143*, 12–17.

Lingard, L., Whyte, S., Espin, S., Baker, G. R, Orser, B., & Doran, D. (2006). Towards safer interprofessional communication: Constructing a model of "utility" from preoperative team briefings. *Journal of Interprofessional Care, 20*, 471–483.

Locatis, C., Williamson, D., Gould-Kabler, C., Zone-Smith, L., Detzler, I., Roberson, J., & Ackerman, M. (2012). Comparing in-person, video, and telephonic medical interpretation. *Journal of General Internal Medicine, 25*, 345–350.

McCabe, M., Gohdes, D., Morgan, F., Eakin, J., & Schmitt, C. (2006). Training effective interpreters for diabetes care and education: A new challenge. *The Diabetes Educator, 32*, 714–720.

McGrath, J. E. (1984). *Groups: Interaction and performance*. Englewood Cliffs, N.J.: Prentice Hall.

McGrath, J. E., & Tschan, F. (2004). *Temporal matters in social psychology: Examining the role of time in the lives of groups and individuals*. Washington, DC: American Psychological Association.

Meeuwesen, L., Twilt, S., ten Thije, J. D., & Harmsen, H. (2010). "Ne diyor?" (What does she say?): Informal interpreting in general practice. *Patient Education and Counseling, 81*, 198–203.

*Mills, P., Neily, J., & Dunn, E. (2008). Teamwork and communication in surgical teams: Implications for patient safety. *Journal of the American College of Surgeons, 206*, 107–112.

Norris, W. M., Wenrich, M. D., Nielsen, E. L., Trece, P. D., Jackson, J. C., & Curtis, J. R. (2005). Communication about end-of-life care between language-discordant patients and clinicians: Insights from medical interpreters. *Journal of Palliative Medicine, 8,* 1016–1024.

Paulsel, M. L., McCroskey, J. C., & Richmond, V. P. (2006). Perceptions of health care professionals' credibility as a predictor of patients' satisfaction with their medical care and physician. *Communication Research Reports, 23,* 69–76.

Poole, M. S., & Real, K. (2003). Groups and teams in health care: Communication and effectiveness. In T. L. Thompson, A. M. Dorsey, K. I. Miller, & R. Parrott (Eds.) *Handbook of health communication* (pp. 369–402). Mahwah, N.J.: Lawrence Erlbaum Publishers.

Poole, M. S., & Roth, J. (1989). Decision development in small groups V: Test of a contigency model. *Human Communication Research, 15,* 549–589.

Poole, M. S., & Van de Ven, A. H. (2004). Central issues in the study of change and innovation. In M. S. Poole & A. H. Van de Ven (Eds.), *Handbook of organizational change and innovation* (pp. 3–31). Oxford: Oxford University Press.

Real, K., & Poole, M. S. (2011). Health care teams: Communication and effectiveness. In T. L. Thompson, R. Parrott, & J. Nussbaum (Eds.) *The Routledge handbook of health communication* (2nd ed., pp. 100–116). New York: Routledge.

*Reddy, M. C., & Jansen, B. J. (2008). A model for understanding collaborative information behavior in context: A study of two healthcare teams. *Information Processing & Management, 44,* 256–273.

Shannon, C., & Weaver, W. (1949). *The mathematical theory of communication.* Illinois: The University of Illinois Press.

Sutcliffe, K. M., Lewton, E., & Rosenthal, M. M. (2004). Communication failures: An insidious contributor to medical mishaps. *Academic Medicine, 79,* 186–194.

The Joint Commission. (2006). *Sentinel Events Statistics,* December 31, 2006. http://www.jointcommission.org/SentinelEvents/Statistics

The Joint Commission. (2012). http://www.jointcommission.org/sentinel_event.aspx

Tuckman, B. W. (1965). Developmental sequence in small groups. *Psychological Bulletin, 63,* 384–399.

Weiland, D., Kramer, B. J., Waite, M. S., & Rubenstein, L. Z. (1996). The interdisciplinary team in geriatric care. *American Behavioral Scientist, 39,* 655–664.

*Williams, R. G., Silverman, R., Schwind, C., Fortune, J. B., Sutyak, J., Horvath, K. D., & Dunnington, G. L. (2007). Surgeon information transfer and communication: Factors affecting quality and efficiency of inpatient care. *Annals of Surgery, 245,* 159–169.

Wittenberg-Lyles, E. (2013). [Figure illustrating the COMFORT Model, July 11. 2013]. *Centering Communication in Palliative Care.* Retrieved from www.clinicalcc.com

Wittenberg-Lyles, E., Goldsmith, J., Ferrell, B., & Ragan, S. L. (in press). *Communication and palliative nursing.* New York: Oxford University Press.

Wittenberg-Lyles, E., Goldsmith, J., & Ragan, S. (2010). The COMFORT initiative: Palliative nursing and the centrality of communication. *Journal of Hospice and Palliative Nursing, 12,* 282–294.

Wittenberg-Lyles, E., Parker Oliver, D., Demiris, G., & Regehr, K. (2010). Interdisciplinary collaboration in hospice team meetings. *Journal of Interprofessional Care, 24*(3), 264–273.

Challenges and Complexities in Health Communication

Factors Affecting the Patient

*Katharine J. Head and
Elisia L. Cohen*

Think about all the times you've gone to see healthcare providers in your life. Every experience was probably slightly different. Maybe you have a primary care physician who is caring and humorous, takes the time to explain health issues to you, and even allows you to email him if you have questions. On the other hand, maybe you have a nurse practitioner who rushes through your appointment, rarely remembers your name, and is not up-to-date with the latest clinical standards for her practice. Just as there are many types of healthcare providers with different skills and personalities, there are also many different types of patients. Patient-centered health communication requires an understanding that patients encounter and enter into the healthcare system from a variety of walks of life. We cannot assume a one-size-fits-all approach to patient–provider communication because it may lead not only to poor healthcare experiences but also to poor health outcomes!

There are many individual patient factors that could present themselves as challenges for a successful healthcare experience. Can you think of some? How about culture? Language? Education? Age? Health insurance? Proximity to a good doctor? Privacy? Embarrassment? Desire to be healthy? While we do not have space to cover all of these factors in this chapter, we do cover some of the most important and well-studied patient factors that might present challenges to effective patient–provider communication. Some of these concepts are covered in other chapters in this book. We present them here, however, in a way that highlights how they may be a challenge for patients.

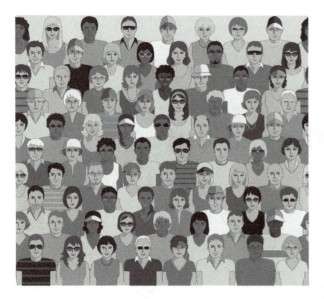

We divide this chapter into two parts. First, we discuss what we label as *internal* challenges for patients. These can also be thought of as personal challenges patients face, as well as things that they might be able to change to address the challenges. Specifically, we explore uncertainty in illness, the role that health literacy and related patient skills play in health and healthcare, and patient participation in healthcare. We then move into the second part of the chapter, where we discuss *external* challenges for patients. One way to think about these challenges is that they are external to the patients' control but can have a major impact on their health. Specifically, we discuss patient demographics like race and gender, community factors like built environment and local culture, and policy issues like the recent national healthcare reform in the United States. As you read this chapter, think about the ways that these internal and external challenges have played a role in your own healthcare experiences or those of your family and friends.

INTERNAL CHALLENGES FOR PATIENTS

Uncertainty in Illness—*What the Heck is Going on?*

When we decide we need to go see a healthcare provider, it is usually because we are inherently *uncertain* about something happening to our body. Sure, we might have some idea of what's going on. A runny nose and fever might signal a bad cold. A tumble on the soccer field resulting in a swollen ankle might indicate a sprain or break. But we go see a healthcare provider to reduce the **uncertainty** we have about our ailment and to find a way to heal.

There are many reasons we are uncertain when it comes to our health and being sick. For example, "people with illness may question their own ability to manage the illness, their provider's diagnostic skills and beliefs about treatment, their relationship with the provider (e.g., paternalistic or consumeristic), and the meaning of tests and procedures in health care" (Brashers, 2001, p. 480). Take a minute and reflect back on your last illness experience (or that of a loved one). What sources of uncertainty were there? Diagnostic? Prognostic? Treatment? Maybe even something as simple as where to park at the hospital? As was probably the case in your experience, uncertainty can pose a challenge for patients as they try to not only make it through the illness and everything that goes with it (including parking) but also make the best decisions about what to do.

Babrow and colleagues outline five dimensions of uncertainty in illness that can help us better understand where uncertainty comes from (Babrow, Kasch, & Ford, 1998). First, there is the **complexity of the illness**. A malignant tumor located in the temporal lobe of the brain is a lot more complex than a broken finger. Second, there is **quality of information** that the patient has access to. This dimension is strongly related to communication and includes factors like clarity of the information, accuracy of the information, and the ambiguity of information patients receive. For example, there might be a lot of ambiguity if a patient receives a second opinion about a diagnosis that conflicts with the first opinion: You would feel very uncertain if one doctor told you that you had a malignant tumor located in the temporal lobe of your brain and another doctor told you there was nothing there! Third, uncertainty can arise from a person's beliefs about the **probability** that something might happen. A woman with no history of breast cancer in her family might feel that it is unlikely she would ever have breast cancer, even if she finds a lump in her breast. Fourth, the **structure of information** and how a patient receives it (another communication issue) can contribute to uncertainty. This includes how information is ordered and how it is integrated into a patient's existing life world. For example, if a patient does find a lump in her breast, a doctor might go ahead and discuss mastectomy before the patient has even had a biopsy. Discussing a mastectomy before discussing smaller procedures (information order), as well as assuming a mastectomy might be necessary (integration), can cause a large amount of uncertainty for a woman. The fifth and final dimension is **lay epistemology**. Epistemology means how someone understands the world. Patients are likely to have a different epistemology than healthcare providers and therefore understand a concept like uncertainty in different ways. For example, to a doctor, a 75% survival rate sounds pretty certain, but to a patient to whom that survival rate is being applied, that uncertainty of falling in the 25% can be awful.

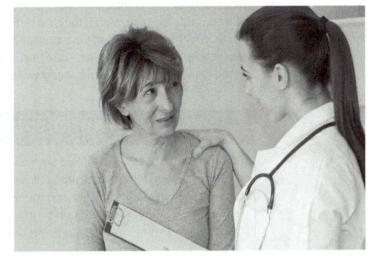

To study uncertainty, health communication scholars use a variety of theories including uncertainty management theory, problematic integration theory, theory of motivated information management, and the risk perception attitude framework, to name a few. At the heart of all of these theories is an understanding that humans will experience uncertainty about a variety of life experiences (including illness), that they will work to manage and process that uncertainty in some way (sometimes good, sometimes bad), and, at least in the field of communication, they often will strive to manage uncertainty through interpersonal communication with family, friends, and healthcare providers. Put simply, we often see **uncertainty management** at play when patients ask questions or receive information from those around them.

One final point. Because feeling uncertain is an uncomfortable state for humans (ever hear a bump in the night while you are home alone?), we assume it is always a bad thing. It definitely serves as a patient challenge that we all face. But feeling uncertain can also be a motivating force in that we want to find ways to reduce that uncertainty. In other words, for some people, feeling uncertain will cause them to take action and ask questions and do research about their illness or treatment. Or, in the case of the bump in the night, you walk into the hallway and realize the noise was just the ice maker in the fridge . . . whew!

In the field of communication, one of the most prolific scholars on the study of uncertainty in illness is the late Dale Brashers. Much of Brashers' work focused on how people diagnosed and living with HIV/AIDS, a highly stigmatized disease, experience uncertainty. As with much communication research exploring uncertainty in illness, Brashers' work falls into the interpretive paradigm where he relies on participant voices and their individual experiences with illness and uncertainty. This paradigmatic perspective allowed Brashers to develop a deep, situated understanding of uncertainty in illness, exploring the different ways HIV positive people experienced their illness and attempted to manage it. (This probably makes sense if you think about your own family or close friends. If a bad cold is going around, there are probably some people who handle it fine and go on with their day, even if they are suffering a little bit and aren't quite sure how soon they will feel better. We, your chapter authors, are this way. However, there are some people, like Katy's brother, Luke, and Elisia's husband, Jeff, who get sick with the same cold and you'd think the world was ending! But, we digress . . .)

PATIENT UNCERTAINTY

Babrow and colleagues identified five sources of uncertainty: complexity of the illness, quality of information, probability of the illness, structure of information, and lay epistemology. Effective communication about illness can help patients to feel more certain about their diagnosis, treatment, and social aspects of their disease, which may lead them to better deal with the challenge of their illness.

In one well-known study, Brashers and his colleagues (2000) conducted focus groups with HIV-infected people and asked them to discuss sources of uncertainty about their illness. The researchers found that in addition to uncertainty about the medical aspect of their illness, the participants also experienced much social and personal uncertainty related to their illness. They also discovered that these people might seek out information and ask questions to reduce this uncertainty, that some communication with providers and friends actually led to more uncertainty, and that some participants actually avoided information in order to maintain uncertainty (i.e., they didn't want to confront the fact that they might have HIV/AIDS). As you can see from this study, communication and information played an important role in how people with HIV/AIDS dealt with their disease.

Now, we don't want patients to stop asking questions, and we don't want healthcare providers or family and friends to stop answering those questions and providing information to patients. But uncertainty research does point to the importance of how and when to share particular information with patients. In other words, this goes back to the structure of information dimension of uncertainty in illness, which includes both the order of when information is presented and how it is integrated into a patient's life world. Another important finding in the Brashers et al. (2000) study is how uncertainty in illness might not be such a good thing for some patients. Some patients might feel that others won't accept them because they have a stigmatized illness, and some might actually not seek treatment or deal with the consequences of the disease because they don't want to face the fact that they are sick. The good thing is that research like this helps us figure out the different ways uncertainty plays out in a person's illness experience, which in turn might help us to develop interventions to assist people in more effectively managing their illness uncertainty.

The field of nursing has also taken an interest in studying uncertainty in illness. This profession-specific interest is likely due to nursing's focus on patient emotional and psychological well-being, in addition to physical health (Clayton & Ellington, 2011). Additionally, as noted by Madar and Bar-Tal (2009), nurses have the most frequent contact with patients and therefore are in a unique position to educate them on their illness, help them maintain hope, and ultimately assist them in managing their uncertainty.

One proponent of studying uncertainty in the field of nursing is Merle Mishel, who began focusing on this topic in the 1980s. Unlike Brashers' work in communication, Mishel's research fits squarely in the scientific paradigm because she's interested in finding patterns of behavior and identifying patients in different categories. For example, in her uncertainty theory, Mishel (1988) focuses on patients' cognitive

COMMUNICATION MATTERS

Sample Items from the Mishel Uncertainty in Illness Scale (Mishel, 1981)

Patients respond on a five-point Likert scale (strongly agree to strongly disagree).

- I don't know what is wrong with me.
- I have a lot of questions without answers.
- I am unsure if my illness is getting better or worse.
- The doctors say things to me that have many meanings.
- It is difficult to know if the treatments or medications I am getting are helping me.

---

scheme for understanding and making sense of illness. She says that patients can end up in one of two camps: (a) the danger appraisal condition, where uncertainty causes stress, or (b) the opportunity appraisal condition, where uncertainty is a preferable state to a negative certainty. Additionally, Mishel (1981) developed a 30-item scale for illness uncertainty so that healthcare providers can identify the level and type of uncertainty a patient is experiencing. We include some sample items from the scale here. The full scale is available from the 1981 publication.

Researchers are testing interventions to see how we can work to reduce uncertainty about specific illnesses and in specific patient populations. For example, Germino and colleagues (2013) studied an uncertainty management program with young Caucasian

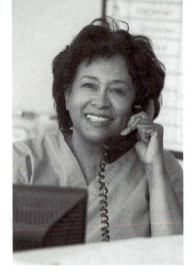

and African-American breast cancer survivors. The program included a CD and booklet with helpful strategies for coping with uncertainty about breast cancer survivorship, as well as four reinforcing phone calls with nurses. The researchers found that participants in the intervention group had less uncertainty, better coping, and more self-efficacy, among other benefits. They also found that African-Americans responded even more positively to the intervention than Caucasians. The authors concluded that in spite of a few limitations to their study, they found this intervention to be very successful and easy to deliver, and they encouraged others working in clinical settings to adopt their program for use with other breast cancer survivors.

Clearly, there are many opportunities for future work in uncertainty. First, because uncertainty is such an encompassing term, it has been studied in various ways. What is needed is a more systematic approach to studying this construct: How do we specifically define uncertainty in illness contexts? What are the major causes of uncertainty in (specific) illness(es)? What challenges do patients face when dealing with different kinds of uncertainty? In adopting a more systematic approach, we can start to understand ways in which we can help patients and their family members manage uncertainty in helpful and healthy ways. Second, we must continue to privilege the role that communication plays in contributing to, managing, and/or reducing uncertainty—and to develop inventions to help patients face the challenge of uncertainty in illness.

Brashers (2001) said, "across contexts, people engage in or avoid communication so that they can manipulate uncertainty to suit their needs ... [research studies] that account for these factors have important consequences for the practice of healthcare" (p. 491). One area for future intervention development that Germino and colleagues (2013) noted was that when we focus on specific populations and how they experience uncertainty in illness, we can also identify specific ways to target them. For example, the researchers noted that younger patients use mobile devices like smart phones and tablets, so we should develop interventions for this patient population that feature these types of technology use in order to "meet them where they are." We wouldn't want to develop an intervention for people that uses technology they are unfamiliar with—that might just cause more uncertainty!

Health Literacy—*I Have What?!*

At the intersection of health and communication lies a skill that is necessary for informed decision making and, ultimately, positive health outcomes. This skill, called **health literacy**, is broadly defined as "the capacity to obtain, process, and understand basic health information and services needed to make appropriate health decisions" (U.S. Department of Health and Human Services [USDHHS], 2012). You can see from this basic definition that health literacy can have a large impact on someone's health. People with low health literacy may not understand health information given to them by their healthcare provider, like a diagnosis. What does, "You have a benign tumor on your femur" mean? They also may not have the skills to know how and where to look up additional information on this diagnosis. For example, it may not occur to them or they may not be able to go home and perform a Google search for the words "benign tumor" and "femur."

Unlike uncertainty, which is a psychological state that people feel, health literacy is a skill that allows patients to do something. And health literacy permeates almost every aspect of healthcare. According to a report by the American Medical Association, a person's health literacy is a stronger predictor of physical and psychological health than education level, demographic factors like race and gender, cultural background,

Health Literacy in Action

Here are some examples of where health literacy comes into play:

- Knowing how to keep yourself healthy
- Knowing when to seek healthcare
- Understanding prescription bottle directions
- Knowing how to accurately fill out a medical form
- Reading and understanding health pamphlets and websites
- Understanding and being able to accurately follow a healthcare provider's directions
- Navigating the healthcare system, including health insurance

and even variables like a patient's self-efficacy (Ad Hoc Committee on Health Literacy for the Council on Scientific Affairs, 1999). Can you think of another single patient factor that has that much of an influence on health?! We sure can't. In sum, a health literate person must possess a variety of skills, including the ability to navigate different information channels and sort through information in order to make an informed health decision.

Because health literacy is so ubiquitous in a patient's healthcare experience, it has been studied extensively and usually from a scientific approach. Health literacy researchers are interested in defining what it means to be health literate and developing field interventions to improve health literacy. But with many cooks in the kitchen, so to speak, comes a body of research that isn't always consistent. For example, there are varying definitions of health literacy because it is such a complex concept (Berkman, Davis, & McCormack, 2010; Ishikawa & Yano, 2008). Some definitions are descriptive in nature, focusing on what health literacy *is*, like the one from the USDHHS listed at the start of this section. Alternatively, some scholars focus on what health literacy *looks like when enacted* by an individual. For example, Zarcadoolas, Pleasant, and Greer (2003) argue that a health literate person should be able to complete certain tasks such as "apply health concepts and information to novel situations" and "participate in ongoing public and private dialogues about health, medicine, scientific knowledge, and cultural beliefs" (p. 119).

HEALTH LITERACY

Health literacy is one of the most important skills patients can have and there has been much communication research about this topic. It is defined as "the capacity to obtain, process, and understand basic health information and services needed to make appropriate health decisions" (U.S. Department of Health and Human Services [USDHHS], 2012).

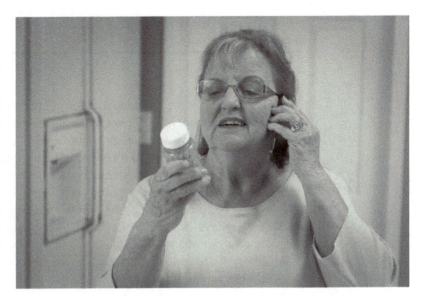

In addition to varying definitions, there are various ways to measure health literacy. Parker, Baker, Williams, and Nurss (1995) developed the **Test of Functional Health Literacy in Adults (TOFHLA)**, which focuses on reading and numerical abilities (numeracy). While this measure proves to be pretty good at indicating a person's health literacy, it only focuses on reading and number tasks; it also is pretty long (50 questions) and has taken patients up to 22 minutes to complete. Alternatively, some researchers have developed health literacy measures that can be used quickly in the clinic to identify patients with low health literacy. For example, Chew, Bradley, and Boyko (2004) developed a health literacy measure to identify adult patients with inadequate health literacy that was easier and more practical to use in the clinic because it only contained 16 questions. Baker, Williams, Parker, Gazmararian, and Nurss (1999) also developed a shorter measure to use in the clinic setting, which they called the Short Test of Functional Health Literacy in Adults (S-TOFHLA). We're including two sample questions from the S-TOFHLA on the next page. Can you answer them correctly?

One final note about defining and measuring a person's health literacy level. While health literacy is a pretty stable construct (some people are just going to be more health literate than others, just like some people are always going to have better hair),

S-TOFHLA

Here are two sample questions from the S-TOFHLA:

The label on your prescription bottle says you should "take medication on empty stomach one hour before or two hours after a meal unless otherwise directed by your doctor." If you eat lunch at 12:00 noon, and you want to take this medicine before lunch, what time should you take it? (Answer: "11:00" or "before 11:00.")

Normal blood sugar is 60–150. Your blood sugar today is 160. If this were your score, would your blood sugar be normal today? (Answer: "No.")

it *can* be context specific, meaning that you might be very health literate in one health situation but have poor health literacy in another situation. This means that even if you are educated and have knowledge about health, you might still have poor health literacy if you find yourself in a new health situation like a cancer diagnosis or an emergency surgery. One primary care physician we work with recently told the story about how, when she was diagnosed with breast cancer, she felt her own health literacy "go out the window." She was a practicing physician herself, but in this particular personal health situation, she felt not only scared and uncertain but also uninformed about what she should do next and where she should search for information. However, the good news is that we can improve our health literacy if we find ourselves in a similar situation.

Because health literacy is such a complex concept, is important in so many different health situations, and can be defined and measured in different ways, we could talk for days on this subject. However, we do not have the space in this one chapter! Therefore, we would like to highlight two important sub-dimensions to health literacy before we move on.

The first sub-dimension is **media literacy**. People are increasingly relying on mediated sources like television and the Internet for information about their health. Have you ever watched a medical drama like *Grey's Anatomy* and wondered if the medical miracles they perform are realistic? How about going on WebMD and researching your symptoms? Developing models of health literacy that consider mediated channels of information is needed, especially when designing health literacy curricula and interventions. As noted by Bergsma and Carney (2008), "Rather than trying to protect [people] from potentially harmful messages, media literacy education to promote health involves them in a critical examination of media messages that influence their perceptions and practices . . ." (p. 523). Such education should provide the "critical thinking skills necessary to ameliorate the influence of these messages and make healthy choices" (p. 523).

The second sub-dimension is **numeracy**, which is a person's basic ability to understand, process, and act on numerical information. Health numeracy also can be thought of as "skills that allow one to understand concepts of risk, probability, and the communication of scientific evidence" (Schapira et al., 2008, p. 502). For example, when talking about probability, a patient may have difficulty understanding the way a certain prognosis is presented by a healthcare provider. Which is clearer to you: "You have a 3 in 5 chance of this skin rash coming back" or "You have a 60% chance of this skin rash coming back"?

Because researchers and healthcare providers alike recognize the important role of health literacy in patient health (Ratzan & Parker, 2006), national attention has been given to developing interventions to improve patient health literacy. Pfizer, along with health researchers in Arizona and North Carolina, developed the Newest Vital Sign program to help healthcare providers identify and address health literacy deficiencies with their individual patients (Pfizer, 2012). Patients are given a food label to read and then asked six questions about the information they saw on the label. Providers can then very quickly assess the patient's health literacy on the basis of their answers; the program also provides clear direction for providers for how to help these patients. For example, the program encourages providers to "rephrase instructions by using simpler words and concepts, and draw pictures if appropriate" when they notice their patient has a quizzical look (Pfizer Clear Health Communication Initiative, 2011).

Another national initiative to increase patient health literacy is the **Ask Me 3** patient education program, which was developed and promoted by the National Patient Safety Foundation (2013). This program offers brochures, posters, and other educational materials that can be used in clinics to encourage patients (and providers) to be asking the right questions about their health. The three questions are easy to remember:

1.   What is my main problem?
2.   What do I need to do?
3.   Why is it important for me to do this?

In addition to encouraging patients to ask these questions, healthcare providers are also encouraged to structure their conversations with patients around these questions.

Overall, researchers and healthcare providers are making great strides in studying—and improving—health literacy. Just raising awareness about this topic is important:

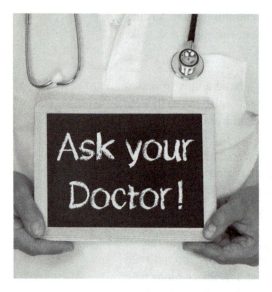

Ten years ago, many people had never even heard the term health literacy, let alone how important it is in health. But improvements can still be made in health literacy work. Cynthia Baur (2010) identifies several important areas for new directions in health literacy work. First, rather than studying health literacy generally, she says that we must study health literacy in specific areas, such as in the disease prevention domain or the ways that policy changes affect health literacy. Second, she advocates that we study health literacy in a way that recognizes it as something developed within social relations. She says, "the health literacy issues for a specific population group and situation must be excavated, made visible, and explicitly addressed in holistic interventions and policies that consider root causes" (p. 48). Third, she says that we must take a public health approach to tracking health literacy information. This means we need to not only consistently measure people's health literacy but also have a system for reporting and tracking that information at a population level. This will help researchers to be able to better develop and deliver appropriately tailored health information to different groups. Additionally, by tracking population health literacy levels, we can more easily see over the years what improvements we are making and where we still have deficiencies.

Patient Participation—*Say What You Need To Say*

John Mayer had it right, at least when it comes to communicating. One of the most important struggles patients face, no matter who they are or even how high their health literacy, is simply talking with their healthcare provider. **Patient participation** is defined as "the extent to which patients produce verbal responses that have the potential to significantly influence the content and structure of the interaction as well as the health care provider's beliefs and behaviors" (Street & Millay, 2001, p. 62). Can you think of some reasons you haven't spoken up during a doctor's visit? For example, have you ever felt rushed by the doctor and left not saying everything you wanted to? Or maybe you felt embarrassed about something and failed to speak up when the nurse was taking your history? (Hey, we've all had an embarrassing rash or wart or both!) Ever been diagnosed with something more serious and felt yourself shut down because you were just trying to process the information? All of these factors (and more) contribute to whether patients participate in their care. Of course, despite these factors, we *want* patients to talk with their healthcare provider because patient participation can improve patient care quality and health outcomes (Street & Millay, 2001).

The relatively recent research emphasis on patient participation reflects the changing role of the patient in the healthcare interaction (Longtin et al., 2010; Sharf & Street, 1997). In the past, the **biomedical** and **paternalistic** models of medicine used a top-down approach, where patients had little input in their own healthcare and were simply told what to do by their healthcare providers. In the last 30 years, healthcare delivery has been changing due to a more **consumerist** approach to medicine, more informed patients, and the understanding that when patients are a part of their own care, they are more satisfied and they have better health outcomes (Longtin et al., 2010). Later in the chapter, we also discuss some of the ways that recent legislation and healthcare reform are affecting the patient's role in similar ways, making them more a part of their own healthcare.

In addition to the changing role of the patient, researchers are also just simply realizing the importance of encouraging patients to speak up. Swain (2008) elucidates the importance and necessity of patients' involvement in their care when she says, "the clinicians bring their knowledge of the condition, prognosis, treatment options and the likely outcome probabilities of those options and that is *complemented* by the patients who brings*[sic]* their own knowledge, that of living with the condition, their attitude to risk and their own values and preferences" (p. 157, emphasis added).

Because of this increased focus on patients participating in their own healthcare, research on the topic is growing. One thing that is clear is that not all patients prefer to participate in their care. Overall, research shows that women, people who are more educated, and people who are healthier tend to prefer participating more in their care than other people (Arora & McHorney, 2000; Levinson, Kao, Kuby, & Thisted, 2005). So if we're working toward developing interventions to promote and facilitate participation, we must be careful about our assumptions regarding who actually wants to participate.

PATIENT PARTICIPATION

Patient participation is especially important in effective health communication between patients and providers. Research reveals that though every patient doesn't participate in the same way, *some* level of participation is needed for an effective interaction.

Another challenge in this research is related to our methods: how we measure patient participation. Some researchers simply ask patients about their participation. For example, Heggland, Øgaard, Mikkelsen, and Hausken (2012) developed a question-naire that measured how much patients participated in decisions about a surgical treatment. They asked questions like did the patient have an opportunity to choose his or her surgeon and did the doctor answer the patient's questions in a clear and understandable manner. Alternatively, some scholars believe that you must measure patient participation as it is enacted during the healthcare visit. These researchers will get permission to audiotape or videotape healthcare interactions between patients and providers and then analyze the amount of participation by the patient (Street & Millay, 2001). You can see from these two examples that patient participation is often studied from a scientific perspective, through self-report and observation. But it may be that an interpretive approach is better suited to "measuring" how an individual patient participates because after all, everyone is different, and participation is a complex thing. Haven't you ever been in a class, and although you don't speak up or go to office hours very often, you were there every day, taking notes, listening, and participating in your own way? Such "tacit" participation may happen with patients, as well.

As previously noted, patient participation in the healthcare encounter complements what the healthcare provider brings to the table. This illuminates the importance of communication being a two-way street. Cegala, Street, and Clinch (2007) studied the effect of patient participation on doctor communication in the primary care setting. They found that doctors provided more information to patients who participated more. Interestingly, they found that doctors not only provided more information when high participation patients asked for it but also *volunteered* more

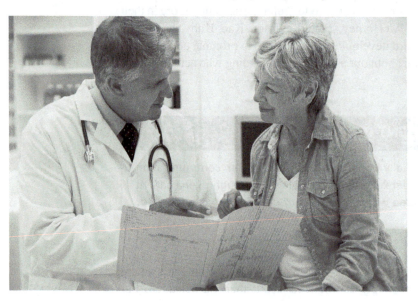

information for high partici-pation patients. In this sense, we can see that by studying patient participation, we start to see the medical interview as a conversation with equal partners. Cegala et al. argue that "high patient participa-tion during a medical inter-view helps the physician to more accurately understand the patient's goals, interests, and concerns, thus allowing the physician to better align his or her communication with the patient's agenda" (p. 181).

In addition to studying the effect of patient participation on healthcare encounters, some researchers have designed **communication skills interventions** to encourage patient participation. Frosch, Rincon, Ochoa, and Mangione (2010) designed an intervention for older people to be more active in their healthcare, especially with regard to chronic disease in this population (e.g., coronary artery disease). Patients in the intervention condition watched videos about patients being involved in their own care and participated in motivational discussions about what they could do in their next healthcare encounter. The researchers found that patients in this intervention condition were more likely to participate in their own care *and* have better health outcomes than those who did not receive any type of intervention.

Although researchers know that patient participation is important for improving the quality of interactions with healthcare practitioners, we also know that sometimes patients don't always participate. Because of that, future research in this area is really important. Don Cegala (2006), one of the most prolific researchers in patient participation, has several suggestions for future directions. First, he says we must focus on more long-term interventions—and long-term effects. He says we must answer the question "of whether patients require periodic reinforcement, or even retraining, to maintain and use effective communication skills with health care professionals" (p. 124). Second, he says we must focus more of our research on underserved populations who may suffer from extra barriers to communication with healthcare professionals. We discuss some of the health disparities research later in this chapter. Third, Cegala says that we must take into account that some patients (e.g., older patients who are used to the paternalistic model of medicine) may not *want* to participate more in their care. While recognizing that we as health communication researchers are operating under the assumption that participation is good, we may need to approach these populations differently and tailor our interventions to their needs. Finally, he says that we must do a better job of tracking how patient participation specifically affects health outcomes.

Up until this point, we've discussed what we've labeled internal challenges for patients: uncertainty, health literacy, and patient participation. In the second half of this chapter, we discuss external challenges for patients.

EXTERNAL CHALLENGES FOR PATIENTS

There are a number of external challenges that can pose unique challenges for effective provider–patient communication and patient navigation of the healthcare system. Just to clarify, when we say "external" challenges, we don't mean the outdoor field day activities you had as a kid. (Man, we both hated the wheel barrow race!) Instead, we mean a number of factors that are external to the patient's control but that may have a large impact on their health. First, the United States looks a lot different than it did in the past, and shifting demographic trends like race, ethnicity, gender, and income/class mean that doctors and patients may come from vastly different backgrounds. Second, there are many community factors, or what we call the "built environment," that can both constrain and facilitate access to healthcare. Finally, though changes in healthcare law and public policy expand access to healthcare, these changes can also create inequalities in the form of gaps in healthcare provider access and availability of services. So, let's dive in and explore some of these external factors a little more.

Demographic Trends—*Is America a Melting Pot?*

General demographic trends in the United States have diversified the patient population in the healthcare system. As the United States becomes more diverse, the pool of available medical practitioners no longer adequately reflects the demographics of the patient population. Researchers argue that culturally competent healthcare systems and providers reflect and respond to the **cultural heterogeneity** or diversity of their patient population (Anderson, Scrimshaw, Fullilove, Fielding, & Normand, 2003); in theory, culture is the most influential of many factors that influence health beliefs and behaviors (Harwood, 1981). There are many different factors that make up one's culture, and in this section, we'll cover just a few.

Race and ethnicity. Whether we want to face it or not, racism exists in our country. And while we often think about race affecting things like education and employment

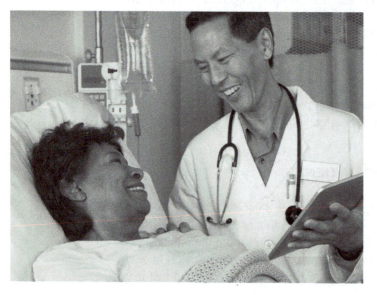

opportunities, it also affects the kind of healthcare a person receives. Sadly, compelling evidence has established disparities in the quality of patient care and health outcomes by race and ethnicity. The Institute of Medicine's (IOM) report, *Unequal Treatment: Confronting Racial and Ethnic Disparities in Health Care*, documented that racial and ethnic minorities receive lower quality healthcare and suffer disproportionally higher rates of disease, disability, and death, even when controlling for access-related factors like health insurance and socioeconomic factors like income (Smedley, Stith, &

Nelson, 2002). Broad evidence also shows that racial and economic minorities and persons with low socioeconomic status receive poorer quality of care than Whites and persons with higher socioeconomic status (Pappas, Queen, Hadden, & Fisher, 1993; Smedley et al., 2002; Weissman, Stern, Fielding, & Epstein, 1991). However, the IOM report also suggests that the patient–practitioner relationship can be an important exacerbating factor to these wide disparities in the U.S. healthcare system. That is, racial differences in health outcomes are not only explained by biological differences but also are in part due to nonclinical factors (e.g., patient preferences in treatment) and clinical factors that may be racially based (e.g., discriminatory treatment). This is clearly not a good thing. But it does allow health communication scholars to work to find ways to improve healthcare for racial and ethnic minorities by improving the patient–provider relationship.

A team of researchers led by Howard S. Gordon has investigated this patient–practitioner relationship and has examined from a scientific perspective whether there are racial differences in doctors' information-giving and patients' participation in the interaction. Gordon and his colleagues studied patient–provider interactions in a Veterans Affairs Medical Center to determine whether there were race-based communication differences. The researchers found that both Black patients and patients in discordant race interactions (i.e., the doctor and the patient were different races) not only received less information from their doctors about their disease but also were less likely to participate in the conversation (Gordon, Street, Sharf, & Souchek, 2006). Therefore, not only did being a Black patient affect the interaction but also being a race different from the doctor affected the patient's care. The researchers concluded that "potential racial variation in doctor-patient communication becomes an issue of concern especially when considering a growing body of research that links patterns of communication to outcomes of care" (p. 1318).

PATIENT DEMOGRAPHICS

Patient demographics like race, ethnicity, gender, and income all play an important role in health communication, especially when the patient and provider come from different backgrounds.

Another researcher who studies race and has dedicated her career toward understanding how race and ethnicity influence the relationship between patients and their primary care practitioners is Lisa A. Cooper. Cooper works with a team of researchers at Johns Hopkins University to examine the potential roles of clinician–community, clinician–clinician, and clinician–self relationships in overcoming disparities in healthcare. She also adopts a very scientific approach to her research. Cooper and Powe's (2004) report for The Commonwealth Fund has identified the effect of patient–provider racial, ethnic, and language concordance (i.e., whether a patient and a provider are the same race, ethnicity, and/or speak the same language) on patient experiences, healthcare processes, and healthcare outcomes. The report identifies how racial and ethnic minorities are represented poorly among physicians and other health-care practitioners and are more likely to find themselves in a "race-discordant" patient–provider relationship. In other words, when racial and ethnic minorities go to a clinic or hospital for healthcare services, they are less likely to encounter healthcare providers who look and sound like them.

Teaching healthcare providers how to use **patient-centered communication skills** to engage their patients is one solution to enhance equity in the provision of healthcare and make sure patients are receiving high quality healthcare, no matter their race or ethnicity. To this end, the U.S. Department of Health and Human Services Office of Minority Health has established standards for **culturally and linguistically appropriate services (CLAS)** as a means to address and correct inequities that exist in the provision of healthcare to culturally and ethnically diverse groups. While there are several categories to the CLAS standards, most if not all of them have a communication element. You can review the CLAS standards at this website: https://www.thinkculturalhealth.hhs.gov/Content/clas.asp

If healthcare providers follow the principles of patient-centered care to deliver CLAS to all patients, we can hopefully start to see less variation in patient experiences based on race and ethnicity. We know that strong evidence links patient-centered care to improvements in patient **adherence** and **health outcomes**; therefore, interventions that enhance communication strategies to improve this dimension of care are prom-ising strategies to reduce racial and ethnic **health disparities** (Beach et al., 2006; Cameron, 2013). Health communication scholars are well positioned to continue research on external factors such as racial and ethnic disparities in healthcare, particu-larly how we can help to reduce some of the health disparities that exist. Cameron (2013) notes, "health communication scholars are poised to collaborate in these efforts to address health disparities . . . through identifying innovative and feasible ways of expanding communication beyond the clinical encounter" (p. 43). Shavers et al. (2012), after examining much of the current research on racial/ethnic disparities, suggest we need "systematic examinations of the patient-physician interactions, particularly as they relate to communication styles and nonverbal behaviors that have the potential to elicit the perception of discrimination among diverse patients" (p. 963). In sum, health communication scholars must be actively involved in future research in this area because discrimination is something that, at its most basic definition, is *communicated.*

Gender. Aspects of gender and gender roles are also important factors to consider as influential on the way that healthcare providers may interact with their patients. Yes, women are from Venus and men are from Mars, but we're not sure we want our healthcare providers to be from different planets. In other words, gender is going to affect communication, but how it affects health communication is an especially important concern.

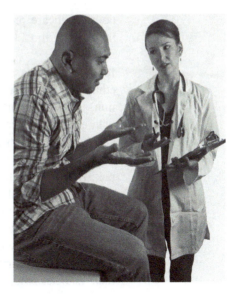

For example, coronary heart disease (CHD) is thought by researchers to be under-diagnosed in women. Experiments that have held patient communication and coronary heart disease symptom presentation factors constant consistently show that physicians' diagnostic and treatment decisions differ by patient sex and gender (Adams et al., 2008; Arber et al., 2006). One possible explanation for this gendered treatment is that there is evidence that providers are less certain about a CHD diagnosis for women than men patients, as men patients demonstrate more "typical" symptoms (Lutfey, Gerstenberger, Link, & McKinlay, 2010; Lutfey & McKinlay, 2009). When confronted with an uncertain diagnosis, providers are less likely to prescribe a CHD medication or tests (Lutfey & McKinlay, 2009). Welch, Lutfey, Gerstenberger, and Grace (2012) conducted an experiment to further examine the effects of patient gender on physician care. The researchers assigned doctors to view different videos in which a patient-actor was discussing his or her symptoms. They then asked doctors to provide a diagnosis and recommend follow-up care. They found that doctors were less certain about the diagnosis for female patients than male patients, which also influenced the follow-up care they recommended.

In looking ahead to future work on this topic, Bertakis (2009) argues that it's not enough to just identify that these differences *do* exist, we have to do something about it. One way to address these gender differences in healthcare is to start at the source: "medical schools, residency training programs, and clinical delivery systems need to incorporate this information into strategies focused on improving the communication between physicians and patients" (p. 359). One group tackling this issue head on is the Department of Veterans Affairs (VA). A traditionally male-centered organization, the VA hospital system has turned its attention to specific female veteran needs through the development of the VA Women's Health Research Consortium, which informs both healthcare provider training and clinical practices (Bastian, Bosworth, Washington, & Yano, 2013).

Income and Class. A third demographic factor that complicates analysis of race, ethnicity, or gender is that of socioeconomic status (income, education, and occupation). In general, an individual's income, education, and occupation are correlated with economic advantage in society; the more economically advantaged individuals are, the better their health. Most recently, researchers have established how the chronic stress associated with low socioeconomic status increases morbidity and mortality risk. Researchers have established three major pathways by which socioeconomic status exerts an influence on health: access to quality health care, environmental exposure, and health behavior (Adler & Newman, 2002). For example, researchers interviewed patients with type 2 diabetes receiving care at safety net clinics (clinics for people with low-income or without insurance) in Southern California to understand persistent barriers to diabetes management. When asked how they managed their diabetes, these patients "described managing diabetes with limited financial resources as often a game of balance and negotiation, whereby purchasing healthy foods is abandoned because of a more pressing concern for their life" (Rendle et al., 2013, p. 3). Although their diabetes management practices were often strategic, these patients often were impeded by "seemingly insurmountable barriers." This patient vantage point was consistent with prior research indicating that patients in safety net clinics are often "less likely than clinicians to identify the systemic and contextual factors contributing to poor diabetes care" (Reichsman, Werner, Cella, Bobiak, & Stange, 2009, p. 4).

Not only may poor patients have difficulty accessing material resources needed for managing their chronic disease (e.g., test strips to measure blood sugar, insulin, and other items that can be costly) but also they might live in an environment where healthy food options are prohibitively expensive or are not easily accessible. Living in such an environment may make them feel economically pressed to choose between expending resources on competing diabetes management health behaviors, such as choosing lower cost, unhealthy food in order to afford diabetes medication or supplies. By engaging with community members to investigate and interpret diabetes management issues related to socioeconomic conditions, health communication researchers have recommended that providers engage in clear, open communication with patients about barriers to managing their diabetes. By tailoring their recommendations and acknowledging the everyday economic realities that patients work within, providers may reduce the burden of external factors on the patient while promoting better chronic disease management and health outcomes. Future research in this area must continue to address the real barriers that patients face; however, changing healthcare policies (discussed below) that directly affect those in lower income brackets may help to also address some of these barriers.

Community Challenges—*How Does My Community Affect My Health?*

Beyond patient demographics, the socio-ecological conditions of the healthcare system that patients have access to also constrain the potential well-being of patients. Place matters for healthcare and communication. For example, we know that areas in the United States that are disparately poor also suffer disparately poorer health than the rest of the nation. When poor residents are also more rural and characterized by low population density and service availability, patients report difficulty accessing high-quality, **evidence-based healthcare**. One of the regions in the United States confronting this challenge is rural Appalachia, where

healthcare networks struggle to build a set of rural services in local settings while ensuring access to specialized services for rural patients. The Rural Appalachian Cancer Demonstration Program sponsored by the Centers for Disease Control and Prevention has found that effective patient–provider communication is critical "in creating either trust or distrust between individuals and families and health care professionals and the health care system" (Behringer & Friedell, 2006, p. 3).

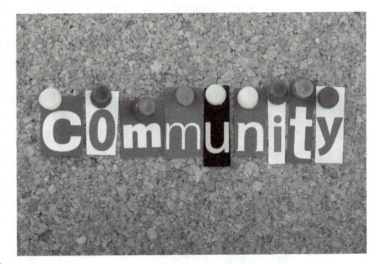

In our research with the University of Kentucky Rural Cancer Prevention Center, we have found that engaging community members involved in community settings such as schools, healthcare systems, non-profit groups, local religious organizations, and even sororities and fraternities can help identify parts of the healthcare and **communication infrastructure** that may be disconnected or in need of intervention to improve or stimulate community conversations about health and well-being. For example, to better understand ways that local communication practices and healthcare systems contributed to misunderstandings about the need for adolescent and young adult vaccination against preventable diseases, our research team interviewed parents, providers, and other stakeholders to identify the local knowledge and attitudes that were related to vaccination behaviors. We found, for example, that even when young adult women (18–26 years of age) were provided with free vouchers for the full Human Papillomavirus (HPV) vaccine series, of 246 women recruited from rural health clinics, only 45% initiated dose one, only 14% of those who received the first dose returned for the second, and only 5% completed the three-dose series (Crosby, Casey, Vanderpool, Collins, & Moore, 2011). Why weren't these women fully using the free vouchers?

Well, we conducted some qualitative, interpretive research to explore why. We identified several barriers to vaccination, including normative maternal and peer influences, insufficient knowledge, vaccination stigma and negative or ambivalent vaccination attitudes, questions about vaccine safety and efficacy, and concerns about cost and anticipated vaccine pain (Head & Cohen, 2012). To address these barriers, we created a targeted educational video called "1-2-3 Pap" that could be delivered in a clinical setting to explain to young adult women the importance of both HPV vaccination and Pap testing as primary and secondary cervical cancer prevention strategies for young adult women (Cohen et al., 2013). We also intervened by offering free and low-cost vaccinations (manufacturer reimbursement programs to provide vaccines) and enhancing standard-of-care procedures that included follow-up phone call reminders and community-based vaccination clinics to optimize HPV vaccination adherence rates. Fundamentally, the study involved credible, local nurses to deliver immunizations in convenient settings, decreasing the burden of accessing healthcare providers and addressing a number of community-level social and economic challenges that had previously depressed HPV vaccination rates for this population (Vanderpool et al., 2013).

The lesson that this case establishes may serve as an example for health communication researchers in other medically underserved communities. Whereas the vaccination completion rate in our study was 31.9% in the comparison condition, nearly half of the women (43.3%) randomized to the DVD intervention completed the vaccination series. These rates were substantially higher than those found in previous studies (e.g., 4.5% in Crosby et al.'s [2011] study of medically underserved women in Appalachian Kentucky; 10% in Dempsey et al.'s [2011] research in Michigan with 19- to 26-year-old women). And although the research strategy was not successful in addressing all barriers to vaccination, the findings suggest the efficacy of community-engaged research that attends to the ways communication strategies may be used to improve the healthcare delivery system in medically underserved communities. Attending specifically to the local health beliefs in Appalachian Kentucky and partnering with credible clinics in the area definitely created a better project for everyone involved and has allowed us to continue working in the area to reduce cancer disparities.

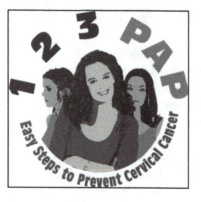

Figure 7.1 The Logo from the "1-2-3 Pap" Intervention.

Public Policy Factors—*What Does Healthcare Reform Mean to Me, Personally?*

A final factor external to the patient that affects healthcare quality and gaps in care is that of public policy. Congressional approval of the **Patient Protection and Affordable Care Act of 2010 (ACA)** effectively expands healthcare access to otherwise medically underserved populations. Great, right? But understanding the new policy and how it affects you is another story. Here we talk about (a) some of the ways that the ACA expands access to different patient populations that previously didn't have health insurance and (b) the development of Patient Centered Medical Homes and their effect on health communication between patients and their providers. The ACA also encompasses some changes in technology use in the healthcare world, which we'll get into in Chapter 12.

HEALTHCARE POLICY

The Patient Protection and Affordable Care Act (ACA) expands healthcare coverage to many individuals who didn't have it before, but it also comes with new challenges.

One immediate implication of the ACA is that it expands health insurance coverage, adding patient demand and potentially pushing the capacity of the medical system, particularly in rural, medically underserved communities. In other words, by increasing access to healthcare, we now have created more "customers" for the healthcare system. In the short term, this has resulted in two major problems. First, as you probably heard on the news, there were some major problems with the government website (HealthCare.gov) where people went to sign up for healthcare coverage. People reported long loading times, the website getting "stuck," being sent to a page that asked them to wait while other customers were served, and, probably the worst, having their data actually being lost after they signed

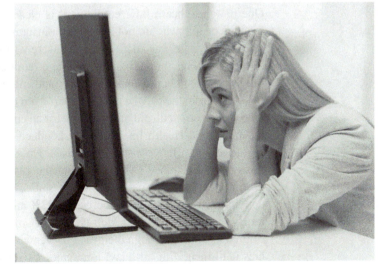

up for coverage. This set of problems not only resulted in thousands of frustrated Americans but even led to a public apology by President Obama and a series of Congressional hearings in which Secretary of Health and Human Services Kathleen Sebelius had to testify about the website situation and how it was being fixed. Not a good start for the ACA. (A few months after the launch and an incredible amount of work dedicated to fixing the site and building back the trust of those Americans who wanted to sign up for coverage, things are looking better.)

Second, a fundamental health communication concern related to the ACA is how to effectively communicate all of the changes in healthcare policy to these new customers. For people without health insurance, what is the best policy for them? For those with health insurance through their employer, should they stick with their health insurance or go to the Health Insurance Marketplace (the website mentioned above) to find better coverage? For those with health insurance whose policies were canceled after the ACA came into effect (because the policies did not meet the new set of higher standards for all health insurance policies), what should they do? Finding ways to effectively communicate information that can aid people's understanding of the ACA and its impact is crucial because national research surveys conducted in 2010 and 2012 (see Gross et al., 2012) suggest that many Americans do not understand healthcare reform and are confused by and often oppose policies that are sometimes falsely thought to be parts of the ACA. However, most people have favored most of the elements of the ACA researchers have examined. Indeed, a team of researchers supported by the Robert Wood Johnson Foundation, GfK, Stanford University, and the Associated Press examined these data and concluded "if education efforts were to correct public misunderstanding of the bill, public favorability might increase considerably" (Gross et al., 2012, p. 19).

One new healthcare law requirement is clear to the uninformed observer: The Act requires people who do not have health insurance to get coverage. The original deadline for coverage was 2013, but as we were writing this chapter, it got pushed back to 2014. Whenever the individual coverage requirement does take effect, the ACA has provisions that should make it easier and more affordable for the uninsured to get insurance from the private market (apart from packages offered by employers). People who are not on Medicaid or who work for an employer not offering insurance must buy insurance in a Health Insurance Marketplace—an insurance exchange that is tightly regulated and offers consumers choices. No one can be turned down for coverage in this new marketplace (which was not the case before the passage of the ACA), be discriminated against based on health status, or be denied coverage for pre-existing conditions. People who earn between 133% and 400% of the federal poverty line will receive tax credits to help defray the cost of coverage. Young adults who are not offered insurance through their job may remain on their parents' health insurance policies until their 27th birthday. For senior citizens who receive government insurance benefits in the form of Medicare, and for poor and low-income families qualifying for Medicaid, these programs will ensure that people can receive preventive care services at no cost. So, that's a lot of changes. Do you know how the ACA will affect you and your family? If not, it's easy to see how effective health communication about this new policy must be used to educate the public about these changes or else the policy has little hope of being effective.

Medical Practice Changes—*Where is my Patient-centered Medical Home?*

Provisions of the ACA also establish and promote the **Patient-Centered Medical Home (PCMH)**. The PCMH concept is a model of care in which patients receive care from a team of healthcare providers led by their personal physician who, in theory, will provide continuous and coordinated care throughout a patient's lifetime to improve health outcomes. The rationale behind this team approach is that it will improve access and communication, reduce problems in the transition of care and care coordination, and ensure care quality and safety. Rittenhouse and Shortell (2009) outline the four cornerstones of the PCMH model, displayed in Table 7.1.

This model is very new. Because of that, there has been very little work by health communication scholars looking specifically at the patient-centered medical home, despite what we believe is a scenario replete with communication issues. Can you think of some? How would you apply health communication principles to studying PCMHs? One thing is certain: Wide-scale adoption of the PCMH model would represent a funda-mental change from the current system of delivering patient care in the United States.

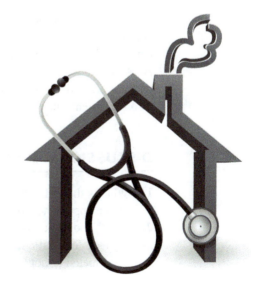

A preliminary evaluation of PCMHs by the Agency for Healthcare Research and Quality (Peikes et al., 2012) revealed that most healthcare systems that said they were using the PCMH model weren't actually using the PCMH in practice, but rather "parts" of it. The authors of the report argue that we must not only have better **implementation** of the PCMH model but also have better **evaluation** of this model, or else "[t]here is a large risk that research currently under way on PCMH . . . will fail to support decisionmakers' information needs" (p. 23). Another challenge facing the healthcare industry—and decidedly a health communication issue—is training and educating new healthcare providers in the PCMH, which will need to start with revamping medical school curricula (Voelker, 2010).

Table 7.1 Cornerstones of PCMH Model

Term	Definition
Primary Care	Comprehensive, first-contact, acute, chronic, and preventive care across the life space
Patient-centered Care	Tailoring care to meet the needs and preferences of the patient; placing the patient at the center of the health care system
New-model Practice	Departure from a "business" healthcare model; this type of evidence-based practice privileges quality improvement, patient safety, transparency, and accountability
Payment Reform	Changes in payment structure to account for this new model; combines fee-for-service, pay-for-performance, and separate payment for care coordination and integration

CONCLUSION

In this chapter, we outlined some important areas in healthcare that might pose challenges for patients. We discussed personal patient factors, or internal challenges, such as the uncertainty patients face with illness, health literacy issues, and the important role of patient participation in their own care. Additionally, we discussed demographics, community challenges, and changes in healthcare policy—factors that are external to the patient but nevertheless affect the quality of patients' interactions with the healthcare delivery system.

The next time you go to the doctor or any healthcare appointment, think about the complexities that we talked about in this chapter. Are you actively participating in your care? Do you understand everything the doctor is telling you? What policies from the ACA do you see affecting your interactions in the doctor's office? As patients begin to take a more active role in their healthcare, it is important for not only researchers but also the patients themselves to be cognizant of these and other challenges.

DISCUSSION QUESTIONS

1. What is the difference between illness uncertainty and low health literacy? How do the approaches for addressing these patient challenges differ?
2. Think about the last time you went to see a healthcare provider. Did you have high or low patient participation? Why? What factors affected whether you participated or not?

3. How might medical education address some of the health communication challenges presented in this chapter?
4. In what ways does the ACA help underserved populations? In what ways might it hurt underserved populations?

IN-CLASS ACTIVITIES

1. Consider the last time you went to see a healthcare provider for a major health issue or illness. Identify five things you were uncertain about and how you worked to reduce that uncertainty. What role did communication play?
2. Consider the measurement issues for health literacy discussed in this chapter. Working in a group, develop your own definition and measurement for health literacy. Think outside the box for this one!
3. Look up the Affordable Care Act and identify three specific ways this healthcare policy will affect you and your family.

RECOMMENDED READINGS

Gaglio, B., Glasgow, R. E., & Bull, S. S. (2012). Do patient preferences for health information vary by health literacy or numeracy? A qualitative assessment. *Journal of Health Communication*, *17*, 109–121.

This article uses a mixed-methods approach, surveys, and qualitative interviews, to determine if cardiovascular patients' level of health literacy and numeracy were related to their health information preferences.

Checton, M. G., & Greene, K. (2011). Beyond initial disclosure: The role of prognosis and symptom uncertainty in patterns of disclosure in relationships. *Health Communication*, *27*, 145–157.

This article examines how a patients' uncertainty about their illnesses affects how they communicate about their illness with other people, including whether they will disclose their illness at all.

Thornton, R. L. J., Powe, N. R., Roter, D., & Cooper, L. A. (2011). Patient–physician social concordance, medical visit communication and patients' perceptions of health care quality. *Patient Education and Counseling*, *85*, e201–e208.

The authors of this article introduce the idea of social concordance between patients and providers (i.e., a combination of social factors like age, race, gender, and education) and the effect that has on patient satisfaction with care.

REFERENCES

Ad Hoc Committee on Health Literacy for the Council on Scientific Affairs, American Medical Association. (1999). Health literacy: Report of the council on scientific affairs. *JAMA*, *281*(6), 552–557.

Adams, A., Buckingham, C. D., Lindenmeyer, A., McKinlay, J. B., Link, C., Marceau, L., & Arber, S. (2008). The influence of patient and doctor gender on diagnosing coronary heart disease. *Sociology of Health and Illness*, *30*, 1–18.

Adler, N. E., & Newman, K. (2002). Socioeconomic disparities in health: Pathways and policies. *Health Affairs*, *21*, 60–76.

Anderson, L. M., Scrimshaw, S. C., Fullilove, M. T., Fielding, J. E., & Normand, J. (2003). Culturally competent healthcare systems: A systematic review. *American Journal of Preventive Medicine*, *24*, 68–79.

Arber, S., McKinlay, J. B., Adams, A., Marceau, L., Link, C., & O'Donnell, A. (2006). Patient characteristics and inequalities in doctors' diagnostic and management strategies relating to CHD: A video-simulation experiment. *Social Science & Medicine*, *62*, 103–115.

Arora, N. K., & McHorney, C. A. (2000). Patient preferences for medical decision making: Who really wants to participate? *Medical Care*, *38*, 335–341.

Babrow, A. S., Kasch, C.R., & Ford, L. A. (1998). The many meanings of uncertainty in illness: Toward a systematic accounting. *Health Communication*, *10*, 1–23.

Baker, D. W., Williams, M. V., Parker, R. M., Gazmararian, J. A., & Nurss, J. (1999). Development of a brief test to measure functional health literacy. *Patient Education and Counseling*, *38*, 33–42.

Bastian, L. A., Bosworth, H. B., Washington, D. L., & Yano, E. M. (2013). Setting the stage: Research to inform interventions, practice and policy to improve women veterans' health and health care. *Journal of General Internal Medicine*, *28*, 491–494.

Baur, C. (2010). New directions in research on public health and health literacy. *Journal of Health Communication*, *15*, 42–50.

Beach, M. C., Gary, T. L., Price, E. G., Robinson, K., Gozu, A., Palacio, A., . . . Cooper, L. A. (2006). Improving health care quality for racial/ethnic minorities: a systematic review of the best evidence regarding provider and organization interventions. *BMC Public Health*, *6*, 104–111.

Behringer, B., & Friedell, G. H. (2006). Appalachia: Where place matters in health. *Preventing Chronic Disease*, *3*, 1–4.

Bergsma, L. J., & Carney, M. E. (2008). Effectiveness of health-promoting media literacy education: a systematic review. *Health Education Research*, *23*, 522–542.

Berkman, N. D., Davis, T. C., & McCormack, L. (2010). Health literacy: What is it? *Journal of Health Communication*, *15*, 9–19.

Bertakis, K. D. (2009). The influence of gender on the doctor–patient interaction. *Patient Education and Counseling*, *76*, 356–360.

Brashers, D. E. (2001). Communication and uncertainty management. *Journal of Communication*, *51*, 477–497.

Brashers, D. E., Neidig, J. L., Haas, S. M., Dobbs, L. K., Cardillo, L. W., & Russell, J. A. (2000). Communication in the management of uncertainty: The case of persons living with HIV or AIDS. *Communication Monographs, 67*, 63–84.

Cameron, K. A. (2013). Advancing equity in clinical preventive services: The role of health communication. *Journal of Communication, 63*, 31–50.

Cegala, D. J. (2006). Emerging trends and future directions in patient communication skills training. *Health Communication, 20*, 123–129.

Cegala, D. J., Street, R. L., & Clinch, C. R. (2007). The Impact of patient participation on physicians' information provision during a primary care medical interview. *Health Communication, 21*, 177–185.

Chew, L. D., Bradley, K. A., & Boyko, E. J. (2004). Brief questions to identify patients with inadequate health literacy. *Family Medicine, 36*, 588–594.

Clayton, M., & Ellington, L. (2011). Beyond primary care providers: A discussion of health communication roles and challenges for health care professionals and others. In T. L. Thompson, R. Parrott & J. F. Nussbaum (Eds.), *The Routledge handbook of health communication* (2nd ed., pp. 69–83). New York: Routledge.

Cohen, E. L., Vanderpool, R. C., Crosby, R. A., Noar, S. M., Bates, W., Collins, T., ... Casey, B. (2013). 1-2-3 Pap: A campaign to prevent cervical cancer in Eastern Kentucky. In M. J. Dutta & G. L. Kreps (Eds.), *Reducing health disparities: Communication interventions* (pp. 158–177). New York: Peter Lang.

Cooper, L. A., & Powe, N. R. (2004). Disparities in patient experiences, health care processes, and outcomes: The role of patient-provider, ethnic, and language concordance. Retrieved from http://www.commonwealthfund.org/programs/minority/cooper_raceconcordance_753.pdf

Crosby, R. A., Casey, B. R., Vanderpool, R., Collins, T., & Moore, G. R. (2011). Uptake of free HPV vaccination among young women: A comparison of rural versus urban rates. *Journal of Rural Health, 27*, 380–384.

Dempsey, A., Cohn, L., Dalton, V., & Ruffin, M. (2011). Worsening disparities in HPV vaccine utilization among 19-26 year old women. *Vaccine, 29*, 528–534.

Frosch, D. L., Rincon, D., Ochoa, S., & Mangione, C. M. (2010). Activating seniors to improve chronic disease care: results from a pilot intervention study. *Journal of the American Geriatrics Society, 58*, 1496–1503.

Germino, B. B., Mishel, M. H., Crandell, J., Porter, L., Blyler, D., Jenerette, C., & Gil, K. M. (2013). Outcomes of an uncertainty management intervention in younger African American and Caucasian breast cancer survivors. *Oncology Nursing Forum, 40*, 82–92.

Gordon, H. S., Street, R. L., Sharf, B. F., & Souchek, J. (2006). Racial differences in doctors' information-giving and patients' participation. *Cancer, 107*, 1313–1320.

Gross, W., Stark, T. H., Krosnick, J., Pasek, J. Sood, G., Tompson, T., . . . Junius, D. (2012). *American's attitudes toward the Affordacle Care Act: Would better public understanding increase or decrease favoribiltiy?* Stanford, CA: Stanford University.

Harwood, A. (1981). *Ethnicity and medical care*. Cambridge, MA: Harvard University Press.

Head, K. J., & Cohen, E. L. (2012). Young women's perspectives on cervical cancer prevention in Appalachian Kentucky. *Qualitative Health Research, 22*, 476–487.

Heggland, L., Øgaard,, T., Mikkelsen, A., & Hausken, K. (2012). Patient participation in surgical treatment decision making from the patients' perspective: Validation of an instrument. *Nursing Research and Practice*, Article ID 939675, 1–8.

Ishikawa, H., & Yano, E. (2008). Patient health literacy and participation in the health-care process. *Health Expectations*, *11*, 113–122.

Levinson, W., Kao, A., Kuby, A., & Thisted, R. A. (2005). Not all patients want to participate in decision making. *Journal of General Internal Medicine*, *20*, 531–535.

Longtin, Y., Sax, H., Leape, L. L., Sheridan, S. E., Donaldson, L., & Pittet, D. (2010). Patient participation: Current knowledge and applicability to patient safety. *Mayo Clinic Proceedings*, *85*, 53–62.

Lutfey, K. E., & McKinlay, J. B. (2009). What happens along the diagnostic pathway to CHD treatment? Qualitative results concerning cognitive processes. *Sociology of Health and Illness*, *31*, 1077–1092.

Lutfey, K., E., Gerstenberger, E. L., Link, C. L., & McKinlay, J. B. (2010). Physician cognitive processing as a source of diagnostic and treatment disparities in coronary heart disease: Results of a factorial priming experiment. *Journal of Health and Social Behavior*, *51*, 16–29.

Madar, H., & Bar-Tal, Y. (2009). The experience of uncertainty among patients having peritoneal dialysis. *Journal of Advanced Nursing*, *65*, 1664–1669.

Mishel, M. H. (1981). The measurement of uncertainty in illness. *Nursing Research*, *30*, 258–263.

Mishel, M. H. (1988). Uncertainty in illness. *Journal of Nursing Scholarship*, *20*, 225–232.

National Patient Safety Foundation. (2013). *Ask Me 3.* Retreived from http://www.npsf.org/for-healthcare-professionals/programs/ask-me-3

Pappas, G., Queen, S., Hadden, W., & Fisher, G. (1993). The increasing disparity in mortality between socioeconomic groups in the United States, 1960 and 1986. *New England Journal of Medicine*, *329*, 103–109.

Parker, R. M., Baker, D. W., Williams, M. V, & Nurss, J. R. (1995). The test of functional health literacy in adults. *Journal of General Internal Medicine*, *10*, 537–541.

Peikes, D., Zutshi, A., Genevro, J., Smith, K., Parchman, M., & Meyers, D. (2012). *Early evidence on the patient-centered medical Home. Final Report.* (AHRQ Publication No. 12-0200-EF). Rockville, MD.

Pfizer. (2012). *The Newest Vital Sign: A new health literacy assessment tool for health care providers.* Retrieved from http://www.pfizerhealthliteracy.com/physicians-providers/newestvitalsign.aspx

Pfizer Clear Health Communication Initiative. (2011). *Help your patient succeed: Tips for improving communication with patients.* Retrieved from http://www.pfizerhealthliteracy.com/asset/pdf/final-why-an-ice-cream-label.pdf

Ratzan, S. C., & Parker, R. M. (2006). Health literacy—Identification and response, Editorial, *Journal of Health Communication*, *11*, 713–715.

Reichsman, A., Werner, J., Cella, P., Bobiak, S., Stange, K. C. (2009). Opportunities for improved diabetes care among patients of safety net practices: A safety net providers' strategic alliance study. *Journal of the National Medical Association*, *101*, 4–11.

Rendle, K. A., May, S. G., Uy, V., Tietbohl, C. K., Mangione, C. M., & Frosch, D. L. (2013). Persistent barriers and strategic practices: Why (asking about) the everyday matters in diabetes care. *Diabetes Education, 39*, 560–567.

Rittenhouse, D. R., & Shortell, S. M. (2009). The patient-centered medical home: Will it stand the test of health reform? *JAMA, 301*, 2038–2040.

Schapira, M. M., Fletcher, K. E., Gilligan, M., King, T. K., Laud, P. W., Matthews, B. A., . . . Hayes, E. (2008). A framework for health numeracy: How patients use quantitative skills in health care. *Journal of Health Communication, 13*, 501–517.

Sharf, B. F., & Street, R. L. (1997). The patient as a central construct: Shifting the emphasis. *Health Communication, 9*, 1–11.

Shavers, V. L., Fagan, P., Jones, D., Klein, W. M. P., Boyington, J., Moten, C., & Rorie, E. (2012). The state of research on racial/ethnic discrimination in the receipt of health care. *American Journal of Public Health, 102,* 953–966.

Smedley, B. D., Stith, A. Y., & Nelson, A. R. (2002). *Unequal treatment: Confronting racial and ethnic disparities in health care.* Institute of Medicine, National Academy Press, Washington, DC.

Street, R. L., & Millay, B. (2001). Analyzing patient participation in medical encounters. *Health Communication, 13*, 61–73.

Swain, D. (2008). Working in partnership with patients: Why do it and what benefits can be realised? *Journal of Communication in Healthcare, 1*, 155–167.

U.S. Department of Health and Human Services (USDHHS). (2012). Health literacy. Retrieved from http://www.health.gov/communication/literacy

Vanderpool, R. C., Cohen, E. L., Crosby, R. A., Jones, M. G., Bates, W., Casey, B. R., & Collins, T. (2013). "1-2-3 Pap" intervention improves HPV vaccine series completion among Appalachian women. *Journal of Communication, 63*, 95–115.

Voelker, R. (2010). Medical education meets health reform. *JAMA, 304*, 2349–2349.

Weissman, J. S., Stern, R., Fielding, S. L., & Epstein, A. M. (1991). Delayed access to health care: risk factors, reasons, and consequences. *Annals of Internal Medicine, 114*, 325–331.

Welch, L. C., Lutfey, K. E., Gerstenberger, E., & Grace, M. (2012). Gendered uncertainty and variation in physicians' decisions for coronary heart disease: The double-edged sword of 'atypical symptoms.' *Journal of Health and Social Behavior, 53*, 313–328.

Zarcadoolas, C., Pleasant, A., & Greer, D. S. (2003). Elaborating a definition of health literacy: A commentary. *Journal of Health Communication, 8*, 119–120.

Socio-cultural Factors in Health Communication

Evelyn Y. Ho

At the 2012 American Public Health Association Conference, more than 12,500 public health professionals and countless other San Franciscans were greeted with large billboards from the nonprofit California Endowment's *Health Happens Here* campaign, making very clear the issue of health disparities. Hung on the side of the building were three separate signs, each over 40 feet tall. The first had a picture of a child and the message "Zip Code 90002 Life Expectancy 73." The second featured a different child and the message "Zip Code 95651 Life Expectancy 82." The take-home message was explicitly stated on the third sign: "Your Zip Code shouldn't predict how long you'll live."

In this chapter about **socio-cultural influences** on health, I will discuss issues that contribute to and frame understandings of health and illness, such as economic class, educational background, race, ethnicity, gender, sex, sexuality, and access. Unfortunately, as the Zip Code campaign demonstrates, we all have very different chances at healthy living, and disparities are a real part of healthcare throughout the world. The scientific, interpretive, and critical–cultural paradigms each approach socio-cultural influences differently. We will examine how each paradigm understands and interrogates culture and explore through exemplar cases how health communication scholars study Chinese medicine. This is a relatively young area of the field, providing numerous opportunities for future research.

HEALTH DISPARITIES

Almost all research about social and cultural influences on health confirms that stark inequalities exist related to race, ethnicity, income, education level, sex/gender, and a variety of other social factors often working in combination. Perhaps the most sobering news is that racial and ethnic minorities, especially African Americans, receive lower quality healthcare even after controlling for insurance, income, age, and co-morbid conditions (Smedley, Stith, & Nelson, 2003). For example, the Centers for Disease Control and Prevention's

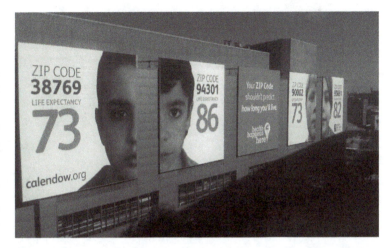

Figure 8.1 Poster Display from the *Health Happens Here* Campaign.

(CDC, 2011) Health Disparities and Inequalities Report (CHDIR) found the following:

- Those with lower socioeconomic circumstances have higher mortality and morbidity and less access to care and lower quality of care.
- The infant mortality rate for Black women is 2.4 times worse than for White women.
- Tobacco use is the leading cause of preventable death, and smoking rates decline with increased income and education.

There are numerous other statistics that speak to **health disparities** both in disease prevalence (also called morbidity) and in treatment disparities. For example, African Americans account for 44% of all new HIV infections among adolescents and adults, despite being only 12–14% of the U.S. population (CDC, 2012), and in their lifetimes an estimated 1 in 32 Black women will be diagnosed with HIV, whereas 1 in 106 Hispanic/Latina women and 1 in 526 White women will be so diagnosed (CDC, 2013). Blacks and Hispanics are less likely to receive the same medications as Whites; Native Americans have four times the rate of end-stage renal disease than Whites; and along with African Americans, Native Americans are less likely to receive kidney transplants or even to be put on the waiting list for a transplant (Geiger, 2002).

Racial or ethnic disparities in healthcare are defined as "differences in the quality of healthcare that are not due to access-related factors or clinic needs, preferences, and

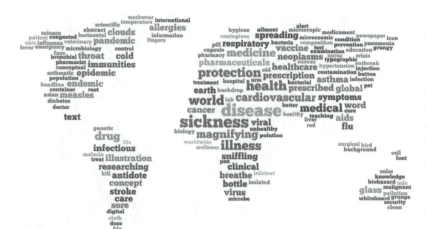

appropriateness of intervention" (Smedley et al., 2003, pp. 3–4). These disparities are caused by individual-level discrimination and bias and systems-level healthcare factors such as language barriers, time pressures, and geographic availability of care. According to the 2010 U.S. Census figures and projections, nearly 37% of Americans are racial/ethnic minorities and Whites will become the minority by 2043 (U.S. Census Bureau, 2012).

The problem, however, is not just a U.S. one. In fact, health disparities are perhaps even greater when comparing health between countries. Medical anthropologist, physician, and founder of the international nonprofit Partners in Health, Paul

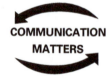

COMMUNICATION MATTERS

UN Universal Declaration of Human Rights

The United Nations Universal Declaration of Human Rights was passed in 1948 following the atrocities of World War II. According to Paul Farmer (2003), this document opened the door to the possibility for not just considering health as a human right but for also for advancing this as a cause for which to strive.

> Article 25.1: Everyone has the right to a standard of living adequate for the health and well-being of himself and of his family, including food, clothing, housing and medical care and necessary social services, and the right to security in the event of unemployment, sickness, disability, widowhood, old age or other lack of livelihood in circumstances beyond his control.

> Article 27.1: Everyone has the right freely to participate in the cultural life of the community, to enjoy the arts and to share in scientific advancement and its benefits.

To see the entire declaration, visit www.un.org/en/documents/udhr/. What would the world (health policy, laws, hospitals, everyday experience) look like if these rights were guaranteed for all?

Farmer, cites the **U.N. Universal Declaration of Human Rights** to make the argument that

> Public health and access to medical care are social and economic rights; they are at least as critical as civil rights. An irony of this global era is that while public health has increasingly sacrificed equity for efficiency, the poor have become well-informed enough to reject separate standards of care.
>
> (Farmer, 2003, pp. 217–218)

The issues that Farmer raises are not just about equity in healthcare but also about how ensuring that equity can itself be a first step in ensuring other human rights.

Communication is understood to play a critical role in reducing health disparities, and the importance of culturally competent care is widely accepted (Betancourt, Green, Carrillo, & Ananeh-Firempong, 2003). While many of the structural level issues in healthcare (such as access to care or insurance) may not easily be solved by communication, there are many areas where communication is essential. In 2013, the *Journal of Communication* dedicated a special issue to communication strategies to reduce health disparities (Harrington, 2013) and in 2006, *American Behavioral Scientist* dedicated a special issue to communication and health care disparities (Perloff, 2006). In the introduction, Perloff explained,

> Yet because communication is malleable, operates on multiple levels of analysis, and fundamentally involves the coordination of meaning, it is a uniquely important focal point for change. Unlike external factors in the environment that cannot be easily altered, communication can be modified, even improved. (p. 757)

In health promotion research, communication messages that attend to the culture-specific needs of a community have been found to increase the effectiveness of those health messages (Dutta, 2007). Similarly, in provider–patient interaction, one important way to ensure culturally competent care is through promoting patient-centered communication (Epner & Baile, 2012). I will discuss these issues more in later sections.

POLICY AND INSTITUTIONAL HISTORY

The **Office of Research on Minority Health (ORMH)** was created in 1990, elevated to a Center in 2000, re-designated an Institute in 2010 (through the Patient Protection Affordable Care Act of 2010—commonly known as *Obamacare*), and is now one of 27 institutes and centers at the **National Institutes of Health (NIH)**. During that same period, the **Department of Health and Human Services (USDHHS)** issued its first ever *Healthy People 2000: National Health Promotion and Disease Prevention Objectives* to set benchmarks and goals for improving the nation's health for the following decade. The report has been repeated every 10 years, and since the very first **Healthy People** publication, an overarching goal has focused on disparities. In 2010, one of two overarching goals was to "eliminate racial and ethnic disparities in health," and for Healthy People 2020 (HP 2020), the goal is to "achieve health equity, eliminate disparities, and improve the health of all groups" (USDHHS, 2010).

Healthy People is used by policy makers, public health officials, health educators and providers, and individuals to guide decision making around health issues, to provide measurable goals and standards, and to raise awareness of determinants of health. HP 2020 uses a **determinants of health** approach, which recognizes that health is affected by a variety of factors, including individual behavior, biology and genetics, access to health services, social interactions and norms, and physical environment (USDHHS, 2012). Such an approach explicitly recognizes that work in health promotion cannot be solely individual-focused in order to succeed.

It is important to note that people have long known about social and cultural influences on health. For example, George Engel (1977) introduced the concept of bio-psychosocial health as a critique of merely recognizing physical health. It has not been until recent times, however, that this conceptualization of health has been at the forefront of health policy.

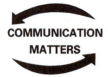

COMMUNICATION MATTERS

National and International Health Agencies

There are numerous U.S. national and international governmental health agencies studying the social and cultural determinants of health and working to reduce health disparities.

- Centers for Disease Control and Prevention's Office of Minority Health & Health Equity (OMHHE) http://www.cdc.gov/minorityhealth/OMHHE.html
- National Institute on Minority Health and Health Disparities http://www.nimhd.nih.gov
- World Health Organization (WHO) http://www.who.int/social_determinants/en

CULTURE AS A VARIABLE: THE SCIENTIFIC PARADIGM

Studies that focus on culture in the area of health communication can be divided into two types. First, culture is treated as a predictive *variable* and is sometimes used synonymously with race or ethnicity. People are categorized based on a variety of cultural variables that impact health and illness. The **culture as variable** approach has been critiqued for neglecting heterogeneity among cultural groups and focusing too much on static (meaning unchanging) cultural variables such as individualism versus collectivism or uncertainty avoidance (Dutta, 2007). Not surprisingly, the bulk of health and medical research could be categorized as scientific with the goal of determining which variables affect the most change resulting in more positive health outcomes. In other words, the goal of research/practice is to create health messages to meet the cultural values, beliefs, and norms (the cultural variables) of a target population, and most health message research falls into this category.

Methodologically, this research is typically quantitative and sometimes experimental. If the goal is to determine what cultural variables are correlated with what positive or negative health outcomes, it makes sense that quantitative methods would be most suitable for this kind of research. The following sections will present important concepts typically studied from a scientific paradigm. However, it is worth noting that these concepts do not have to be studied this way, and the sections on interpretive and critical research will address some of these issues as well.

Cultural Competency

Cultural competency has been defined as "a set of congruent behaviors, attitudes, and policies that come together in a system, agency, or among professionals that enables effective work in cross-cultural situations" (OMH, 2005). Cultural competency requires work on the organizational, structural, and clinical levels, and unfortunately barriers often exist at each of these levels (Betancourt et al., 2003). For example, a lack of racial/ethnic minority healthcare workers (organizational), a lack of interpreter services (structural), or poor provider attitudes (clinical) can all be barriers to culturally competent care.

In 2001, the U.S. Department of Health and Human Services (USDHHS) and the Office of Minority Health (OMH) introduced national standards for **culturally and linguistically appropriate services** or **CLAS** (USDHHS & OMH, 2001). The standard establishes a total of 14 mandates, guidelines, and recommendations in the areas of culturally competent care, language access services, and organizational supports for cultural competence. The four required mandates are in the area of language access services and

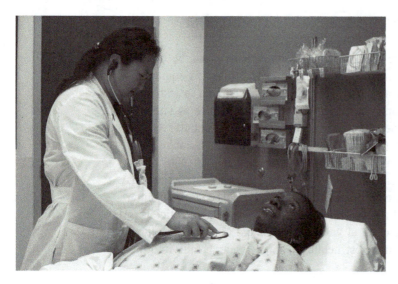

include provisions that patients must be provided with competent interpreters (or language services) free of charge during all hours of operation and that this service and all signs be advertised in the languages of commonly encountered groups in the area. The recommendations and guidelines are set for promoting culturally competent care and organizational supports including items like the following: Healthcare organizations should (a) recruit and retain diverse staff and leadership, (b) provide respectful care compatible with cultural health beliefs, (c) develop strategic plans around CLAS, and (d) develop participatory, collaborative community partnerships. CLAS is especially important given research that demonstrates that language barriers and language discrimination may be a greater detriment to people's health than just their race/ethnicity (Sentell & Braun, 2012).

The term cultural competency can imply that there is a point at which people become *competent*. But when would this realistically occur? As some scholars have argued, perhaps cultural competency is better described as a process (and ongoing practice) rather than an endpoint (Perloff, Bonder, Ray, Ray, & Siminoff, 2006). Theoretically, increased cultural competency should relate to more positive outcomes for providers and patients, but the research is mixed. Cultural competence training and racial and ethnic **concordance** have been correlated with patient satisfaction and health promotion, and education programs that use culturally sensitive practices and appropriate language practices (such as using translations and interpreters) are associated with increased patient knowledge, program completion, and participation (Fortier & Bishop, 2003). However, in a review of patient-centered care models incorporating cultural competency, while practitioners increased their cultural sensitivity and patients were more satisfied, patient health outcomes did not improve (Renzaho, Romios, Crock, & Sønderlund, 2013). In other words, while providers and patients may be happier with culturally competent care, it may not make a difference to the health disparities already discussed.

One institution that is poised to make a difference is the Center for Advancing Equity in Clinical Preventive Services at Northwestern University's Feinberg

School of Medicine. One of only three Centers of Excellence funded by the **Agency for Healthcare Research and Quality (AHRQ)**, the Center has developed a variety of multimedia patient education and outreach programs for ethnic minorities (Cameron, 2013). For example, to promote breast cancer screening among Latinas, researchers conducted focus group interviews to learn about barriers to breast cancer screening. They then created Spanish and English videos addressing those barriers, resulting in increased knowledge and more positive attitudes after the intervention.

Race and Ethnicity

When discussing culture and health communication, what often emerges is research about communicating with racial and ethnic minorities. While culture is often associated with race and ethnicity, the three concepts are not identical (Ford & Harawa, 2010), and oftentimes people of the same racial and ethnic groups have vastly different cultural experiences of health. I will discuss this in further detail in future sections. Although ethnic minorities are certainly not the only ones with cultural beliefs that affect healthcare, many racial and ethnic minorities face differences in healthcare because of their experience and because of their race/ethnicity.

Studying the shared cultural variables of particular ethnic groups can be helpful in establishing clinically practical suggestions for culturally sensitive health communication. However, this is an area where researchers may disagree because when variables are generated in order to create a prescribed list of do's and don'ts for how to communicate with ethnic minorities, this practice can marginalize or *other* ethnic minority groups (Johnson et al., 2004). **Othering** occurs when a dominant group and its characteristics, beliefs, and practices are considered the norm or standard by which any differences from that standard are marked as deficient. Regarding ethnic minorities, othering can occur in two important and related ways. First, ethnic minority groups can be othered through standardizing dominant White cultural beliefs and practices as the unquestioned norm. Second, an overreliance on defining cultural variables associated with particular ethnic minority groups can create a **deficit model of cultural differences**: "From this viewpoint, patients' problems with access, communication, and compliance are seen as occurring because customs and traditions conflict with mainstream medical practices" (Johnson et al., 2004, p. 255).

Johnson et al. (2004) call this process *culturalism*, or the tendency to treat problems as a matter of cultural differences. To avoid this deficit model and overly stereotyping patients, researchers have addressed cultural competency through improvements in overall communication skills rather than address communication skills only when working with ethnic minorities. Some authors have called this patient-centered care and drawn attention to how patient-centeredness can lead to cultural competency

(Epner & Baile, 2012). Therefore, skills such as focusing on understanding a patient's style of communication, finding out the role of family, and recognizing the impact of social and economic factors are important in all health encounters (Betancourt et al., 2003) and can minimize the othering of ethnic minority groups.

Ethnicity is often difficult to define without overgeneralizing. Ford and Harawa (2010) propose that ethnicity comprises two dimensions: "The attributional dimension describes the unique sociocultural characteristics (e.g., culture, diet) of groups while the relational dimension captures characteristics of the relationship between an ethnically defined group and the society in which it is situated" (p. 252). While a vast majority of research regarding health communication and culture, especially from a scientific paradigm, has examined the attributional dimension, people are not just grouped together based on their cultural similarities, beliefs, or practices. In fact, one similarity among ethnic minorities is shared experiences of racism and discrimination in healthcare (Johnson et al., 2004).

Recognizing how particular ethnic groups are situated in society and how that may affect particular individuals requires context-specific examinations of ethnicity. One way to recognize what aspects of ethnicity are important and relevant to actual people is to include the people themselves in various stages of the research process (Dutta, 2007). I will present these alternatives in further detail in the following sections about culture as context.

Finally, it is worth mentioning that when discussing race and ethnicity in healthcare, many scholars have been calling for increased attention to the heterogeneity among groups and for disaggregating data sets that may gloss over such differences. This can be illustrated through two examples. First, in an article about the history of diabetes, Tuchman (2011) argues that current findings that diabetes disproportionately affects Native Americans, Hispanics/Latinos, and Blacks make invisible the fact that in parts of Appalachia, Whites have higher rates of diabetes than Latinos/Hispanics. In other words, overemphasis on race obscures class-based disparities.

A second example looks at "Asian American/Native Hawaiian/Pacific Islander" populations (or AAPI for Asian American Pacific Islander). The 2000 U.S. Census was the first to separate Native Hawaiians and Pacific Islanders from Asian Americans (Stafford, 2010). While some Asian American groups score relatively high on various health indicators, the relatively small number of Native Hawaiian and other Pacific Islanders means those disparities in socioeconomic status (SES), morbidity, and mortality get lost in aggregated data. Not only does aggregated data make invisible these health disparities but also high profile Pacific Islander athletes give a false image that all Pacific Islanders are ready to burst onto the football field in good health

(Stafford, 2010), when in reality obesity and diabetes disproportionately affect this group (Tuchman, 2011).

Takeuchi and Gage (2003) explain that in the 1980s and 1990s health researchers' attention to race waned in favor of examining SES variables instead. This happened, they explain, for four reasons. First, because some still treated race as a biological phenomenon, many social scientists were uncomfortable with the idea that racial disparities would then require biological explanations. Second, social scientists worried that race-based explanations would lead to victim blaming. Third, Asians and Latinos did not fit neatly in the Black/White dichotomy. And finally, policy makers saw benefits to poor people as holding more political appeal than racial justice. It wasn't until the 2000s that attention was brought back to race and issues of racism. The next section will discuss the ties between racism, discrimination, and health.

Racism, Discrimination, and Health

There are two important and related concepts to explain the deleterious physical and psychological effects of everyday discrimination. From public health is the concept of *weathering*, and originally from education and counseling psychology but now used in many disciplines is the concept of *microaggressions*.

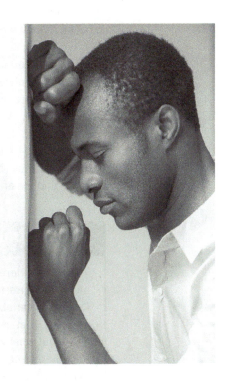

Weathering. A public health study in 1990 found that Blacks living in Harlem had worse death rates than those living in Bangladesh (McCord & Freeman, 1990). This discrepancy could partially be explained by SES differences, but another explanation became known as *weathering*. **Weathering** is defined as the cumulative effect of social, economic, and political exclusion and the physical burden of attempting to deal with these exclusions over time (Keene & Geronimus, 2011). Research on weathering has argued that while racism and race-based structural inequalities might typically be thought of as merely a social problem, these experiences of discrimination actually have deleterious *physical* effects (Geronimus, Hicken, Keene, & Bound, 2006).

In a study of allostatic loads (a measure of long-term physiological burden of stress), Blacks (in all income levels) were equivalent to Whites who were 10 years older (Geronimus et al., 2006). In other words, a typical 60-year-old Black man in the study had the physicality of a typical 70-year-old White man. In fact, non-poor Blacks had worse numbers than poor Whites, and Black women had the strongest disparities, leading the authors to conclude that race and sex, and not just income-level, have a pervasive impact on health. A similar study demonstrated that homicide deaths among Black men and preventable chronic diseases have increased so dramatically that young Black males living in urban neighborhoods had only a 50–62% chance of reaching age 65 compared to those living in rural areas (62–67%) and to Whites overall (80%; Geronimus, Bound, & Colen, 2011).

Microaggressions. Similar to the weathering hypothesis, microaggressions can accumulate over time. **Microaggressions** are "The brief and commonplace daily verbal, behavioral, and environmental indignities, whether intentional or unintentional, that communicate hostile, derogatory, or negative racial, gender, sexual-orientation, and religious slights and insults to the target person or group" (Sue et al., 2007, p. 271).

Microaggresive insults may seem harmless. For example, telling a Latino person "your English is so good" may seem like a compliment, but it implies that you did not expect that they would speak English very well, if at all.

Research has found important correlations between increased exposure to microaggressions and deleterious health. For example, microaggression frequency is correlated with more depressive and somatic symptoms in Latino and Asian American youth (Huynh, 2012). African American graduate students showed psychological distress that was correlated with underestimation of personal ability (Torres, Driscoll, & Burrow, 2010). LGBTQ people in therapeutic relationships report both overt and covert microaggressions (Nadal et al., 2011) that negatively affect the relationship with their therapist and the effectiveness of therapy (Shelton & Delgado-Romero, 2011).

CULTURE AS VARIABLE VS. CULTURE AS CONTEXT

The main differences between these two approaches to culture are what they believe culture to consist of and how culture is supposed to relate to health. Culture as variable says that culture is a fixed entity, such as race or ethnic identity label, that can help predict health outcomes. The goal of this research is to figure out what variables to change to make certain cultural groups healthier. On the other hand, culture as context believes that culture is created and sustained in interaction and is the meanings, understandings, and ways of speaking used by people. The goal of this research is to understand what people mean by health or illness and how those understandings figure into their overall lives.

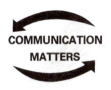

Web Resources Regarding Microaggressions

There are a variety of microaggression compilations on the Internet demonstrating the pervasiveness of microaggressions and reminding readers of how these seemingly small messages can add up to systematic consequences. These also function as public spaces to talk about people's experiences of microaggressions. Here are two websites you can visit to learn more:

http://www.microaggressions.com
http://microaggressions.tumblr.com

Also, researchers Derald Wing Sue and David P. Rivera write this blog about microaggressions:

http://www.psychologytoday.com/blog/microaggressions-in-everyday-life

CULTURE AS CONTEXT: INTERPRETIVE AND CRITICAL PARADIGMS

Despite many advances in healthcare and medicine and a recognition of the importance of culture, some scholars have argued that perhaps traditional scientific approaches to the study of health and culture are problematic because not everyone views illness universally (Kleinman, Eisenberg, & Good, 1978). In this vein, culture has also been understood as a *context* for understanding a person's health experience (Dutta, 2007). This approach to health and culture tends to focus on meanings and understandings and recognizes that culture can only be understood in conversations with the actual people involved. Generally qualitative and either interpretive or critical, this research is by definition more specific to particular contexts and has been less generalizable.

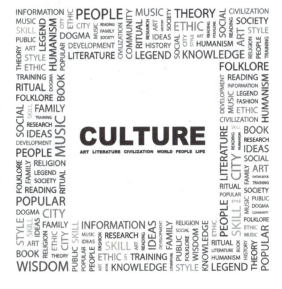

While newer in the field of health communication, the **culture as context** approach draws from related research in the cultural study of communication, medical anthropology, and medical sociology. As Zoller and Kline (2008) explain, much of the interpretive and critical push in health communication came from scholars and theorists outside of the field such as Michel Foucault,

Susan Sontag, Deborah Lupton, and others. The interpretive and critical models in health communication have been important in breaking down biased theories of culture that tend to homogenize and overgeneralize and focus solely on medicalized definitions of effectiveness. While the interpretive and critical approaches share similar goals of the scientific perspective to reduce health disparities and increase health and well-being, research in these areas takes a step back to first determine what health or illness even means from culture to culture.

Interpretive Paradigm

The interpretive approach to the study of socio-cultural influences on health communication builds out of medical anthropology, medical sociology, and social construction approaches in health communication. As Sharf and Vanderford (2003) explain, health communication should, "unpack the sociocultural sources of symbolic usage in health care" (p. 12). Rather than view health as merely having a physical component, interpretive studies recognize that people interpret and make meaning of bodily, physical, and psychological states often in very culturally specific ways. These explanations of illness, also called **explanatory models**, not only are important for diagnosis but also affect how people understand what is happening to them, how they approach treatment, and how others around them (and society) understand their health and illness identity (Kleinman et al., 1978). Methodologically, ethnography is useful for studying explanatory models. Ethnographic (participant-observation) research is typically done on a long-term basis, and researchers can study illness and health as part of a person's overall life experience and not just in a medical environment. Because the interpretive approach is interested in learning about meaning and understanding, the qualitative methodologies such as phenomenology, discourse analysis, and narrative analysis fit well.

Explanatory models can be seen clearly in examining cross-cultural understandings of health and illness, exploring illnesses that are sometimes called **culture-bound illnesses** or **folk illnesses**. Note that in naming illnesses in this way, researchers imply that scientifically understood illnesses like hypertension are not culture-bound, but rather, universally understood. An example of a folk illness is *susto* (or fright), in which a person's spirit may become detached from her body after a frightening experience resulting in a listlessness, restlessness, and indifference to food and hygiene (Rubel, 1984). Typically associated with Mexico, it also is found in a variety of people in North and South America, the Philippines, India, China, and Taiwan. While some may believe that *susto* is just stress, depression, or even PTSD under a different name, others argue that paying close attention to the cultural tenants of *susto* demonstrates how different it is from anything found in biomedicine.

Two important types of explanatory models are **disease** and **illness**. These words are often used interchangeably, but scholars make the distinction between the professional medical diagnosis and description of a disorder—*disease*—and the experience, perception, and meaning of those symptoms—*illness* (Kleinman et al., 1978). Illnesses, because they are everyday people's experiences, can often begin long before a formal disease designation is made.

An example to illustrate the distinction can be seen in the recent discussions around the American Psychiatric Association's (APA) update of the Diagnostic and Statistical Manual of Mental Disorders (DSM-5). The proposal of a new category, autism spectrum disorder (ASD), should better distinguish ASD from language disorders, attention deficit

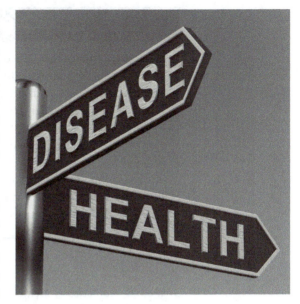

hyperactivity disorder, and others (Huerta, Bishop, Duncan, Hus, & Lord, 2012). In a study testing the proposed DSM-5 criteria versus the current DSM-IV, only nine percent of children studied who have DSM-IV pervasive developmental disorders would be identified as having ASD using the DSM-5 criteria (Huerta et al., 2012). An explanation of this is that diagnostic specificity has improved, and from a *disease*

perspective, it is important to determine exactly who has what disease. From an *illness* perspective, however, a mother may still notice a child's "unusual sensory behaviors" or "repetitive behaviors," but they may not be acknowledged symptoms of a disease. A diagnosis of ASD carries with it not only the potential for stigma or shame but also the potential to secure health treatments and assistance only open to those with a medical diagnosis.

A major distinction between disease and illness is the medical professional framing versus a lay or everyday person's experience. While some have named this distinction **medical health beliefs** versus **lay health beliefs** (Lupton, 2003), others have used the terms **voice of medicine (VOM)** versus the **voice of the lifeworld** (VOL; Mishler, 1984). In the now famous text, *The Discourse of*

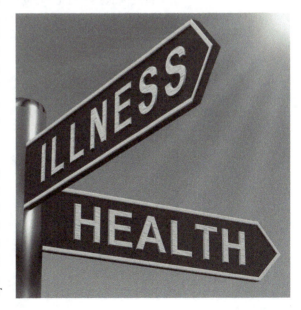

DISEASE VS. ILLNESS

What is the difference between a disease and an illness? Disease focuses on the medicalized understanding, whereas illness is a person's experience of a being sick. Why is this distinction important to make if the goal is to get people healthier? A good example to illustrate the distinction is Chronic Fatigue Syndrome. A person might experience an illness of debilitating fatigue. However, doctors and medical science can't really explain what it is, what causes it, or how to cure it. Before this name was given to this illness experience, patients were just told that it was all in their head or that it couldn't be that bad. Because it was not a recognized disease, healthcare providers had no guidance on how to address this and many people got little help.

Medicine: Dialectics of Medical Interviewing, social psychologist Elliot Mishler uses conversation analysis to understand provider–patient interaction. By audio-recording actual physician–patient interviews, Mishler was able to transcribe the interviews using a special transcription system that acknowledges the way people actually talk, including false starts, overlaps, ungrammatical phrasing, etc.

In the analysis, Mishler introduced the idea of voices to "specify relationships between talk and speakers' underlying frameworks of meaning" (p. 14), with the VOM focused on the technical-scientific assumptions of medicine and the VOL focused on the natural attitude of everyday life. Patients and providers can move from the VOM to

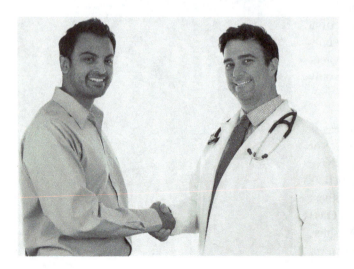

the VOL at various moments during a medical encounter, and patients and providers may oftentimes vie for positioning one voice over the other. Structurally, however, the way typical provider meetings are set up, the flow of questions between physicians and patients has a tendency to bring conversations back to the VOM (Mishler, 1984). In fact, some have argued that the culture of medicine and the medical gaze systematically ignore important patient experiences leading to health disparities (Good, Good, & Becker, 2002). For example, one could argue that the entire purpose of the medical interview is to transform and translate patient narratives from the VOL into the VOM; doctors can do this by addressing only the medically useful parts and ignoring those parts of the VOL (including cultural health beliefs) that are less medically relevant. Mishler's argument is that doctors who can move into the VOL will have more humane interactions. However, some scholars question this assumption of humanity. One study found that it was the *match* in voices that was more important than the use of the VOL (Barry, Stevenson, Britten, Barber, & Bradley, 2001). Conversations had better outcomes when the doctor and patient remained in either the VOM or the VOL than when patients attempted to speak in the VOL and were either ignored or moved back to VOM by the doctor.

Critical Paradigm

One of the earliest critical pieces in health communication came from Deborah Lupton (1994), a medical sociologist, calling for more critical work. In the neighboring disciplines of medical anthropology and sociology, scholars in the 1990s began studying the culture, taken-for-grantedness, and the power of biomedicine itself (e.g. Rhodes, 1996). Beginning perhaps a decade later, the critical approach to health communication has emerged (Zoller & Kline, 2008).

One popularly used critical approach to the study of health and culture from health communication is the **culture-centered approach (CCA)** created by Mohan Dutta (Dutta, 2007). CCA emerges out of other critical approaches used in health promotion research such as the **PEN-3 model**, which was designed because the health promotion ideas from "the West" were not working in non-Western countries (Airhihenbuwa, 1995). The PEN-3 model acknowledges three dimensions of health belief and behavior that are interrelated: health education, educational diagnosis of health behavior, and cultural appropriateness of health behavior. Within each of these dimensions are three P-E-N categories (e.g., person, extended family, and neighborhood are part of the health education dimension).

One difference in how PEN-3 is used as opposed to some of the more scientific models of health promotion is in how a researcher approaches the participants/people. For example, the model was used in 1990 at the African Regional Child Survival Workshop in Nigeria (see Airhihenbuwa, 1995). To begin, stakeholders and people from the various countries and organizations involved participated in workshops to generate lists of health beliefs and interview questions to be taken back to the community to determine whom the intervention (health education) should address (educational diagnosis of health behavior). A second workshop was held with the trainers of village health workers to further refine the lists of health beliefs into positive, existential, and negative (cultural appropriateness). Finally, local village health workers participated in a workshop to determine which of the beliefs were deeply rooted in culture and which were more superficial. Not surprisingly, these findings differed in each local community.

Moving beyond just health promotion, the CCA also takes seriously the participation and health beliefs of local populations. However, it differs from the cultural sensitivity approaches of the scientific paradigm in that it does not focus on tailoring messages to change individual beliefs and behavior. Rather, it focuses on changing social structures through dialogue with marginalized voices (Dutta, 2007). Similar to interpretive research, CCA recognizes that science does not necessarily have the correct answer to health understandings. Differentiating itself, critical research recognizes that health decisions are made within a social structure in which some understandings are privileged more than others (leading to some voices being marginalized), some resources are more available than others, and health practices are unequally distributed, which leads to unequal health decision making and outcomes. As Dutta and Basu (2011) explain, the CCA's focus is on social change, whereas interpretive ethnographic approaches have the goal of cultural status quo. For example, in a study of rural West Bengal, Dutta (2012) concludes that health, for rural Bengalis, is about food, and the pain of hunger and irregular access to enough food defines their experiences of health. Contrast this hunger with not only plentiful food for middle-class Bengalis (of which Dutta claims membership) but also the diseases of excess such as obesity, diabetes, and heart disease, and the result is what some call structural violence (Farmer, 1999).

Key to this work is **Community-Based Participatory Research (CBPR**; Minkler & Wallerstein, 2003) or **Participatory Action Research (PAR)**. Also used in interpretive research, these approaches are based on working and serving *with* partners in communities. Instead of academic researchers or policy makers determining what is best or most relevant for a given community, community members work together to determine the agenda and purpose for research. For example, researchers used partici-

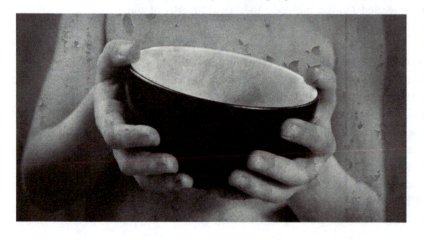

patory research methods in developing a prenatal education class for Latina mothers-to-be that included not just the pregnant women but also community health workers and researchers (Auger, DeCoster, & Colindres, 2008).

CBPR work, although theoretically democratizing and necessarily applied and practical, can also carry with it various paradoxes and dialectics (McDermott, Oetzel, & White, 2008). For example, although the research should be community driven, oftentimes the original project idea comes from a researcher who often brings the funding, which then brings its own constraints. Other tensions exist along the lines of who gets to participate (and who chooses), how to deal with conflicting goals, and how long a project will last.

EXEMPLAR STUDIES OF CHINESE MEDICINE
WHAT IS CULTURAL HERE?

To better understand the complexity of socio-cultural influences on health, this next section will review exemplar studies from a variety of perspectives and paradigms about Chinese medicine. I present these studies to draw connections between the topics already presented. At this point, you might be thinking, "What do you mean by Chinese medicine?" Is it that the medicine is Chinese—as in acupuncture or Tai Qi? Or is it the people using the medicine who are Chinese—as in ethnically Chinese? Does it matter if the person using acupuncture is also Chinese? These questions are inherently both cultural and communicative.

Chinese (American) Patients

Wang, Schwartz, Luta, Maxwell, and Mandelblatt (2012) were concerned with health literacy among Chinese Americans. According to U.S. Census figures, Asian Americans are the fastest growing racial group and Chinese Americans (CAs) are the largest Asian ethnic group (U.S. Census Bureau News, 2012). The 2007 California Health Interview Survey found that 27.4% of the Chinese Americans surveyed reported **low English proficiency (LEP)**, and of those, 68.3% also had low health literacy (Sentell & Braun, 2012). In their study, Wang and colleagues designed two different health education videos to promote mammograms in Chinese American women who did not currently follow mammogram guidelines. The purpose was to test the effectiveness of a culturally targeted video versus a generic video about mammography screening. This purpose falls within the scientific paradigm with a goal to predict and control behavior.

The study used a CBPR framework in which Chinese American women were interviewed in focus groups to determine their preferences for this kind of educational video. From these interviews, the researchers determined that a soap opera style story and a recommendation from a female physician would be most acceptable. To create a culturally targeted video, a Chinese breast cancer survivor drafted the script and worked with the research team to finalize the video. In this way, the study also drew from interpretive and critical paradigms involving patients and taking community voices seriously in the design of the study. The culturally targeted video used Chinese actors who discussed culturally based Chinese beliefs such as fatalism toward cancer and yin-yang balance. The actors also demonstrated hesitancy toward Western examinations and the importance of social and family support. The video setting was a birthday party of a breast cancer survivor with people speaking Chinese, eating Chinese foods, and listening to Chinese music. In contrast, the generic video used a multi-ethnic cast speaking English during a lunch. The only Chinese actress (playing a restaurant owner) joins a lunchtime conversation about breast cancer and expresses having no time or insurance to get a mammogram. The generic video was dubbed into Chinese and was thus linguistically appropriate. In both videos a female physician gives mammogram recommendations.

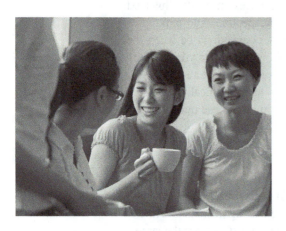

To test the effect of the videos, participants were randomized into the culturally targeted video group, the generic/linguistically appropriate video group, or a control group who read a handout about mammograms. Participants filled out surveys with scales measuring their knowledge, Eastern cultural views of health (including fatalism and self-care preferences), health beliefs (perceived susceptibility, severity, benefit and barriers), screening intention, socio-demographics (such as age, education, time in U.S., insurance status, etc.), and English proficiency. Using quantitative bivariate analysis, the researchers found that both video groups increased knowledge and intention to get a mammogram. However, unexpectedly, for women age 50–64 the generic video led to greater intention to get a mammogram and changed their cultural views more than the cultural video. While the authors acknowledged that these results were surprising, they concluded that perhaps the generic video's acknowledgment of and solutions to barriers resonated with this particular group.

There are some real strengths and weaknesses in this study. For one, the study is itself an intervention and therefore applied in the real world with real women who may get mammography screening when they previously would not. Second, the study demonstrably shows that a health communication intervention leads to changes in knowledge, attitude, and beliefs—a hallmark set of criteria for measuring change. Third, the study took seriously the input of Chinese American women themselves. However, theoretically and methodologically, some researchers would find fault with the notions of culture being measured in this study. For example, because health studies need quick measures of culture, scales such as the Chinese Cultural Views of Healthcare scale are developed. This includes a nine-item scale measuring fatalism and a four-item scale measuring self-care. Similarly, the health belief scale measures those variables important to the health belief model. These scales leave out much of the nuance to cultural health beliefs that other methods may be better able to discern. For example, an analysis of the script of the video shows that the cultural video does not seem to discuss Chinese medicine or food/health beliefs stemming from Chinese medicine such as balance, yin-yang, qi, hot-cold, etc. This is probably a significant omission.

Chinese (American) Medicine

As the previous study demonstrates, what is Chinese about health beliefs and treatment is not always clear. Does Chinese mean a preference for family support? Chinese language? Seeing a Chinese actor? In the next two exemplar studies, I will examine exactly what is meant by Chinese medicine because it does not always mean it is also ethnically Chinese. Indeed, scholars have written about the Americanization of Chinese medicine in the United States (e.g., Hare, 1993).

In the first study, Ho and Bylund (2008) used the case of an acupuncture clinic to examine the difference between health models and health delivery. First, the authors differentiate between the **biomedical model**, which is widely used in medicine; the **biopsychosocial model**, which takes into account a person's illness experience as a part of their larger emotional, cognitive, and social life; and the **holistic model**, which is not unique to Chinese medicine but understands health and illness as a balance of the whole person—body, mind, and spirit. What we typically think of as Western medicine can fit within any of the three models. On the other hand, acupuncture, if it is a part of Chinese medicine, is normally considered holistic. These medical models are separate from models of provider–patient interaction or health delivery. Here the main models are the paternalistic (doctor knows best), the collaborative or partnership model (mutual negotiation), and the consumerist model (patient shopping for services).

After reviewing the models, Ho and Bylund (2008) then presented numerous examples of the acupuncture clinic using a holistic model of health and a variety of different models of health interaction. They used data collected from ethnographic participant observation and from audio-recordings of naturally occurring talk in the acupuncture clinic to tease out, from an interpretive paradigm, exactly how acupuncturists make claims about the appropriate way to approach health and interaction. While all of the acupuncturists presented acupuncture as a holistic medicine that took into account a whole person to heal, the practitioners differed on whether holism also meant that acupuncturists were more collaborative in their interactions.

In one example, a client, Carol, told the acupuncturist, Jean, that she is her favorite because Jean always hits the points correctly and she helps Carol understand what's going on in her body from a Chinese medicine perspective. When Jean responds, she

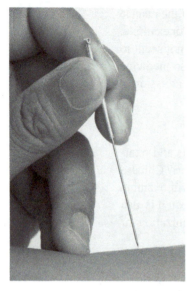

only focuses on the fact that she hits "that spot" instead of the other aspects of what could be seen as a more collaborative relationship. Later in the same conversation, Carol says that she feels she is "in harmony" with Jean. Jean responds by saying "don't want to cut down on our treatment time" and then moves on to Carol's headache. Ho and Bylund conclude that in these (and other) examples, while clients may think a holistic health model equates with a more collaborative provider–patient interaction model, there are many instances in which what is holistic about Chinese medicine is its approach to medicine, not its provider–patient relationship model. This is a wonderful case study of a single acupuncture clinic. However, as with many interpretive studies, we do not know if these findings are idiosyncratic or if such findings are more generalizable. To determine exactly how other patients engage with Chinese medicine requires much more study.

The final study comes from a critical, culture-centered approach to Chinese medicine. Ho and Robles (2011) also used a community-based participatory research model in their intervention study of HIV-related neuropathy. In this case, the intervention was to use acupuncture and massage therapy to treat a painful and sometimes debilitating side effect of HIV medication. The communication component here comes in the form of eliciting health narratives and talk about treatment decision making. The authors conducted focus group and individual interviews at the beginning and end of the series of 10 treatment sessions to find out about patients' treatment experiences. The study used a culture-centered approach to elicit the marginalized voices of those with HIV-related neuropathy and their preferences for non-drug treatments.

Participants reported not only that the treatments offered them temporary relief but also that the clinic itself and the providers were different, more caring, more open, and listened better. Despite Ho and Bylund's (2008) argument that Chinese medicine's *healthcare model* should be understood separately from its *models of interaction*, Ho and Robles (2011) found that the neuropathy clients understood their treatments to be both holistic and collaborative. The participants reported that unlike the physical pills of biomedicine, the holistic/alternative therapies gave them an option to participate in their healthcare. They sometimes opted for drug interruptions even though they knew it could be physically dangerous to do so and in those moments used acupuncture and massage therapy to cope at least temporarily. In this study, the *Chineseness* of the practice seems least relevant to the people's experiences. What is relevant instead is the alterative and holistic nature of both the medicine itself and the expectation of a different kind of provider–patient relationship that goes along with it.

What makes this study critical is its acknowledgment of structural inequalities in care. Participants faced real challenges in how they would pay for alternatives, often because they lost their jobs and health insurance due to their neuropathy. Facing multiple forms of marginalization (they were HIV-positive, many were low-income, and they often chose alternative medicines over scientific biomedicine), many participants felt like they had no choices in how to approach their own health. As an intervention study, this study was able to provide treatments that may not otherwise have been available, even if only for a limited amount of time. However, judged from a scientific perspective, the authors could not show (in a statistically significant way) that the acupuncture and massage therapy worked to improve people's health. From an interpretive/critical perspective, though, what the participants said was that they experienced temporary relief and they felt heard and acknowledged in their health decision making. Each paradigm uses different criteria from which to judge success and failure, and this study shows that while one paradigm may not yield useful results, we can still learn something important about cultural influences on health.

DIRECTIONS FOR FUTURE RESEARCH

As this chapter has demonstrated, there are an almost endless number of possibilities for future research in the area of socio-cultural influences on health. Given such terrible health disparities, any efforts that can lead to health improvement, especially for marginalized populations throughout the world, can make a real difference. As the world shrinks with globalization, international health disparities will become even more consequential. To promote global health equality, I present a few directions for future research.

First, as the exemplar studies demonstrated, health communication research that focuses on socio-cultural influences needs to take into account research from all three paradigms and pragmatically integrate them. To determine what health and illness mean to local communities, one needs to be interpretive. To ensure that all voices are heard and that our work does not further oppress marginalized populations, a critical approach is necessary. Finally, in order to measure if changes have actually made a difference, a scientific approach is useful. This means that research in health communication should look beyond hospitals and into alternative health settings and everyday lives. In addition, cross-paradigmatic work will also determine what aspects of culture are most relevant in any given setting. For example, a priori determination of what is meant by "Chinese" does not take into account all the various ways in which Chineseness can be applied to health. In addition, research must recognize the interaction of people's simultaneous and overlapping social identities such as race/ethnicity, SES, gender/sex/sexuality, geography, etc. if it is to understand the complexity of culture.

Health research is increasingly taking seriously qualitative research, and health communication scholars are well-trained to fulfill this role on interdisciplinary teams. This is the second direction for research. The best health research is interdisciplinary in nature. Health communication students and researchers need to read across disciplines, and communication scholars need to stake a claim for what we can offer the conversation. As stated earlier, sometimes the most changeable aspects of a health situation are the communicative ones. Health policy makers promoting patient-centered care, cultural competency, and health literacy are all essentially arguing for the promotion of better health communication.

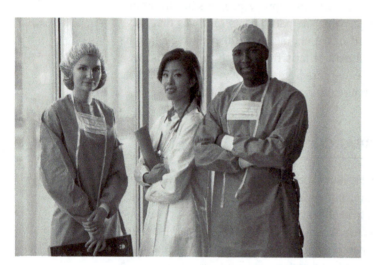

This leads to the third area of future research. Health communication research needs to be more applied if health communication scholars want to have our voices heard. Health research is by nature applied, and our research should be no different. As health communication scholars, we can study how communication itself can improve health outcomes. In addition, we do not have to accept that physical health outcomes are the only measures of success. Psychological, emotional, spiritual, and other more holistic measures of well-being may also be examined.

CONCLUSION

I will end this chapter with a note of hope and a challenge. Given how stark health disparities are, it would be easy to throw up one's hands and give up. However, the glass-is-half-full perspective means that we have plenty of room to be able to make real differences in the lives of real people precisely because the disparities are currently so great and because communication is so central to that change. Are you ready to play a role in reducing health disparities through health communication research?

DISCUSSION QUESTIONS

1. The rates of HIV among African Americans are disproportionately higher than other Americans. How might a scientific, interpretive, or critical researcher approach solving this health disparity? What goals would each have?

2. If health is a human right, what role does communication serve in advancing that right?

3. What do you think is more Chinese? A German person using acupuncture to treat lower back pain or a Chinese person using surgery to relieve back pain? What cultural issues are involved in both of these situations as they relate to health?

IN-CLASS ACTIVITIES

1. How do you cure hiccups? What happens if you go to sleep with your hair wet? To help students internalize the cultural nature of illness experience, investigate a common "illness" (like hiccups) with no clear treatment or an everyday "health warning" (like avoiding sleeping with wet hair). Have students interview each other in class about the causes, treatments, consequences, and sources of information for the illness/warning. Compile all the answers to see how culturally similar or different people are.

2. Health disparities are found not only across different countries but also within countries. Ask students to share health disparities that they are aware of in the United States. Choose one or two examples and pose ideas for overcoming these health disparities within the United States.

RECOMMENDED READINGS

Culhane-Pera, K. A., Vawter, D. E., Xiong, P., Babbitt, B., & Solberg, M. M. (Eds.). (2003). *Healing by heart: Clinical and ethical case stories of Hmong families and Western providers*. Nashville, TN: Vanderbilt University Press.

This book includes an extensive introductory chapter about Hmong culture and beliefs and then includes numerous case studies and commentaries from Hmong people and biomedical providers to discuss ethics and clinical ramifications of culture. It is a useful companion to the now classic book about Hmong health beliefs told through the story of a Hmong girl with epilepsy or *quag dab peg*: Fadiman, A. (1997). *The spirit catches you and you fall down*. New York: Farrar, Straus and Giroux.

Hsieh, E. (2010). Provider-interpreter collaboration in bilingual health care: competitions of control over interpreter-mediated interactions. *Patient Education & Counseling, 78*(2), 154–159.

This is a focus group study of professional medical interpreters and their communicative competition with health providers over different speech conventions, controlling other's narratives and overstepping expertise and role boundaries.

Koenig, C. J., Dutta, M. J., Kandula, N., & Palaniappan, L. (2012). "All of those things we don't eat": A culture-centered approach to dietary health meanings for Asian Indians living in the United States. *Health Communication, 27*(8), 818–828.

This study uses a culture-centered approach to understand how Asian Indians with type 2 diabetes understand food, eating, and dietary recommendations that often conflict with biomedical diet suggestions.

REFERENCES

Airhihenbuwa, C. O. (1995). *Health and culture: Beyond the western paradigm.* Thousand Oaks, CA: Sage.

Auger, S. J., DeCoster, M. E., & Colindres, M. D. (2008). Teach-with-stories method for prenatal education. In H. M. Zoller & M. J. Dutta (Eds.), *Emerging perspectives in health communication: Meaning, culture, and power* (pp. 155–181). New York: Routledge.

Barry, C. A., Stevenson, F. A., Britten, N., Barber, N., & Bradley, C. P. (2001). Giving voice to the lifeworld. More humane, more effective medical care? A qualitative study of doctor-patient communication in general practice. *Social Science & Medicine, 53*(4), 487–505.

Betancourt, J. R., Green, A. R., Carrillo, J. E., & Ananeh-Firempong, O., II. (2003). Defining cultural competence: A practical framework for addressing racial/ethnic disparities in health and health care. *Public Health Reports, 118*(4), 293–302.

Cameron, K. A. (2013). Advancing equity in clinical preventive services: The role of health communication. *Journal of Communication, 63*(1), 31–50.

Centers for Disease Control and Prevention. (2011, January 14). *Health disparities and inequalities report.* Morbidity and Mortality Weekly Report Supplement/Vol. 60. Retrieved from http://www.cdc.gov/hiv/topics/surveillance/resources/reports/-supplemental

Centers for Disease Control and Prevention. (2012, December). *Estimated HIV incidence in the United States, 2007–2010.* HIV Surveillance Supplemental Report 2012, Volume 17, Number 4. Retrieved from http://www.cdc.gov/hiv/surveillance/resources/reports/2010supp_vol17no4/index.htm

Centers for Disease Control and Prevention. (2013, March 8). *HIV among women.* Retrieved from http://www.cdc.gov/hiv/topics/women/print/index.htm

Dutta, M. J. (2007). Communicating about culture and health: Theorizing culture-centered and cultural sensitivity approaches. *Communication Theory, 17*(3), 304–328.

Dutta, M. J. (2012). Hunger as health: Culture-centered interrogations of alternative rationalities of health. *Communication Monographs, 79*(3), 366–384.

Dutta, M. J., & Basu, A. (2011). Culture, communication, and health. In T. L. Thompson, R. Parrott & J. F. Nussbaum (Eds.), *The Routledge handbook of health communication* (2nd ed., pp. 320–334). New York and London: Routledge.

Engel, G. (1977). The need for a new medical model: A challenge for biomedicine. *Science, 196*, 129–196.

Epner, D. E., & Baile, W. F. (2012). Patient-centered care: the key to cultural competence. *Annals of Oncology, 23*(suppl 3), 33–42.

Farmer, P. (1999). *Infections and inequalities*. Berkeley, CA: University of California Press.

Farmer, P. (2003). *Pathologies of power*. Berkeley, CA: University of California Press.

Ford, C. L., & Harawa, N. T. (2010). A new conceptualization of ethnicity for social epidemiologic and health equity research. *Social Science & Medicine, 71*(2), 251–258.

Fortier, J. P., & Bishop, D. (2003). *Setting the agenda for research on cultural competence in health care: final report.* Edited by C. Brach. Rockville, MD: U.S. Department of Health and Human Services Office of Minority Health and Agency for Healthcare Research and Quality.

Geiger, H. J. (2002). Racial and ethnic disparities in diagnosis and treatment: A review of the evidence and a consideration of causes. In B. D. Smedley, A. Y. Stith & A. R. Nelson (Eds.), *Unequal treatment: Confronting racial and ethnic disparities in health care* (pp. 417–454): The National Academies Press.

Geronimus, A. T., Bound, J., & Colen, C. G. (2011). Excess black mortality in the United States and in selected black and white high-poverty areas, 1980–2000. *American Journal of Public Health, 101*(4), 720–729.

Geronimus, A. T., Hicken, M., Keene, D., & Bound, J. (2006). "Weathering" and age patterns of allostatic load scores among blacks and whites in the United States. *American Journal of Public Health, 96*(5), 826–833.

Good, M.-J. D., Good, B., & Becker, A. (2002). The culture of medicine and racial, ethnic, and class disparities in healthcare. In B. D. Smedley, A. Y. Stith & A. R. Nelson (Eds.), *Unequal treatment: Confronting racial and ethnic disparities in health care* (pp. 594–625): The National Academies Press.

Hare, M. L. (1993). The emergence of an urban U.S. Chinese medicine. *Medical Anthropology Quarterly, 7*, 30–49.

Harrington, N. G. (2013). Introduction to the special issue: Communication strategies to reduce health disparities. *Journal of Communication, 63*(1), 1–7.

Ho, E. Y., & Bylund, C. L. (2008). Models of health and models of interaction in the practitioner-client relationship in acupuncture. *Health Communication, 23*(6), 506–515.

Ho, E. Y., & Robles, J. S. (2011). Cultural resources for health participation: Examining biomedicine, acupuncture, and massage therapy for HIV-related peripheral neuropathy. *Health Communication, 26*(2), 135–146.

Huerta, M., Bishop, S. L., Duncan, A., Hus, V., & Lord, C. (2012). Application of DSM-5 criteria for autism spectrum disorder to three samples of children with DSM-IV diagnoses of pervasive developmental disorders. *The American Journal of Psychiatry, 169*(10), 1056–1064.

Huynh, V. W. (2012). Ethnic microaggressions and the depressive and somatic symptoms of Latino and Asian American adolescents. *Journal of Youth and Adolescence, 41*(7), 831–846.

Johnson, J. L., Bottorff, J. L., Browne, A. J., Grewal, S., Hilton, B. A., & Clarke, H. (2004). Othering and being othered in the context of health care services. *Health Communication, 16*(2), 253–271.

Keene, D. E., & Geronimus, A. T. (2011). "Weathering" HOPE VI: The importance of evaluating the population health impact of public housing demolition and displacement. *Journal of Urban Health, 88*(3), 417–435.

Kleinman, A., Eisenberg, L., & Good, B. (1978). Culture, illness and care: Clinical lessons from Anthropologic and cross-cultural research. *Annals of Internal Medicine, 88,* 251–258.

Lupton, D. (1994). Toward the development of critical health communication praxis. *Health Communication, 6,* 55–67.

Lupton, D. (2003). *Medicine as culture: Illness, disease and the body in western societies* (2nd ed.). Thousand Oaks, CA: Sage.

McCord, C., & Freeman, H. P. (1990). Excess mortality in Harlem. *New England Journal of Medicine, 322*(3), 173–177.

McDermott, V. M., Oetzel, J. G., & White, K. (2008). Ethical paradoxes in community-based participatory research. In H. M. Zoller & M. J. Dutta (Eds.), *Emerging perspectives in health communication: Meaning, culture, and power* (pp. 180–202). New York: Routledge.

Minkler, M., & Wallerstein, N. (Eds.). (2003). *Community-based participatory research for health.* San Francisco, CA: Jossey-Bass.

Mishler, E. G. (1984). *The discourse of medicine: Dialectics of medical interviews.* Norwood, NJ: Ablex.

Nadal, K. L., Issa, M.-A., Leon, J., Meterko, V., Wideman, M., & Wong, Y. (2011). Sexual orientation microaggressions: "Death by a thousand cuts" for lesbian, gay, and bisexual youth. *Journal of LGBT Youth, 8*(3), 234–259.

Office of Minority Health. (2005, October 19). What is cultural competency? Retrieved from http://minorityhealth.hhs.gov/templates/browse.aspx?lvl=2&lvlID=11

Perloff, R. M. (2006). Introduction: Communication and health care disparities. *American Behavioral Scientist, 49*(6), 755–759.

Perloff, R. M., Bonder, B., Ray, G. B., Ray, E. B., & Siminoff, L. A. (2006). Doctor-patient communication, cultural competence, and minority health. *American Behavioral Scientist, 49,* 835–852.

Renzaho, A. M. N., Romios, P., Crock, C., & Sønderlund, A. L. (2013). The effectiveness of cultural competence programs in ethnic minority patient-centered health care—a systematic review of the literature. *International Journal for Quality in Health Care, 25*(3), 261–269.

Rhodes, L. A. (1996). Studying biomedicine as a cultural system. In C. F. Sargent & T. M. Johnson (Eds.), *Medical anthropology: Contemporary theory and method* (pp. 165–180). Westport, CT: Praeger.

Rubel, A. J. (1984). *Susto: A folk illness.* Berkeley and Los Angeles, CA: University of California Press.

Sentell, T., & Braun, K. L. (2012). Low health literacy, limited English proficiency, and health status in Asians, Latinos, and other racial/ethnic groups in California. *Journal of Health Communication, 17,* 82–99.

Sharf, B. F., & Vanderford, M. L. (2003). Illness narratives and the social construction of health. In T. L. Thompson, A. M. Dorsey, K. Miller & R. Parrott (Eds.), *Handbook of Health Communication* (pp. 9–34). Mahwah, NJ: Erlbaum.

Shelton, K., & Delgado-Romero, E. A. (2011). Sexual orientation microaggressions: The experience of lesbian, gay, bisexual, and queer clients in psychotherapy. *Journal of Counseling Psychology, 58*(2), 210–221.

Smedley, B. D., Stith, A. Y., & Nelson, A. R. (Eds.). (2003). *Unequal treatment: Confronting racial and ethnic disparities in health care*: Washington, DC: The National Academies Press.

Stafford, S. (2010). Caught between "The Rock" and a hard place. *American Journal of Public Health, 100*(5), 784–789.

Sue, D. W., Capodilupo, C. M., Torino, G. C., Bucceri, J. M., Holder, A. M. B., Nadal, K. L., & Esquilin, M. (2007). Racial microaggressions in everyday life: Implications for clinical practice. *American Psychologist, 62*(4), 271–286.

Takeuchi, D. T., & Gage, S. J. (2003). What to do with race? Changing notions of race in the social sciences. *Culture, Medicine and Psychiatry, 27*(4), 435–445.

Torres, L., Driscoll, M. W., & Burrow, A. L. (2010). Racial microaggressions and psychological functioning among highly achieving African-Americans: A mixed-methods approach. *Journal of Social and Clinical Psychology, 29*(10), 1074–1099.

Tuchman, A. M. (2011). Diabetes and race: A historical perspective. *American Journal of Public Health, 101*(1), 24–33.

U.S. Census Bureau (2012, December 12). *U.S. Census Bureau projections show a slower growing, older, more diverse nation in half a century from now*. Retrieved from http://www.census.gov/newsroom/releases/archives/population/cb12-243.html

U.S. Census Bureau News. (2012). *Facts for features Asian/Pacific American Heritage Month: May 2012*. Retrieved from http://www.census.gov/newsroom/releases/archives/facts_for_features_special_editions/cb12-ff09.html

U.S. Department of Health and Human Services. (2010, December 29). *Disparities*. Retrieved from http://www.healthypeople.gov/2020/about/DisparitiesAbout.aspx

U.S. Department of Health and Human Services. (2012, September 20). *Determinants of health*. Retrieved from http://www.healthypeople.gov/2020/about/DOHAbout.aspx

U.S. Department of Health and Human Services & Office of Minority Health (2001). *National Standards for Culturally and Linguistically Appropriate Services in Health Care*. Rockville, MD: Author.

Wang, J. H., Schwartz, M. D., Luta, G., Maxwell, A. E., & Mandelblatt, J. S. (2012). Intervention tailoring for Chinese American women: Comparing the effects of two videos on knowledge, attitudes and intentions to obtain a mammogram. *Health Education Research, 27*(3), 523–536.

Zoller, H. M., & Kline, K. N. (2008). Theoretical contributions of interpretive and critical research in health communication. In C. S. Beck (Ed.), *Communication Yearbook 32* (pp. 89–135). New York: Routledge.

CHAPTER

9

Risky Health Behaviors Among Adolescents and Young Adults

Pamela K. Cupp, Matthew W. Savage, Katharine Atwood, and Melissa H. Abadi

The focus of this chapter is contemporary health and social issues that often affect adolescents and young adults. In your high school health class, you may have studied some of these behaviors. However, in this chapter we will not only discuss the behaviors themselves but also examine some of the research that guides the development of the curricula that address them. First, we will review the current literature on four sets of behaviors that often result in negative health outcomes: (a) substance use, (b) risky sexual behavior, (c) gender-based violence, and (d) cyberbullying. Then we will discuss several highly recognized theories that inform health communication research and explore how they have been used either to provide an understanding of who is at greatest risk of engaging in these behaviors or to inform the development and/or dissemination of interventions that promote healthy or reduce harmful behaviors. And as you know by now from reading previous chapters, we also will address conflicting research results and areas for future research.

SUBSTANCE USE

Substance use remains a key public health issue among youth and young adults in the United States. As youth age, they are faced with tough decisions about alcohol and drug use that center around a number of developmental milestones, such as first relationships and school dances, and achievements, such as graduation and winning football seasons. Youths' decision to use substances and subsequent opportunities to use them can be linked to many factors, including greater exposure to risky situations and social influences (Jessor, 1998). Studies show that family and community influences (e.g., parent's involvement, family relationships) weigh heavily on adolescents' decisions to use substances, with peer and school factors (e.g., peer drug use, school involvement) becoming more influential as youth age. The ever-increasing desire for independence, greater access to alcohol and illegal drugs, less monitoring by adult role models, and the need to fit in socially all contribute to risky substance use behaviors (Fleming, Catalano, Haggerty, & Abbott, 2010).

The **National Institute on Drug Abuse Monitoring the Future (MTF)** report indicates use of alcohol, tobacco, marijuana, and other illicit substances doubles from 8th grade to 12th grade and continues to increase into young adulthood (Johnston, O'Malley, Bachman, & Schulenberg, 2009). In the past few years, nonmedical use of prescription drugs (NMUPD) and use of synthetic drugs (also known as "K–2," "spice," or "bath salts") have become increasingly popular among youth, largely because of misperceptions that there is little harm associated with these drugs (Johnston, O'Malley, Bachman, & Schulenberg, 2013).

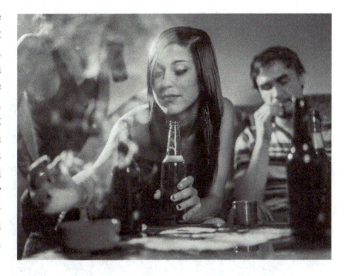

Early onset of substance use in adolescence often leads to substance use problems later in life, including more frequent use, experimentation with other types of drugs, multiple drug use, and substance use disorders (Palmer et al., 2009). There are a number of serious health consequences associated with substance abuse and addiction, including lung and cardiovascular disease, stroke, cancer, limited brain functioning, and mental health disorders (Volkow, 2010). Also, due to the lowering of inhibitions and impaired judgment, substance use has been linked with risky sexual behavior, which in turn can lead to sexually transmitted infections (STIs), HIV/AIDS, and unwanted pregnancy. Other serious outcomes of impaired judgment or other physical limitations brought on by substance use include driving while intoxicated, violence, and participation in criminal activities.

RISKY SEXUAL BEHAVIOR

Although education and prevention programs have made great strides in reducing sexual risk behaviors that place adolescents and young adults at risk for STIs, HIV/

AIDS, and unplanned pregnancy, there is still much work to be done. According to the **Youth Risk Behavior Survey**, a national bi-annual survey of high school students, the prevalence of high school students "ever having sex" and "having four or more partners" declined between 1991–2001: from 54.1% to 45.6% for "ever having sex," and from 18.7% to 14.2% for "having four or more partners." These percentages haven't changed significantly, however, from 2001 to 2011 (CDC, 2012a). The percentage of youth reporting condom use with their most recent sex partner increased from 46.2% in 1991 to 60.2% in 2011, but the percentage has not changed significantly since 2003 (63.0%; CDC, 2012a). Research also shows that there are persistent disparities in sexual risk taking behaviors, particularly among Hispanic and African-American youth, whose rates are much higher than other racial/ethnic groups (CDC, 2012a). (Chapter 8 addresses health disparities in greater detail.)

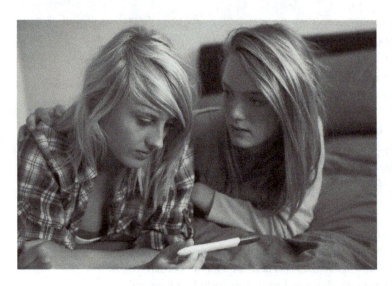

Risky sexual behaviors among youth and young adults can lead to negative health consequences such as STIs, HIV, and unplanned pregnancy. In fact, it may startle you to know that young people ages 15–24 account for almost 50% of the 19 million new STI cases detected in the United States each year (CDC, 2012b). As with sexual risk taking behavior, there are significant health disparities in infection rates that are often related to social and economic inequalities (e.g., education, health services, access to insurance). For example, chlamydia rates for African-American females are six times higher and rates for African American males are 11 times higher than their Caucasian counterparts, while rates for Hispanics are twice that of Caucasians (CDC, 2012b).

Adolescents and young adults also account for 34% of the 56,300 people infected with HIV in the United States each year (CDC, 2012c). Those at greatest risk of HIV infection are young men who have sex with men (YMSM). Ninety-one percent of those diagnosed with HIV between the ages of 13 and 19 became infected from male-to-male sexual contact (CDC, 2012c). However, females are also at risk. In 2010, 25% of all people living with HIV in the United States were female, and 20% of all new cases reported that year were among women (CDC, 2013a). Most new infections among women are the result of having heterosexual contact with a high risk sexual partner.

Similar to statistics for other STIs, the likelihood of contracting HIV is 20 times higher for African-American women and four times higher for Hispanic women than for Caucasian women (CDC, 2013a). Elevated rates of HIV and STIs among racial and ethnic subgroups are not well understood, but they may have *less* to do with differences in sexual risk behaviors and *more* to do with the fact that sexual contact often occurs within sexual networks that are already experiencing elevated HIV and STI rates. Unfortunately, sexual networks of minorities are less likely to be reached with effective prevention and treatment interventions (Millett, Flores, Peterson, & Bakeman, 2007).

Teen pregnancy rates actually declined from 2010 to 2011 by about eight percent among girls aged 15–17 (CDC, 2012d). In addition, the teen birth rate dropped to the lowest in the 70 years that these data have been collected in the United States (Planned Parenthood Federation of America, 2012). But, there is still work to be done. The United States has the highest birth rate among teens in the developed world. Furthermore, one in five teen births in United States is a second birth, underscoring the need for effective interventions and greater access to birth control. Nonetheless, this recent drop is good news given that teen pregnancy results in substantial emotional, educational, and economic costs both to the child and to the family unit. Less than half of teen mothers complete high school by age 22, whereas 90% of their similarly aged child-free peers graduate (Perper, Peterson, & Manlove, 2010). In addition, children of teen mothers are more likely to grow up in poverty, be raised in a single parent household, have reduced educational attainment, and become teen parents themselves (Hoffman, 2008). The **Centers for Disease Control and Prevention** has designated reductions in teen pregnancy as one of the "winnable" health challenges for the United States (CDC, 2012d), encouraging the use of evidence-based interventions among at-risk youth.

What is an Evidence-based Intervention?

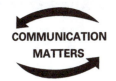

COMMUNICATION MATTERS

Programs exist to convince smokers to quit, to encourage alcohol drinkers to do so in moderation, and to discourage adolescents from bullying their peers, either face-to-face or online. What distinguishes evidence-based interventions from other programs is that they frequently draw on previously validated theories and have been tested scientifically to determine whether they achieve their proposed goals. To conduct a scientifically valid test of an intervention, you should use recognized study procedures and statistical strategies that have been developed over time as a result of many scientific trials. If you would like to better understand what a scientifically valid evaluation strategy for testing interventions might look like, you may begin by examining the CONSORT model (Schulz, Altman, Moher, & the CONSORT Group, 2010). This model was developed to encourage researchers to follow accepted procedures in both designing and reporting on their studies.

GENDER-BASED VIOLENCE

Gender-based violence (GBV) is a worldwide epidemic that involves rape or sexual assault, physical or mental abuse, or economic deprivation (Garcia-Moreno, Jansen, Ellsberg, Heise, & Watts, 2006). GBV is usually the result of socially ascribed gender differences, norms that perpetuate inequality, and the need to exert power or influence over individuals of the other gender. In most (but not all) cases, the victims of GBV are female. GBV takes many forms, including intimate partner violence, acquaintance rape, stranger rape, domestic violence, forced prostitution or human trafficking, and genital mutilation (Gender Based Violence Area of Responsibility Working Group, 2010). In this chapter we are going to focus on two types of GBV: intimate partner violence and rape.

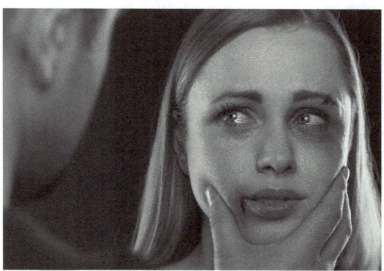

Intimate partner violence (IPV) is defined as violence that "includes physical, sexual and psychological abuse (or threat thereof) by current or former" intimate partners (Wong, Huang, DiGangi, Thompson, & Smith, 2008, p. 57). The worldwide reported rates of IPV against women ranges by country from 15% to 71% (Garcia-Moreno et al., 2006). The CDC (2013b) reports that about four percent of the U.S. population (almost 12 million people) is raped, battered, or stalked by an intimate partner each year. About one out of four women (24.8%) and one in seven men (13.8%) have been beaten or physically abused by an intimate partner at some point in their lives. Of adults who report being victims of IPV, 22% of women and 15% of men indicate the first occasion was when they were between 11 and 17 years old (CDC, 2013b), with nine percent of high school students reporting they had been hit, slapped, or beaten by a partner in the last year (CDC, 2012f). IPV puts victims at risk for many negative outcomes, including physical injury or death, psychological distress, and lost productivity and wages. For perpetrators, the results can involve incarceration, estrangement from children and other family members, fines and penalties, and lost wages.

Rape, whether by an intimate partner, acquaintance, or stranger, is an enormous problem. About one million women are raped each year in the United States, a statistic that should be particularly alarming to young women. Almost 80% of all female rape victims are under 25 years of age, with 42% being less than 18 years old (CDC, 2013b). Acquaintance violence and rape are most common among high school and college students. We choose to use the term **acquaintance rape** instead of date rape because in more than 85% of circumstances the individuals are not on an actual date but are at a party, in a private space studying, or in another social situation (CDC, 2012e). While alcohol is not the cause of these acquaintance rapes (or any other violent behavior), it is often present in those situations. Alcohol is commonly perceived to reduce inhibitions and impair judgment and physical responses, all of which lead to poor decision making. In addition, beliefs about how alcohol will cause a person to act and social norms supporting the dominant role of males may be involved. Males may supply females with alcohol because they believe it will result in either the female's consent to or inability to oppose having sex; they may also perceive females who are intoxicated as "deserving" of sexual assault or rape (Sampson, 2002). However, a recent case in Ohio, where two male teens were convicted of raping an extremely intoxicated female student, demonstrated that having sex with a person so drunk that she or he does not have the capacity to say "no" *is* considered rape. For more information about this case, you may access http://www.cnn.com/2013/03/17/justice/ohio-steubenville-case.

CYBERBULLYING

Many of us have heard the tragic story of Tyler Clementi. He was a smart and talented young man, celebrated for his accomplishments as a violinist. As Tyler began college at Rutgers University, he began to share his sexuality with those close to him. Sadly, he soon became a victim of cyberbullying. **Cyberbullying** is bullying through technology, such as sending threatening text messages or spreading embarrassing photos or nasty rumors via social media. His college roommate invaded his privacy by setting up a webcam to spy on him in his dorm room during an intimate act; the roommate invited others to view this online. Many joined in and publicly mocked Tyler using social media outlets. Tyler discovered he had been publicly ridiculed. When he found out that his abusers were planning a second attempt, he ended his life by jumping off the George Washington Bridge. Tyler was only 18 years old. You can learn more by visiting the website of the Rutgers University Tyler Clementi Center (tylerclementi.org).

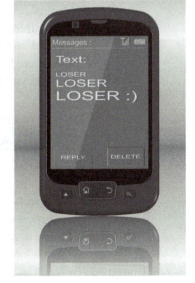

When compared to research on substance abuse, risky sexual behavior, and gender-based violence, the research base on cyberbullying is less developed. As communication technology finds its way into all sectors of adolescents' and teens' daily lives, the need for cyberbullying research, however, becomes more urgent. The Pew Internet and American Life Project (2013) has tracked teens' use of communication technology since 2001. One of the project's findings is that most people get their first cell phone at 12–13 years of age. In addition, 95% of teens now report using the Internet. Another study conducted in 2008 found that 58% of teens reported having a social networking profile and 71% of teens reported owning a cell phone. With such prevalence, the opportunity for harm is increased. Indeed, a review of empirical studies shows that large proportions of adolescents report being victims of cyberbullying. Results of studies that survey youth indicate 20% to 40% of participants reported being victimized by a cyberbully (Dehue, Bolman, & Vollink, 2008; Li, 2007; Smith et al., 2008), while 15% of adolescents reported they cyberbullied others (Kowalski & Limber, 2007).

Tyler Clementi's story can help us explore nuances among cyberbullying studies, and it suggests the need for future cyberbullying research. First, although Tyler was an adult and a college student when he was cyberbullied, the majority of researchers focus on cyberbullying as a problem for middle and high school students. Tyler's story, however, cautions us that cyberbullying may occur during later periods of adolescence and into early adulthood. Recognizing this fact, more researchers have recently begun to examine cyberbullying among college students. Second, although Tyler's story ended in suicide, researchers such as LeBlanc (2012) remind us that cyberbullying is associated with multiple harmful outcomes besides suicide. Victims have reported lower self-esteem (Patchin & Hinduja, 2010), as well as higher levels of depression and more significant life challenges (Ybarra, Mitchell, Wolak, & Finkelhor, 2006), than non-victims. Further, victims hold internalized negative affect toward the cyberbully (Patchin & Hinduja, 2011). The physical and psychosocial problems that emerge in conjunction with cyberbullying underscore the need for health communication research that aims to deter perpetration and help victims.

RISKY BEHAVIOR

Substance use, risky sexual behavior, gender-based violence, and cyberbullying are behaviors that put the health of adolescents and young adults at particular risk. Tracking data from credible sources such as the Centers for Disease Control and Prevention and the National Institute on Drug Abuse help us to understand the prevalence of some of these behaviors and, in part, assess the effectiveness of interventions designed to reduce them.

THEORIES USED IN HEALTH COMMUNICATION STUDIES OF RISKY BEHAVIOR

As mentioned earlier, whereas the beginning of the chapter provides an overview of the current state of the literature about our four targeted risk behaviors and their potential negative consequences, this section focuses on several theories that can help identify people who are at high risk, guide program or intervention development, and determine how to best disseminate messages for optimal effectiveness. We also will include examples of how these theories have been used in research. Each of the theories presented here is consistent with the scientific paradigm. As you will see as you read through this section, the theories (which are paired with appropriate scientific methods) are used in both developing interventions and measuring their effectiveness. Data is collected using quantitative methods, most often in the form of self-report surveys. The underlying assumption is that, while we are all unique, there are identifiable patterns in our behaviors and physiological responses that will help to inform harm reduction or health promotion programs. For instance, using drugs or alcohol consistently increases the chances of addiction and related negative outcomes such as broken relationships or job loss regardless of personal characteristics.

Depending on the goal of the study, data may be collected either from groups that are thought to be at greatest risk or from the general population. In an intervention study (when researchers test whether a particular program works or not), data typically is collected both before and after program implementation. In addition to collecting data from the intervention or experimental group (those receiving the program), data is also collected from a comparison group (made up of people with characteristics similar to the intervention group but who have not received the program). The expectation is that those in the intervention group will report safer behaviors after the implementation of the program than will those in the comparison group. If this expectation is met, researchers have evidence that the program is successful and is worthy of additional study and possible implementation in real world settings (translational research). If the expectation is not met, researchers do not deem the program successful, and they either need to abandon the program or, if possible, conduct additional data analyses to determine how the program could be improved.

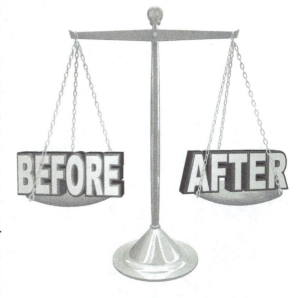

Theories, Models, and Variables That Help Us Identify and Reach At-risk Populations

Sensation seeking. Individual difference variables, also called personality variables, are generally defined as those stable traits or attributes that help to describe a person. Over the past century, some social scientists have searched for systems and principles that explain the regularities of human behavior, while others have been motivated to understand why individuals act differently in seemingly similar circumstances. Understanding and explaining these differences is critical in predicting and changing human behavior, a major goal within the scientific paradigm.

One important individual difference variable that is strongly related to risky behavior is **sensation seeking**. Marvin Zuckerman, the "father" of sensation seeking, describes it as, "the need for varied, novel, and complex sensations and experiences and the willingness to take physical and social risks for the sake of such experiences" (1979, p. 10). Many studies confirm that it is possible to predict which people will be most likely to engage in risky behaviors such as drug or alcohol use, having multiple sex partners, or initiating sexual activity at an early age by using the sensation seeking scale (Zuckerman, Kolin, Price, & Zoo, 1964). Naturally, not all people who score high on the sensation seeking scale, described as high sensation seekers (HSS), will engage in illegal, illicit, or unsafe behaviors; likewise, low scores on the scale do not mean the low sensation seekers (LSS) won't do something wild. However, there is strong evidence that sensation seeking is a good predictor of many problem behaviors, particularly in adolescence.

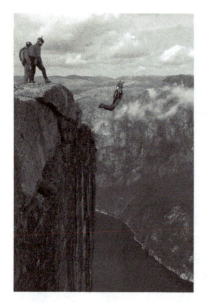

Sensation seeking has four dimensions:

1. *Thrill and Adventure Seeking:* a preference for activities such as bungee jumping, skydiving, or the use of drugs and alcohol.
2. *Experience Seeking:* a fondness for travel, listening to new music, or trying new types of food.
3. *Disinhibition:* an inclination to ignore or challenge social norms, rules, or the law.
4. *Boredom Susceptibility:* a tendency to become bored in situations or with people.

The original scale consisted of 40 "forced choice" items, which required people to pick which of two items was more like them (Zuckerman et al., 1964). For example, which of the following would you choose: (A) I like wild, uninhibited parties. (B) I like parties where people mostly sit around and talk. If you chose (A), that would be one point in the HSS column for you. Over the years, researchers worked to take this arguably inconvenient scale and transform it into something more user friendly. Researchers at the University of Kentucky got it down to an eight item Likert scale, in fact, and made sure the language was simpler and more current. This "brief" sensation seeking scale (Hoyle, Stephenson, Palmgreen, Lorch, & Donohew, 2002) appears below. How do you score? If you score above 24, we'd probably call you a high sensation seeker.

Brief Sensation Seeking Scale

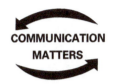

Interest and Preference Survey

Instructions: Please circle the number that best matches how much you agree or disagree with each statement.

1. I would like to explore strange places.

1	2	3	4	5
Strongly Disagree	Disagree	Neither Disagree Nor Agree	Agree	Strongly Agree

2. I get restless when I spend too much time at home.

1	2	3	4	5
Strongly Disagree	Disagree	Neither Disagree Nor Agree	Agree	Strongly Agree

3. I like to do frightening things.

1	2	3	4	5
Strongly Disagree	Disagree	Neither Disagree Nor Agree	Agree	Strongly Agree

4. I like wild parties.

1	2	3	4	5
Strongly Disagree	Disagree	Neither Disagree Nor Agree	Agree	Strongly Agree

5. I would like to take off on a trip with no pre-planned routes or timetables.

1	2	3	4	5
Strongly Disagree	Disagree	Neither Disagree Nor Agree	Agree	Strongly Agree

6. I prefer friends who are excitingly unpredictable.

1	2	3	4	5
Strongly Disagree	Disagree	Neither Disagree Nor Agree	Agree	Strongly Agree

7. I would like to try bungee jumping.

1	2	3	4	5
Strongly Disagree	Disagree	Neither Disagree Nor Agree	Agree	Strongly Agree

8. I would love to have new and exciting experiences, even if they are illegal.

1	2	3	4	5
Strongly Disagree	Disagree	Neither Disagree Nor Agree	Agree	Strongly Agree

From Hoyle et al. (2002).

The focus of many health communication studies is to identify and effectively reach HSS, the people most likely to engage in problem behaviors, such as substance abuse or high risk sexual activity. For instance, a large body of research links sensation seeking to problem drinking and other substance use and abuse. Many studies have shown that HSS are not only more likely to engage in substance use but also more likely to do so at an earlier age and with a variety of substances (Donohew, 1990; Zuckerman, 1979). In terms of sex, a meta-analysis (generally, a study that examines the results of a large body of previous studies on a specific topic) found consistent evidence to support an association between sensation seeking and sexual risk taking behaviors, including number of partners, unprotected sex, and high risk sexual encounters (Hoyle, Fejfar, & Miller, 2000).

While there is a link between high sensation seeking and some of the behaviors believed to be related to IPV (e.g., substance use and engaging multiple sex partners), there is not strong scientific evidence of a direct link between sensation seeking and IPV. Similarly, in a recent study of high school seniors, researchers found that some of the behaviors correlated with high sensation seeking (such as smoking cigarettes, drinking alcohol, and getting in trouble at school) are also related to the likelihood of perpetrating cyberbullying (Roberto, Eden, Savage, Ramos-Salavar, & Deiss, 2014). In addition, verbal aggression, engaging in risky behaviors, and prior cyberbullying victimization predict a person's likelihood to perpetrate cyberbullying. These studies suggest that future research should examine the association between sensation seeking and violent tendencies and behaviors such as IPV and cyberbullying.

Activation model of information exposure. In addition to helping to identity and understand who may be most likely to engage in a variety of risk behaviors, the construct of sensation seeking was used to frame a theory of arousal, and ultimately, inform message design (Donohew, Lorch, & Palmgreen, 1998). Donohew and colleagues point out that most models of communication propose an overly rational approach to human decision making and action. These researchers believe that humans tend not to be that rational at all, at least not most of the time. Instead, these researchers claim that ". . . individuals often are only dimly aware—if at all—of the choices they are making" (Donohew, Nair, & Finn, 1984, p. 267). Their **activation model of information exposure (AMIE)** takes this into account. It states that people vary in their willingness to attend to a message and that variance is related to their differing needs for novelty and sensation (Donohew et al., 1984). If a message "matches" a person's need for novelty and sensation, that person will likely pay attention to and stick with the message. If not, they won't. This is oversimplifying things a little, of course. Sometimes you have to pay attention to a message even if you don't really want to. But in the daily mix of persuasive health messages you might encounter, when you *do* have a choice to pay attention or not, a message's "sensation value" matters.

Several studies examining the effectiveness of health promotion public service announcements (PSAs) have shown that HSS do pay greater attention to messages that appeal to emotions and are fast-paced than messages that are slow moving, preachy, require thinking, and not very novel (Donohew, Lorch, & Palmgreen, 1991). Thus, it appears that how messages make HSS feel is very important. Interestingly, research has shown that LSS like the messages designed for HSS almost as much as they like the ones designed for them (Donohew et al., 1991). This is an important finding, given that it allows prevention specialists to target messages to the riskiest segment of the population without ignoring those at lower, but still some, risk. As a side note, this is an excellent example of interdisciplinary research. Donohew and colleagues, a mix of communication and psychology scholars, provided a communication-oriented application to the important work on sensation seeking coming from researchers in psychology.

We mentioned earlier that researchers have used the construct of sensation seeking to guide message design. One example of such a study is work by Zimmerman and colleagues, who used the AMIE framework to tailor a classroom-based pregnancy and HIV prevention curriculum to HSS youth. In this study with ninth graders in two midwestern cities, Zimmerman and colleagues modified an evidence-based HIV prevention curriculum (*Reducing the Risk*; Kirby, Barth, Leland, & Fetro, 1991) to increase its sensation value by including novel and exciting videos, dramatic peer speakers who were living with HIV or

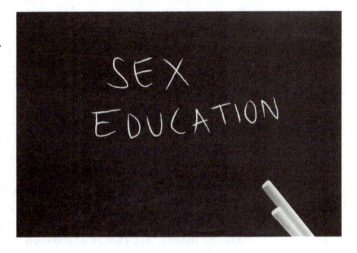

AIDS, and classroom prizes and games (Zimmerman et al., 2008). The researchers found larger delays in initiation of sexual intercourse among participants receiving either the original curriculum or the one modified for high sensation seekers than the participants who received the standard health textbook, indicating that the adapted program was successful but not significantly better than the original one. Their findings suggest additional work is needed to identify which curriculum components were sufficiently high in sensation value and which needed greater enhancement.

Theories That Inform Intervention Design

In the last section, where we reviewed theories that help us understand who is at greater risk for problem behaviors and what message characteristics they find appealing, we concentrated on the affective or emotional appeal of messages. In this section, we are going to examine theories that guide the development of the content of prevention messages. Remember, a goal of health communication research is to design and implement messages that influence the target behavior.

SENTAR. The previous section included a description of how AMIE helps us to understand that message characteristics should match the individual differences of the receiver in order to be effective. Researchers subsequently drew from AMIE to inform a model of message design called **SENTAR**, which stands for SENsation seeking TARgeting (Stephenson, 2003). SENTAR recognizes the need for messages to be novel in order to increase the likelihood that they will be noticed and processed by HSS persons. SENTAR has been used to inform several mass media campaigns designed to deter adolescents from smoking marijuana. For each campaign, the researchers (a) used sensation seeking to segment their audience, (b) conducted elicitation research (in this case, focus groups with both LSS and HSS adolescents and young adults) to determine which messages would appeal to HSS, (c) developed PSAs for television based on this input, and (d) aired these PSAs during programs that high sensation seekers liked. Results of one study with adolescents demonstrated a decrease in 30-day marijuana use among HSS youth (Palmgreen, Donohew, Lorch, Hoyle, & Stephenson, 2001; Stephenson, 2003). The SENTAR model has informed a considerable body of research and has been credited with influencing a national anti-drug campaign sponsored by the **Office of National Drug Control Policy** (Palmgreen & Donohew, 2010).

Theory of reasoned action. Since its inception in the mid–1970s, the **theory of reasoned action (TRA**; Fishbein & Ajzen, 1975) has proven to be an effective model for predicting and changing behavior (Perloff, 2001), has been applied to a broad spectrum of preventive health interventions, and has been the basis for two subsequent theories, the **theory of planned behavior (TPB**; Ajzen & Madden, 1986) and the **integrative model of behavior change** (Fishbein, 2000). The TRA predicts behavior by considering a person's beliefs, attitudes, norms, and intentions. A description of these interim steps, called mediating variables, follows.

1. **Beliefs** are representations of how an attitude, norm, or behavior is viewed in a person's world. For instance, while many people use condoms for protection against pregnancy and disease, some religions forbid such a practice. Thus, religious beliefs may influence a person's individual belief system about birth control and STI prevention.
2. **Attitudes** are more specific than beliefs and relate to how you feel about performing a particular behavior. *An overall negative attitude about cyberbullying* may be too general to actually predict behavior; to be predictive, the attitude would need to relate to the specific event. A positive attitude about

supporting a victim of cyberbullying by speaking out against such cruelty to the cyberbullies would be more likely to predict a specific action.

3. **Subjective norms** are (a) the perceptions you have of how others feel about a behavior and (b) how motivated you are to comply with, or be influenced by, the attitudes of others about the behavior in question. For instance, a young woman's decision to have unprotected sex may be influenced by (a) what her mother thinks of her engaging in unprotected sex and (b) how motivated she is to comply with her mother's wishes.

4. Finally, **intentions** to perform a behavior have been found to be the most significant predictor of actually engaging in the behavior. Intentions should have a direct correspondence to the behavior in question. A drinking intention might be *to say no (action) to drinking at the party (context) on Saturday (time) because someone needs to be the driver.* A highly specified intention like this one is much more likely to predict behavior than a general claim to never drink inappropriately.

Social cognitive theory. Imagine if you had to learn everything by direct personal experience. That sure would be cumbersome and sometimes dangerous. Bandura (1977) recognized this as he was developing his **social cognitive theory (SCT)**. He recognized that much of what we learn comes from observing the trials, and sometimes failures, of others. By experiencing mistakes vicariously, rather than directly, people are able to avoid many painful experiences (like avoiding tequila after seeing what happened to a friend who did several shots at a party). In addition, modeling the appropriate behavior of others may also lead to rapid learning of positive or creative approaches to situations or problems. Ultimately, SCT suggests that a person's learning is a product of a continuous interaction between these cognitive, behavioral, and environmental factors (Bandura, 1986).

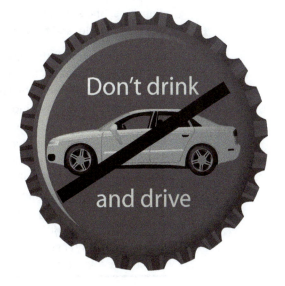

SCT proposes not only that people learn from watching others but also that the larger social environment influences our judgments about our own capabilities. This informal assessment of ability, referred to as **self-efficacy**, is context specific and usually relates to the performance of a specific behavior. An example of a self-efficacy statement might be, "I am confident that I could engage in a civil conversation instead of becoming verbally abusive even if my girlfriend tried to make me angry by flirting with someone else at a party."

Both the TRA (and subsequent theories that have grown out of this framework) and SCT have been used independently and together to effectively inform behavior change interventions in many areas of health promotion. One of the most notable prevention interventions for adolescent tobacco (Botvin, Eng, & Williams, 1980) and other substance use (Botvin & Kantor, 2000) prevention, called *Life Skills Training* (LST), is based in part on SCT. This program concentrates on improving an adolescent's abilities to cope with challenges in the social environment and on developing resilience.

The classroom-based HIV prevention intervention study we mentioned earlier by Zimmerman and colleagues drew not only on the AMIE model but also on SCT and the TRA. *Reducing the Risk* (RTR; Kirby et al., 1991), a classroom-based pregnancy

---

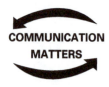

COMMUNICATION MATTERS

I See Myself . . . **Theory in Practice**

Carol (name changed), a popular high school student, excelled academically. She also cheered for her school, hung out with her friends, and dated some of her classmates. She planned to become a doctor and volunteered at a local clinic in preparation. She dated one guy for most of her freshman and sophomore college years, but they broke up . . . perhaps because she heard he had been cheating on her. Before her college graduation, she became engaged to a guy whom she loved and respected. However, when she went to the clinic where she had been volunteering to take the HIV test required for their marriage license, she learned she was HIV positive. She was stunned. She took the test again, but she received the same diagnosis. She and her sweetheart married, but the pressure proved to be more than he could handle, and they soon divorced.

This all happened in the 1990s, before the development of effective drug regimens that allow HIV patients to live longer and healthier lives, and Carol's health deteriorated rapidly. She spent the last two years of her life working to get the HIV prevention message out to young people. Her contributions to the study conducted by Zimmerman and colleagues (2008) were invaluable. She worked with students to increase their positive *attitudes* about waiting to have sex and about using condoms. Students hung on her every word (even those who usually did not pay attention in class), and they learned about negative *peer norms* and pressures to have unprotected sex. She would help students practice sexual refusal skills to increase their *self-efficacy* at refusing unwanted advances. She asked them to look in the mirror and see the face of HIV. Then she would quietly turn to the research team and say, "I look at them, and I see myself." Carol would say, "Learn from my mistakes and live to achieve your dreams."

and STI prevention program, also relied on these theories in program development and evaluation. RTR focused on increasing positive attitudes about waiting to have sex and using condoms, challenging peer norms about teenage sex, and improving self-efficacy by using role plays to work through potential scenarios in which a partner is insisting on unprotected sex.

Roberto, Meyer, Boster, and Roberto (2003) used the TRA to successfully change verbal and physical aggression among junior high school students. These findings might suggest future directions for cyberbullying prevention efforts. Consistent with the TRA, analysis revealed that attitudes and subjective norms predicted behavioral intent, and intent predicted behavior in terms of watching a fight, spreading rumors about a fight, and insulting others. For actual fighting, attitudes predicted behavioral intentions and intentions predicted behavior, but surprisingly, subjective norms did not significantly predict behavioral intentions. There are two possible explanations for this interesting finding. First, it might be due to how subjective norms about fighting were measured in the study. There are many referent groups that participants could be asked to consider (e.g., close friends, all peers, people at the fight). Perhaps the researchers didn't assess the most relevant referent group. Second, it might be related to the active and spontaneous nature of fighting. That is, fighting may be such a sporadic event, and less thoughtful than other risky behaviors, that norms might not be as strongly considered as they are with other risky behaviors. Because cyberbullying is more like spreading rumors about a fight and insulting others than actual physical fighting, Roberto and Eden (2010) suggest using the TRA to inform future cyberbullying prevention efforts, which should aim to influence attitudes and subjective norms in order to change behavioral intentions.

While Roberto and Eden (2010) offered suggestions for preventing cyberbullying perpetration, Savage and Deiss (2010) used SCT to study how victims of cyberbullying might be persuaded to use recommended responses to cyberbullying. Recommended responses include (a) not retaliating, (b) seeking social support, (c) saving evidence, and (d) reporting the incident. The researchers constructed messages using SCT components to persuade participants to adopt these four recommended responses. These messages altered participants' perceptions of threat and efficacy while also influencing attitudes and intentions in expected directions for all the recommended responses except not retaliating. Although well-rounded cyberbullying interventions are still being developed, studies like those reviewed here remind us that theories such as TRA and SCT offer useful frameworks to design these efforts.

Theories to Guide the Distribution of Interventions

The final theory that we are going to examine has been used to distribute messages so that the intended audience is likely to listen to, consider, and adopt the recommended behavior(s). **Diffusion of innovations theory** (**DOI**; Rogers, 1983) provides an understanding of how information about a new idea or innovation is communicated within an organization, community, or society, as well as how decisions are made whether to adopt the new approach or product. DOI explains why and how new behaviors, attitudes, or technologies become trendy and are adopted by a large group. The late Everett Rogers, the primary theorist behind DOI, proposed that there are four elements in the diffusion of new ideas (Rogers, 1983). First, there has to be an innovation—a new product, idea, or way of behaving. Second, this new innovation must be communicated through identified channels. Third, the innovation must be given time to diffuse beyond the original channels, to the larger community. Last, there must be a network of people to consider, test, and adopt the innovation. For an innovation to be successfully diffused and adopted, it is important that community members who are well liked and respected support the innovation.

THEORIES. MODELS. AND VARIABLES THAT INFORM HEALTH COMMUNICATION PREVENTION EFFORTS

<u>Understanding the Audience</u>

   Sensation Seeking
   Activation Model of Information Exposure

<u>Designing the Message</u>

   SENTAR
   Theory of Reasoned Action
   Social Cognitive Theory

<u>Disseminating the Message</u>

   Diffusion of Innovations

EXEMPLAR STUDIES IN RISKY HEALTH BEHAVIOR

Although we have examined several intervention studies in passing, below you will find more detailed descriptions of three important intervention studies. They demonstrate the application of theory and adherence to rigorous scientific guidelines in the development and evaluation of programs that are widely recognized and respected.

Substance Abuse

Translational research in health communication allows us to take what is learned in basic research and apply it to everyday situations and realities. The multicultural evidence-based substance use prevention program *keepin' it REAL* is an example of how translational research can have a major impact (Hecht & Miller-Day, 2007). The development of *keepin' it REAL* started with participatory research, which involved gathering narratives from adolescents on the who, when, why, and where of substance use offers and refusals in order to better understand youth perspectives. The researchers were among the first to study the communicative processes among youth in drug offers and refusals, as well as ethnic similarities and differences in these processes.

The analyses found four core refusal strategies, which represent the name of the program: Resist (simple no), Explain (no with explanation), Avoid (avoid the offer or the place where the offer will be made), and Leave (leave the place). Using communication competence and social cognitive theories, the researchers translated the narrative research into a 10-lesson prevention curriculum for middle-school students that reflected the real-life situations, cultures, and identities of the targeted youth. Before program implementation, the researchers conducted additional participatory research with community stakeholders, and they further translated the research and program goals into accessible and actionable language for teachers and students. Pilot test results showed that the program was successful in reducing substance use and impacting norms, expectations, and resistance strategies.

These program effects led the **U.S. Substance Abuse and Mental Health Services Administration** to name *keepin' it REAL* a model program for the **National Registry of Effective Prevention Programs**. The next phase of translational research involved widespread dissemination of the program, which demonstrated continued effects with various populations, and eventually led to a collaboration with D.A.R.E. America. And now, *keepin' it REAL* is the most widely disseminated substance use prevention program in the world (Hecht, Colby, & Miller-Day, 2010). The developers have also begun using branding perspectives and SCT to examine the mechanisms and components of the program that contribute to successful outcomes and to further assess how branding equity can improve health communication messages (Lee & Hecht, 2011).

Sexual Activity

School-based program. Jemmott and colleagues used both SCT and the theory of planned behavior (TPB, which is an extension of the TRA described earlier) to guide the development of an HIV prevention intervention for African-American inner-city adolescents (Jemmott, Jemmott, & Fong, 1998). They called their curriculum *Be Proud! Be Responsible!* The program sought to strengthen attitudes supporting condom use by reducing fears that condoms would compromise sexual enjoyment and to increase behavioral control or self-efficacy in correctly using and negotiating condom use with potential sex partners. The researchers conducted a randomized controlled three-arm trial, testing the efficacy of their curriculum against an abstinence-only and a general health curriculum (Jemmott et al., 1998). They found that their curriculum had a greater impact on increasing condom use at the six and 12 month follow-up periods than the abstinence only and general health conditions. Similar findings on condom use have been achieved in randomized trials with African-American inner-city males (Jemmott, 1992) and among youth in Liberia (Atwood, Kennedy, Shamblen, Teglee, & Shannon, 2012). The intervention has also been replicated among 86 community organizations, with similar impact on increasing condom use (Jemmott, Jemmott, Braverman, & Fong, 2005). *Be Proud! Be Responsible!* is now commercially available and is used by many schools and community groups; thus, it is another great example of translational research.

Community-based program. Researchers have used DOI to guide the development of popular peer opinion leader approaches to HIV prevention. Remember, DOI suggests that HIV prevention messages can be diffused through a community if community members who are considered popular, credible, and influential are identified and trained to adopt, support, and promote the specific behavior change innovation (Kelly, 2004). Kelly and colleagues (1997) drew on this principle in a series of studies involving men who frequented gay bars. The researchers asked bartenders to identify natural opinion leaders. Bartenders used their knowledge of the social networks to identify "trend setters" who then served as "agents for behavior change."

In a randomized community level trial, four cities received the natural opinion leader intervention and four control cities were provided with education materials only (Kelly et al., 1997). The intervention involved opinion leaders initiating informal discussions at the bar with their friends/peers about condom use and other safer sex practices. This was a good time to have these discussions because patrons leaving the bar were often heading out to have sex with either their regular or a new partner. Results at the one-year follow-up period showed that participants in the intervention cities had unprotected sex less frequently and greater increases in the mean percentage of protected sex than participants in control cities (Kelly et al., 1997).

Using similar strategies for identifying, recruiting, and training popular peer opinion leaders, studies have found similar reductions in high risk sexual behaviors among male commercial sex workers (Miller, Klotz, & Eckholdt, 1998), young gay males (Kegeles, Hays, & Coates, 1996), and inner-city women (Sikkema et al., 2000). Given the success of the natural opinion leader program in the United States, the **National Institute of Mental Health (NIMH)** sponsored a large, five-country trial of the program. The participating countries were China, India, Peru, Russia, and Zimbabwe. More than 18,147 research subjects from 138 venues participated overall. While participants in the intervention condition received the peer opinion leader intervention program, those in the comparison condition were provided educational materials in the form of brochures and pamphlets, as well as information about and access to voluntary counseling and testing.

Unfortunately, across the sample the difference between participants in the intervention and comparison conditions was not statistically significant at follow-up (NIMH Collaborative HIV/STD Prevention Trial Group, 2010). However, it was because there was positive change in both groups, not because no change occurred at all. In fact, both groups reported significant and clinically relevant reductions in unprotected sex (30%) and in STD incidence (20%). These similar results were surprising. The authors provide several plausible explanations, including the fact that the participants in the comparison condition actually received an intervention (which included a community-wide educational intervention, HIV/STD counseling and testing, and an interview during which they were asked to reflect on their own HIV risk behaviors) that was deemed more effective than the typical "standard of care" program. While you could argue that this is a more rigorous test of the experimental intervention, it actually compares the effectiveness of the two programs instead of conducting an independent test to see whether the natural opinion leader program works.

Intimate Partner Violence

Understanding the problem of dating violence among teens in the United States, researchers at the University of North Carolina developed a theory-based intervention targeting young adolescents (Foshee et al., 1998). This program, *Safe Dates*, is designed to (a) prevent the initiation of psychological, physical, or sexual intimate partner violence and (b) reduce or eliminate the incidence of on-going violence by providing skills and social support. The program includes both school- and community-based activities. School activities include a peer-led play, a 10-unit

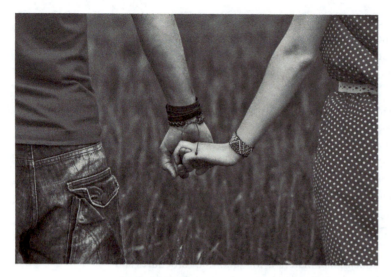

curriculum, and a poster contest. At the community level, training in dating violence for community service providers and a crisis line, support groups, and informational materials for parents are offered. In a randomized controlled trial, 14 schools were assigned to either the intervention or comparison condition. While students in the intervention schools received both the school- and community-level programs, students in the comparison schools received only the community-level services. At follow-up, students in the intervention condition who had never experienced partner violence were less likely to report psychological abuse perpetration than were students in the comparison condition. For those students who reported experiencing violence at baseline, those in the intervention condition reported less psychological abuse and sexual violence perpetration at follow-up. The CDC is currently conducting additional intervention effectiveness and implementation feasibility trials of *Safe Dates*. They are also examining the economic cost of program delivery. If all of the evaluation outcomes are positive, it is likely they will recommend *Safe Dates* as a program that can help prevent dating violence (both perpetration and victimization) among adolescents.

CONFLICTS IN RESEARCH ON RISKY BEHAVIOR PREVENTION

In this section, we want to highlight two issues that are important in research that seeks to design interventions to reduce risky behavior prevention. These are methodological issues and, frankly, they're important to any research that develops and tests interventions. The first issue is choosing the appropriate comparison group, and the second issue is testing competing theoretical explanations.

Well-designed research needs to provide a rigorous but fair test of any intervention. In research design, we have choices among different kinds of groups to which to compare an intervention. We could compare adolescents receiving our intervention to adolescents who receive absolutely nothing (a true "control" group), to adolescents who receive "standard of care" (or what currently is being offered), or to some other experimental program maybe in a "head-to-head" competition. The Zimmerman et al. (2008) study, for example, modified an existing effective curriculum to make it higher in sensation value and tested the modified curriculum against the standard version. Similarly, in the five-country trial of the peer opinion leader intervention (NIMH Collaborative HIV/STD Prevention Trial Group, 2010), both the experimental and comparison interventions provided education and social support, just in different formats. In both of these studies, researchers found no differences between the effects of the experimental and comparison interventions. It wasn't that the experimental versions did not work, they just didn't work *better than* the comparison programs. Testing a new program against an existing successful program is a perfectly reasonable research design, and in fact, it allows researchers to be sensitive to the ethical imperative to provide critical health information to all research participants. Our point is that research design needs to be very sensitive to the goals of the study and be able to detect intervention effects when they are present.

Arguably the most intriguing scientific research is that which tests competing theoretical explanations for effects. We know *that* something happens, but *why* precisely is it happening? In research using AMIE to guide message design to attract and hold the attention of HSS, we have just such a situation. As we mentioned earlier, according to AMIE message features act as a source of stimulation that can help audience members meet their optimal level of arousal; therefore, effectively targeted messages can attract and hold the attention of a target audience. Attention is just the first step of the persuasion process, however. Some theoretical perspectives suggest that "flashy" message features may compromise message processing, acting as distractors that would impede the ability to centrally process message arguments (ELM; Petty & Cacioppo, 1986) or as drains on limited cognitive resources that would reduce the ability to encode and store message arguments (Lang, 2000). In both of these cases, message receivers would be less likely to counter-argue the persuasive messages and, therefore, more likely to accept them. Same outcome; different theoretical explanation. We do not currently have a definitive answer to this question, but it is one in which scholars are very interested.

DIRECTIONS FOR FUTURE RESEARCH

There is reluctance in the United States to directly confront issues related to adolescent risk, particularly risky sexual behavior. Part of the reluctance is due to the "kids will be kids" viewpoint, which tacitly concedes that any strategies proposed to reduce risky behavior are doomed to failure. Another perspective could be defined as the "see no problem, treat no problem" denialist approach, which promotes stating the rules and then condemning those who break them. The prevention research perspective takes the stance that risky behavior can be prevented and that well-designed interdisciplinary

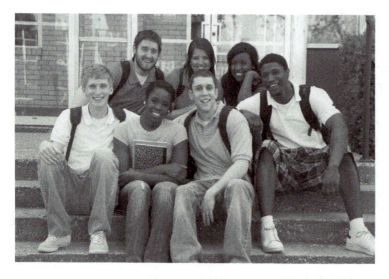

research can show us the best way to do so.

Researchers in health communication need to continue to advance the study of adolescent and young adult risk behavior and how to prevent it, including (a) understanding the underlying motivation(s), (b) developing prevention and treatment messages, interventions, or systemic strategies grounded in theory and sound methodology, and (c) contributing to public policy discussions that continue to advocate for communication-based approaches to dealing with poor decision making and conflict. For instance, studies that examine whether there is a direct link between sensation seeking and cyberbullying or intimate partner violence would be a contribution in that it would help in understanding how to design the most effective prevention messages, including content, format, and channel. Continued research to demonstrate that exposure to interventions such as those described in this chapter lead to improved health outcomes, not to increased risk, are critical in persuading our leaders to continue to fund prevention science and health education.

CONCLUSION

This chapter has provided an overview of four risk behaviors and their potential consequences. In addition, we have covered a number of theories that researchers use to inform prevention interventions and have provided examples of effective programs. To maximize scarce resources and have the greatest impact on the target audience, educators and policy makers need to select evidence-based programs that have strong theoretical bases and have been tested using appropriate scientific methods and statistical procedures.

DISCUSSION QUESTIONS

1. Describe self-efficacy. What theory did it originate from and how is it important in prevention interventions? What communication strategies can you think of to improve self-efficacy? What theories can inform these strategies?

2. Why do you think that natural opinion leaders were effective in delivering prevention messages in gay bars? Describe another situation where you think natural opinion leaders might be effective.
3. Watch a public service announcement on television. Do you think it was good? Why? Why not? Would it appeal to high sensation seekers?
4. What is an evidence-based intervention? Why is it important to adopt evidence-based interventions? What factors might you need to consider in adopting an evidence-based intervention?
5. Do you think cyberbullying might have played a role in causing Tyler Clementi to take his life? How might friends and acquaintances respond if they know someone who is the victim of cyberbullying?

IN-CLASS ACTIVITIES

1. Develop (individually or in small groups) a PSA script about the negative consequences of drinking and driving, tailoring it to the needs of a high sensation seeker OR develop a PSA script promoting safer sex (abstinence, being faithful to one's partner, or condom use) that includes a message that relies on self-efficacy (*I am capable of performing this action*) or behavioral intentions *(I plan to do or not to do a specific activity tonight or sometime in the future)*. Share these with the class.
2. Bullying is a serious problem in the United States. In small groups, have the students share ideas and strategies for addressing the problem of bullying online and offline, as well as in and out of school.

RECOMMENDED READINGS

Hecht, M. L., & Miller-Day, M. (2007). The drug resistance strategies project as translational research. *Journal of Applied Communication Research, 35*, 343–349.

This article is a good example of translational research.

Lee, J. K., & Hecht, M. L. (2011). Examining the protective effects of brand equity in the *keepin' it REAL* substance use prevention curriculum. *Health Communication, 26*, 605–614.

This article demonstrates how a communication strategy (branding) can be important in public health interventions.

Foshee, V., Bauman, K., Arriaga, I., Helms, R., Koch, G., & Linder, G. (1998). An evaluation of *Safe Dates*, an adolescent dating violence prevention program. *American Journal of Public Health, 88*(1), 45–50.

This article provides both a good description of a randomized controlled trial and describes both a school-based and a community-wide intervention.

REFERENCES

Ajzen, I., & Madden, T. (1986). The prediction of goal directed behavior: Attitudes, intentions, and perceived behavioral control. *Journal of Experimental Social Psychology*, *22*, 453–474.

Atwood, K.A., Kennedy, S.B., Shamblen, S. Teglee, J., & Shannon, F. (2012) Impact of school based HIV prevention program in post-conflict Liberia. *AIDS Education and Prevention*, *24*(1), 67–76.

Bandura, A. (1977). *Social learning theory*. Englewood Cliffs, NJ: Prentice-Hall.

Bandura, A. (1986). *Social foundations of thought and action: A social cognitive theory*. Englewood Cliffs, NJ: Prentice-Hall.

Botvin, G., Eng, A., & Williams, C. (1980). Preventing the onset of cigarette smoking through life skills training. *Preventive Medicine*, *9*(1), 135–143.

Botvin, G. J., & Kantor, L. W. (2000). Preventing alcohol and tobacco use through life skills training. *Alcohol Research and Health*, *24*(4), 250–257.

CDC. (2012a). Trends in HIV-related risk behaviors among high school students – United States, 1991–2011. *Morbidity and Mortality Weekly Report*, *61*, 556–560

CDC. (2012b). *Sexually Transmitted Disease Surveillance 2011*. Atlanta: U.S. Department of Health and Human Services.

CDC. (2012c). *HIV and young men who have sex with men*. Atlanta: Division of Adolescent and School Health.

CDC. (2012d). *Teen pregnancy*. Atlanta, GA: Division of Reproductive Health. Retrieved from http://www.cdc.gov/teenpregnancy/aboutteenpreg.htm

CDC. (2012e). *Understanding intimate partner violence factsheet*. Atlanta, GA: Division of Injury Prevention and Control. Retrieved from http://www.cdc.gov/violenceprevention/pdf/ipv_factsheet2012-a.pdf

CDC. (2012f). *Understanding teen dating violence factsheet*. Atlanta, GA: Division of Injury Prevention and Control. Retrieved from http://www.cdc.gov/violenceprevention/pdf/ipv_factsheet2012-a.pdf

CDC. (2013a). *HIV among women factsheet*. Atlanta, GA: Division of HIV/AIDS. Retrieved from http://www.cdc.gov/hiv/topics/women/index.htm

CDC. (2013b). *The National Intimate Partner and Sexual Violence Survey*. Atlanta, GA.. Division of Injury Prevention and Control. Retrieved from http://www.cdc.gov/violenceprevention/nisvs

Dehue, F., Bolman, C., & Vollink, T. (2008). Cyberbullying: Youngsters' experiences and parental perception. *CyberPsychology & Behavior*, *11*, 217–223.

Donohew, L. (1990). Public health campaigns: Individual message strategies and a model. In E. B. Ray & L. Donohew (Eds.), *Communication and health: Systems and applications* (pp. 136–152). Hillsdale, NJ: Erlbaum.

Donohew, L., Lorch, E., & Palmgreen, P. (1991). Sensation seeking and targeting of televised anti-drug PSAs. In L. Donohew, H. Sypher, & W. Bukoski (Eds.), *Persuasive communication and drug abuse prevention* (pp. 209–226). Hillsdale, NJ: Erlbaum.

Donohew, L., Lorch, E., & Palmgreen, P. (1998). Applications of a theoretic model of information exposure to health interventions. *Human Communication Research, 24,* 454–468.

Donohew, L., Nair, M., & Finn, S. (1984). Automaticity, arousal, and information exposure. In R. Bostrom (Ed.), *Communication yearbook 8* (pp. 267–284). Newbury Park, CA: Sage.

Fishbein, M. (2000). The role of theory in HIV prevention. *AIDS Care, 12,* 273–278.

Fishbein, M., & Ajzen, I. (1975). *Belief, attitude, intention, and behavior: An introduction to theory and research.* Reading, MA: Addison-Wesley.

Fleming, C. B., Catalano, R. F., Haggerty, K. P., & Abbott, R. D. (2010). Relationships between level and change in family, school, and peer factors during two periods of adolescence and problem behavior at age 19. *Journal of Youth and Adolescence, 39,* 670–682.

Foshee, V., Bauman, K., Arriaga, I., Helms, R., Koch, G., & Linder, G. (1998). An evaluation of *Safe Dates,* an adolescent dating violence prevention program. *American Journal of Public Health, 88*(1), 45–50.

Garcia-Moreno, C., Jansen, H. A. F. M., Ellsberg, M., Heise, L., & Watts, C. (2006). Prevalence of intimate partner violence: Findings from the WHO multi-country study on women's health and domestic violence. *The Lancet, 368,* 1260–1269.

Gender Based Violence Area of Responsibility Working Group. (2010). *Handbook for coordinating gender based violence in humanitarian settings.* Retrieved from http://gbvaor.net/wp-content/uploads/2012/10/Handbook-for-Coordinating-Gender-based-Violence-in-Humanitarian-Settings-GBV-AoR–2010-ENGLISH.pdf

Hecht, M. L., Colby, M., & Miller-Day, M. (2007). The dissemination of keepin' it REAL through D.A.R.E. America: A lesson in disseminating health messages. *Health Communication, 25,* 585–586.

Hecht, M. L., & Miller-Day, M. (2007). The drug resistance strategies project as translational research. *Journal of Applied Communication Research, 35,* 343–349.

Hoffman, S. D. (2008). *Kids having kids: Economic costs and social consequences of teen pregnancy.* Washington, DC: The Urban Institute Press.

Hoyle, R. H., Fejfar, M. C, & Miller, J. D. (2000). Personality and sexual risk taking: A quantitative review. *Journal of Personality, 68,* 1203–1231.

Hoyle, R. H., Stephenson, M. T., Palmgreen, P., Lorch, E. P., & Donohew, R. L. (2002). Reliability and validity of a brief measure of sensation seeking. *Personality and Individual Differences, 32,* 401–414.

Jemmott, J. B. (1992). Reductions in HIV risk-associated sexual behaviors among black male adolescents: Effects of an AIDS prevention intervention. *American Journal of Public Health, 82*(3), 372–377.

Jemmott, J. B., Jemmott, L. S., Braverman, P. K. & Fong, G. T. (2005). HIV/STD risk reduction interventions for African American and Latino adolescent girls at an adolescent medicine clinic. *Archives of Pediatric Adolescent Medicine, 159,* 440–449.

Jemmott, J. B., Jemmott, L. S. & Fong, G. T. (1998). Abstinence and safer sex HIV risk-reduction interventions for African American adolescents. *JAMA, 279*(19), 1529–1536.

Jessor, R. (1998). *New perspectives on adolescent risk behavior*. Cambridge: Cambridge University Press.

Johnston, L. D., O'Malley, P. M., Bachman, J. G., & Schulenberg, J. E. (2009). *Monitoring the Future national survey results on drug use, 1975–2009: Volume II – College students and adults ages 19–50 (NIH Publication No. 09–7403)*. Bethesda, MD: National Institute on Drug Abuse.

Johnston, L. D., O'Malley, P. M., Bachman, J. G., & Schulenberg, J. E. (2013). *Monitoring theFFuture national results on drug use: 2012 overview, key findings on adolescent drug use*. Ann Arbor: Institute for Social Research at The University of Michigan.

Kegeles, S. M., Hays, R. B., & Coates, T. J. (1996). The MPowerment Project: a community-level HIV prevention intervention for young gay men. *American Journal of Public Health, 86*, 1129–1136.

Kelly, J. A. (2004). Popular opinion leaders and HIV prevention peer education: Resolving discrepant findings, and implications for the development of effective community programmes. *AIDS Care, 16*(2), 139–150.

Kelly, J. A., Murphy, D. A., Sikkema, K. J., McAuliffe, T. L., Roffman, R.A., Soloman, L. J., Winett, R., & Kalichman, S. C., (1997). Randomized, controlled, community-level HIV prevention intervention for sexual risk behaviour among homosexual men in U.S. Community HIV Prevention Research Collaborative. *The Lancet, 350*, 1500–1505.

Kirby, D., Barth, R., Leland, N., & Fetro, J. (1991). *Reducing the Risk:* Impact of a new curriculum on sexual risk taking. *Family Planning Perspectives, 23*(6), 253–263.

Kowalski, R. M., & Limber, P. (2007). Electronic bullying among middle school students. *Journal of Adolescent Health, 41*, S22–S30.

Lang, A. (2000). The limited capacity model of mediated message processing. *Journal of Communication, 50*, 46–70.

LeBlanc, J. C. (2012). *Cyberbullying and suicide: A retrospective analysis of 22 cases*. Paper presented at the 2012 meeting of the American Academy of Pediatrics National Conference and Exhibition, New Orleans, LA.

Lee, J. K. & Hecht, M. L. (2011). Examining the protective effects of brand equity in the *keepin' it REAL* substance use prevention curriculum. *Health Communication, 26*, 605–614.

Li, Q. (2007). Bullying in the new playground: Research into cyberbullying and cyber victimization. *Australasian Journal of Educational Technology, 23*, 435–454.

Miller, R. L., Klotz, D., & Eckholdt, H. M. (1998). HIV prevention with male prostitutes and patrons of hustler bars: replication of an HIV prevention intervention. *American Journal of Community Psychology, 26*, 97–131.

Millett, G., Flores, F., Peterson, J. L., & Bakeman, R. (2007). Explaining disparities in HIV infection among black and white men who have sex with men: a meta-analysis of HIV risk behaviors. *AIDS, 21*, 2083–2091.

NIMH Collaborative HIV/STD Prevention Trial Group. (2010). Results of the NIMH Collaborative HIV/STD Prevention Trial of a Community Popular Opinion Leader Intervention. *Journal of Acquired Immune Deficiency Syndrome, 54*(2), 204–214.

Palmer, R. H. C., Young, S. E., Hopfer, C. J., Corley, R. P., Stallings, M. C., Crowley, T. J., & Hewitt, J. K. (2009). Developmental epidemiology of drug use and abuse in adolescence and young adulthood: Evidence of generalized risk. *Drug and Alcohol Dependence, 102,* 78–87.

Palmgreen, P., & Donohew, L. (2010). Impact of SENTAR on prevention campaign policy and practice. *Health Communication, 25,* 609–610.

Palmgreen, P., Donohew, L., Lorch, E. P., Hoyle, R. H., & Stephenson, M. T. (2001). Television campaigns and adolescent marijuana use: Tests of sensation seeking targeting. *American Journal of Public Health, 91*(2), 292–296.

Patchin, J. W., & Hinduja, S. (2010). Cyberbullying and self-esteem. *Journal of School Health, 80*(12), 614–621.

Patchin, J., & Hinduja, S. (2011). Traditional and nontraditional bullying among youth: A test of general strain theory. *Youth and Society, 43*(2), 727–751.

Perloff, R. (2001). *Persuading people to have safer sex.* Mahwah, NJ: Erlbaum.

Perper, K., Peterson, K., & Manlove, J. (2010). Diploma attainment among teen mothers. *Child Trends, Fact Sheet,* Publication #2010–01: Washington, DC: Child Trends.

Petty, R. E., & Cacioppo, J. T. (1986). *Communication and persuasion: Central and peripheral routes to attitude change.* New York, NY: Springer-Verlag.

Pew Internet & American Life Project (2013). *Demographics of internet users.* Retrieved February 1, 2013, from http://www.pewinternet.org

Planned Parenthood Federation of America (2012). *Pregnancy and childbearing among U.S. teens.* New York. Retrieved from http://www.plannedparenthood.org/files/PPFA/pregnancy_and_childbearing.pdf

Roberto, A. J., & Eden, J. (2010). Cyberbullying: Aggressive communication in the digital age. In T. A. Avtgis & A. S. Rancer (Eds.), Arguments, aggression, and conflict: New directions in theory and research (pp. 198–216). New York: Routledge.

Roberto, A. J., Eden, J., Savage, M., Ramos-Salazar, L., & Deiss, D. (2014). Prevalence and predictors of cyberbullying perpetration by high school seniors. *Communication Quarterly, 67,* 97–114.

Roberto, A. J., Meyer, G., Boster, F. J., & Roberto, H. L. (2003). Adolescents' decisions about verbal and physical aggression. *Human Communication Research, 29*(1), 135–147.

Rogers, E. M. (1983). *Diffusion of innovations.* New York: Free Press.

Sampson, R. (2002). Acquaintance rape of college students. Problem Oriented Guides for Police, Series 17. Washington, DC: U.S. Department of Justice.

Savage, M. W., & Deiss, D. M. (2010, November). *Sticks and stones might break my bones, but typed words will really hurt me: Testing a cyberbullying victimization intervention.* Paper presented at the 96th annual National Communication Association Convention, San Francisco, CA.

Schulz, K., Altman, D., Moher, D. & the CONSORT Group (2010). CONSORT 2010 Statement: updated guidelines for reporting parallel group randomized trials. *BMC Medicine, 8*(18), 2–9.

Sikkema, K. J., Kelly, J. A., Winett, R. A., Solomon, L. J., Cargill, V. A., Roffman, R.A., . . . Mercer, M. B. (2000). Outcomes of a randomized community-level HIV prevention intervention for women living in 18 low income housing developments. *American Journal of Public Health, 90,* 57–63.

Smith, P. K., Mahdavi, J., Carvalho, M., Fisher, S., Russell, S., & Tippett, N. (2008). Cyber-bullying: Its nature and impact in secondary school pupils. *Journal of Child Psychology and Psychiatry*, *49*, 376–385.

Stephenson, M. T. (2003). Mass media targeting high sensation seekers: What works and why. *American Journal of Health Behavior*, *3*, 233–239.

Volkow, N. (2010). *Drugs, brains, and behavior: the science of addiction* (NIH Pub No. 105605). Bethesda, MD: National Institute on Drug Abuse.

Wong, F., Huang, J., DiGangi, J., Thompson, E., & Smith, B. (2008). Gender differences in intimate partner violence on substance abuse, sexual risks, and depression among a sample of South Africans in Cape Town, South Africa. *AIDS Education and Prevention*, *20*(1), 56–64.

Ybarra, M. L., & Mitchell, K. J. Wolak, J. & Finkelhor, D. (2006). Examining characteristics and associated distress related to Internet harassment: Findings from the Second Youth Internet Safety Survey. *JAMA*, *118*(4), 1169–77.

Zimmerman, R. S., Cupp, P. K., Donohew, L., Sionean, C. K, Feist-Price, S., & Helme, D. (2008). Effects of a school-based theory driven HIV and pregnancy prevention curriculum. *Perspective on Sexual and Reproductive Health*, *40*(1), 42–51.

Zuckerman, M. (1979). *Sensation seeking: Beyond the optimal level of arousal*. Hillsdale, NJ: Erlbaum.

Zuckerman, M., Kolin, E., Price, L., & Zoob, I. (1964). Development of a sensation seeking scale. *Journal of Consulting Psychology*, *28*, 477–482.

Mental Health and Illness

*Nancy Grant Harrington and
Ashley P. Duggan*

I feel sad and rejected and I can't concentrate in my studies. I find faults in all the people around me and I feel lonely and alone. I blame people around me for my sadness; I soak my pillow with tears. I leave my school for home and miss my lectures. I look moody all day and I don't answer my phone calls and avoid friends.
Joy, 19–24-year-old female patient

Anxiety has affected my life in such a way that I can no longer go outside for long periods of time. I also have difficulty sleeping because I try to concentrate on fighting it off and yes you can fight it off but it really depends on the person and symptoms. I've also had anxiety attacks far away from home, and I didn't know what to do. I'm 23 and I'm too young for this to disrupt everything so early in life. I tell my friends that I'm always suffering and sick but, they just say suck it up buddy lets go out and have some fun it's all in your head. What people don't seem to realize is how bad anxiety can truly be until they get it if at all.
Al, 19–24-year-old male patient

I began having an eating disorder when I was 14. I'm going to be 17 in two weeks and I still find myself sometimes struggling. I was anorexic/purge and restrictive type. I used to cut myself due to emotional issues I did not face. Last year, I went to treatment and now I have a new perspective of life. Although I still struggle sometimes, I find myself much, much happier. I am at a healthy goal weight and I no longer feel like I have to hurt myself. To girls with eating disorders or those who are thinking about purging, restricting, or cutting: It may seem worth it now, but in the end, I can promise you it will be your biggest regret. It is a disease. Don't test the hands of fate. Seek help.

StayingStrong, 13–18-year-old female patient

These quotes come from young people who have various forms of mental illness. They share their experiences on MedicineNet.com, a website that provides medical information on a host of physical and mental illnesses. Through reading their comments, you can get a sense of the pain and suffering they go through because of their mental illness. They are not alone.

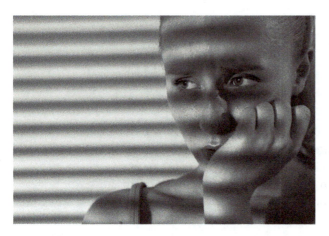

Mental illness affects literally billions of people worldwide. It is defined as any diagnosable disorder that impairs a person's mood, thoughts, and/or behaviors (Centers for Disease Control and Prevention [CDC], 2013). Mental illness can impair a person's ability to establish and maintain satisfying friend and family relationships and the ability to function effectively in the workplace. It also is related to chronic physical illness such as heart disease and diabetes, and it can even lead to premature death. In the United States alone, the cost of mental illness to society is estimated to be approximately $300 billion (CDC, 2013).

Mental illness can affect anyone, from children to the elderly. Manifestation of mental illness can occur at any point along a person's life course, depending on the illness. Attention-deficit/hyperactivity disorder, for example, typically appears in childhood;

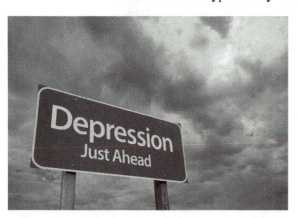

schizophrenia appears in young adulthood; dementia most often manifests in the elderly. Approximately 25% of the American adult population suffers from some form of mental illness at any given time, and nearly 50% will be affected at some point during their lifetime (CDC, 2013). Mood disorders such as anxiety and depression are the most common form (CDC, 2013). These days, mental illness among college students is of particular concern, with increased demand for services being seen on college campuses across the nation (Watkins, Hunt, & Eisenberg, 2011).

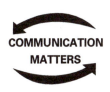

Mental Health Resources: Where to Get Help

NIMH Resources: http://www.nimh.nih.gov/health/topics/depression/index.shtml

Here you can find a description of several mental illnesses, including the causes, signs and symptoms, risk factors, diagnosis, treatments, and what to do to get help. There is also information on clinical trials.

Web MD Health Centers: http://www.webmd.com/

Under "Health A-Z," you can click on any one of numerous health conditions, including mental illnesses, to find a tremendous variety of resources to help with diagnosis and treatment, finding sources of support, and healthy living. The site even has videos that illustrate what various conditions, such as depression, look like.

American Mental Health Counselors Association: http://www.amhca.org/

Here you can find resources connected to mental health counseling. This organization focuses on counseling in mental health as a specific context rather than counseling more generally.

Your College's or University's Student Health Center

Check with your instructor to find out where on campus students can go for mental health services.

In this chapter, we address mental health and illness. As you can imagine, there is a tremendous amount of research on communication and mental illness, not just within the communication discipline but also across numerous other disciplines such as psychology, nursing, medicine, and social work. This work reflects multiparadigmatic perspectives, with research from scientific, interpretive, and critical–cultural traditions. In our review, we'll be focusing on research from the scientific and interpretive perspectives. We'll begin with some basic conceptual issues and then move on to consider research on how mental illness is portrayed in the media and how it affects communication in interpersonal relationships. We'll also address approaches to treatment of mental disorders.

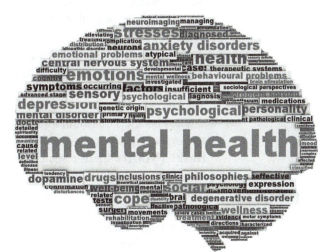

PARADIGMATIC APPROACHES TO THE STUDY OF MENTAL HEALTH AND ILLNESS

Research from the scientific paradigm investigates observable/measurable variables associated with the incidence, prevalence, and impact of mental illness. Research from the interpretive paradigm focuses on uncovering and understanding the subjective, situated meanings of mental illness and related behavior.

Before we begin, though, we want to make two very important observations: First, whereas physical illness may or may not have a direct impact on communication, most mental illnesses do have such a direct impact, which makes the topic especially important to communication scholars. If you have ever communicated with someone suffering from depression or social anxiety, for example, or if you suffer from such a disorder yourself, you'll know what we're talking about. Second, because human beings are social animals, communication is directly relevant to establishing and maintaining good mental health and preventing and treating mental illness (Fisher et al., 2012). Keep these points in mind as you consider the research we present in this chapter.

CONCEPTUAL ISSUES IN MENTAL HEALTH AND ILLNESS

The ways we understand mental illness and its symptoms, causes, and treatments comes from research. Even if we have firsthand experience with symptoms of mental illness, research shapes our understanding of the symptoms by giving us language for diagnosis and explanation. In addition, we understand mental health treatment from health education programs, policies, and materials that also are connected to research. Research to define mental health and illness is often sponsored or funded by large government organizations such as the **National Institutes of Health** (NIH). In addition to funding research across multiple disciplines, such as communication, psychology, and neurology, divisions of NIH share research findings and produce detailed booklets on health topics that affect individual people or segments of groups within the larger population. One division of NIH, the **National Institute of Mental Health (NIMH),** funds research on mental health and illness and produces summary documents that provide credible sources of information on the different forms of mental illness, signs and symptoms, causes and treatment, and suggestions for how to find help, either for a family member or friend or for yourself. In Table 10.1, we present major categories of mental disorders and provide brief descriptions. You can find more information at http://www.nimh.nih.gov

Table 10.1 Categories of Mental Illnesses

Disorder	Description
Anxiety disorders	
Agoraphobia	Fear of any place or situation where escape might be difficult.
Generalized Anxiety Disorder (GAD)	Excessive, exaggerated anxiety and worry about everyday life events for no obvious reason.
Obsessive Compulsive Disorder (OCD)	The need to check things repeatedly or the tendency to have certain thoughts or perform routines and rituals repeatedly, causing distress and interfering with daily life.
Panic Disorder	Fear of disaster or of losing control when there is no real danger.
Post-Traumatic Stress Disorder (PTSD)	A mental disorder triggered by a disturbing outside event that leads to psychological and biological changes, resulting in an impaired "flight or fight" response.
Social Phobia	Fear of being humiliated in public.
Specific Phobia	Fear and avoidance of a specific object or situation.
Attention-Deficit/ Hyperactivity Disorder	Extreme inattentiveness, hyperactivity, and impulsiveness that interfere with the ability to function effectively in daily life.
Autism Spectrum Disorder (ASD)	A developmental brain disorder, ranging from mild impairment to severe disability, associated with difficulty communicating with and relating to other people.
Dementia/Alzheimer's Disease	Significant global loss of cognitive abilities such as attention, memory, language, logical reasoning, and problem-solving severe enough to interfere with social or occupational functioning.
Eating Disorders	
Anorexia Nervosa	Intense fear of gaining weight, associated with severely restricted food intake and extreme weight loss.
Binge Eating Disorder	Uncontrollable eating and associated weight gain.
Bulimia Nervosa	Eating a large amount of food in a short time followed by purging the body of food, usually through vomiting or laxative use.
Mood Disorders	
Bipolar Disorder	Brain disorder that causes unusual shifts in mood, energy, activity levels, and the ability to carry out day-to-day tasks.
Dysthymic Disorder	Chronic, mild depression.
Major Depressive Disorder	Feelings of intense sadness, hopelessness, worthlessness, and fatigue, and diminished interest or pleasure in almost all activities; depression increases risk of suicide.

(Continued)

Table 10.1 Continued

Disorder	Description
Personality Disorders	
Antisocial Personality Disorder	Disregard for social rules and cultural norms, impulsive behavior, and indifference to the rights and feelings of others.
Avoidant Personality Disorder	Extreme social inhibition, sensitivity to negative evaluation, and feelings of inadequacy.
Borderline Personality Disorder	Problems with regulating emotions and thoughts, maintaining stable relationships, and engaging in impulsive behavior.
Schizophrenia	Chronic, severe, and disabling brain disorder whose symptoms include distorted thoughts and hallucinations.

Compiled from NIMH, http://www.nimh.nih.gov/statistics/index.shtml; CDC, http://www.cdc.gov/mental-health/basics/mental-illness.htm; and WebMD, http://www.webmd.com

The terminology we use to discuss mental health and illness matters because how we label something bestows meaning. Communication students know this all too well. So, should we talk about mental health, with an emphasis on health promotion and illness prevention, or should we talk about mental illness, with an emphasis on diagnosis and treatment? When we refer to someone in a diagnostic sense, do we refer to a mentally ill person or a person who is mentally ill? For example, do we refer to a schizophrenic or a person with schizophrenia? A person with borderline personality disorder or a narcissist? The language we choose will emphasize either the person or the disorder, and emphasizing the disorder has considerable implications for stigma (Shattell, 2009).

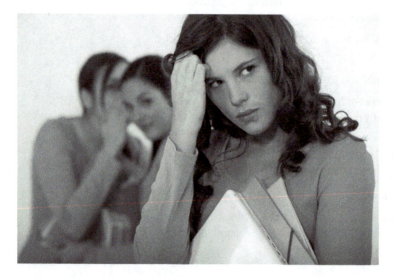

Indeed, **stigma** is a huge concern in mental illness. The concept of stigma as studied in the social sciences stems from the work of Erving Goffman, a sociologist. Goffman (1963) argued that stigma resulted from a person's possessing a "deeply discrediting" characteristic that makes that person different from what the community considers normal in terms of physical characteristics, personal traits, or group membership. Within the communication discipline, Rachel Smith developed a model of stigma communication that describes how messages (a) identify and categorize people as stigmatized, (b) suggest that stigmatized people pose risks to others, and (c) imply that stigmatized people are responsible for their stigma. These messages then lead to negative cognitive and emotional reactions in others. These negative reactions in turn result in negative attitude and stereotype formation, sharing of stigma messages within the community, and rejection of the stigmatized people (Smith, 2007).

STIGMA AND MENTAL ILLNESS

Smith's (2007) model of stigma communication describes how messages (a) identify and categorize people as stigmatized, (b) suggest that stigmatized people pose risks to others, and (c) imply that stigmatized people are responsible for their stigma. These messages lead to negative cognitive and emotional reactions, which result in negative attitude and stereotype formation, sharing of stigma messages within the community, and rejection of the stigmatized people. The World Health Organization is working to reduce mental illness stigma worldwide.

If you've ever felt stigmatized because you are "different" for some reason, you know how painful and limiting stigma can be. The problem is particularly pronounced with mental illness. Indeed, in its 2001 report "Mental Health: New Understanding, New Hope," the **World Health Organization** (WHO) presented a comprehensive review of the burden of mental illness worldwide, discussed approaches to prevention and treatment, and addressed policy and service provision implications (WHO, 2001). The report also offered 10 recommendations for next steps and presented specific strategies depending on the level of resources available. Many of the strategies addressed the reduction of stigma around mental health. As Director General Dr. Gro Harlem Brundtland wrote, "As the world's leading public health agency, WHO has one, and only one option—to ensure that ours will be the last generation that allows shame and stigma to rule over science and reason" (WHO, 2001, p. x).

MEDIA PORTRAYALS AND REPORTING OF MENTAL ILLNESS

Unfortunately, reducing the burden of stigma surrounding mental illness is particularly challenging in light of its portrayal in the media. Extensive research within the scientific paradigm documents the extent to which the mentally ill and aspects of mental illness are portrayed negatively in print, advertising, television, and film.

(Chapter 13 also covers media images of health.) As Stuart (2006) observed, "People with mental disorders and their families are acutely aware of negative images of mental illness in the entertainment and news media. Most directly blame the media, citing images linking mental illness to violence as a central source of stigma" (p. 102). Let's take a closer look at the images of mental illness in the media.

Pirkis, Blood, Francis, and McCallum (2006) conducted an extensive review of the literature on how mental illness is portrayed in fictional film and television. They asked three research questions:

1. What is the extent and nature of portrayal of mental illness in fictional film and television programs?
2. Is there evidence that portrayal of mental illness in fictional films and television programs can have harmful effects?
3. Is there evidence that portrayal of mental illness in fictional films and television programs can have positive effects? (p. 524)

The researchers identified 71 publications and categorized them according to which research question(s) the articles could answer (some articles could answer more than one of the research questions). They also classified the articles as reporting "small-scale descriptive studies, anecdotal reports, and commentaries," "larger-scale descriptive studies," or "larger-scale experimental studies." The numbers and percentages of articles across categories appear in Table 10.2.

As you can see, most of the studies were of the smaller, descriptive variety, and most addressed how mental illness was portrayed. Relatively few studies considered the positive effects of portrayals of mental illness, and there were only five experimental studies, all of which explored the negative effects of the portrayal of mental illness in film and on television.

Table 10.2 Categorization of Literature Reviewed by Pirkis et al. (2006)

Research Question	Small-scale Study	Larger-scale Descriptive Study	Larger-scale Experimental Study	Total[a]
Extent of Portrayal	24 (33.8%)	17 (23.9%)	0 (0.0%)	41 (57.7%)
Negative Effects	13 (18.3%)	8 (11.3%)	5 (7.0%)	26 (36.6%)
Positive Effects	16 (22.5%)	2 (2.8%)	0 (0.0%)	18 (25.3%)

[a]Column totals more than 100% because 14 studies were classified in more than one category.

In terms of how mental illness was portrayed, Pirkis et al. (2006) wrote, "Overwhelmingly, studies in this area have shown that such portrayal is negative, and perpetuates stereotypes about mental illness" (p. 528). Drawing on the research they reviewed, the authors provided a list of categories into which mentally ill persons could be classified based on how they appear in film and television: homicidal maniac, rebellious free spirit, enlightened member of society, female patient as seductress, narcissistic parasite, zoo specimen, simpleton, and "the failure" or victim. The names of these categories alone tell you that the characterizations of the mentally ill are biased and negative; although "rebellious free spirit" and "enlightened member of society" may sound positive, these descriptors hardly present an accurate portrayal of the mentally ill and instead cultivate misperceptions.

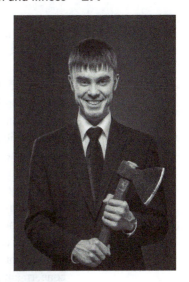

MEDIA IMAGES OF MENTAL ILLNESS

Extensive research documents the extent to which the mentally ill and aspects of mental illness are portrayed negatively in print, advertising, television, and film. Mentally ill people often are portrayed as violent and dangerous. Mental health professionals and treatments are depicted unrealistically. Communication campaigns can have positive effects on reducing stigma and encouraging people to seek help.

Mental health professionals also are portrayed in misleading ways. Again drawing on the research they reviewed, Pirkis et al. (2006) detailed how mental health professionals are categorized into one of five types: "Dr. Dippy," the comic character; "Dr. Evil," the sinister scientist; "Dr. Wonderful," who is perfect in every way, including being available for the patient 24/7; "Dr. Sexy," whose competence is related more to her (sexual) relationships with her patients than her competence as a medical professional; and the "rationalist foil," who relies on "scientific arguments and psychodynamic formulations to explain supernatural phenomena, only to be proved wrong as the plot unfolds" (Pirkis et al., 2006, p. 532).

It should come as no surprise that the treatment of mental illness also appears to be presented in a biased way in film and television. Pirkis et al. (2006) point out that "only those treatments that serve a filmic purpose are depicted" (p. 532). So, we see a whole lot of psychotherapy, which allows for character development, and a whole lot of electroconvulsive (ECT or "shock") therapy, which allows for high drama. Indeed, an in-depth study of how ECT has been portrayed revealed incredible inaccuracies—

including that the most common side-effect was being turned into a zombie (we kid you not; see Pirkis et al., 2006, p. 533).

In terms of finding evidence that portrayal of mental illness is related to harmful effects, Pirkis et al. (2006) found a great deal. Studies show that attitudes toward the mentally ill primarily stem from images in the media more so than real life experience and that fictional portrayals are more powerful than news reports. Further, there is some evidence for a "dose-response" effect, which means that the more people are exposed to media images of mental illness, the more negative their attitudes are. This effect may be moderated by the perceived realism of the portrayal (keeping in mind that perceived realism does not necessarily equate to actual realism). Equally pernicious is the possibility that inaccurate portrayal of mental health professionals and treatment for mental illness may influence willingness to seek treatment. Although there is not a great deal of empirical evidence for this, Pirkis et al. did find it to be a concern among several of the commentary articles they reviewed.

So are there any positive effects from the coverage of mental illness in fictional film and television? Well, the potential seems to be in using these media as either teaching tools or counseling tools. For example, such media can be used as a teaching tool for mental health professionals. Robinson's (2003) book *Reel Psychiatry: Movie Portrayals of Psychiatric Conditions* uses characters from films to present examples of diagnoses of various mental illnesses; importantly, the book "explicitly discusses the degree of accuracy of the given portrayal" (Pirkis et al., 2006, p. 535). Still, opinions on using films for instruction are divided, with some authors arguing that the potential for harmful effects of negative portrayals is just too great. The jury is actually out on this question, though, because there have been no evaluation studies of the effectiveness of using television and film in instruction of mental health professionals (Pirkis et al., 2006).

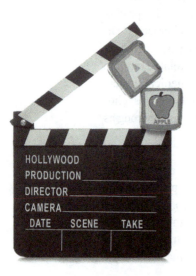

Another potential positive outcome can come from using film and television to complement psychotherapy for people with mental illness. Hesley and Hesley's (2001) book *Rent Two Films and Let's Talk in the Morning: Using Popular Movies in Psychotherapy* offers a list of films that therapists can use to prompt discussion with their clients. Once again, however, the effectiveness of using the films in therapy has not been evaluated (Pirkis et al., 2006).

An empirically supported example of how the media can have a positive impact on perceptions of mental illness comes from outside entertainment television and film: use of public communication campaigns designed to reduce stigma toward mental illness, increase **mental health literacy**, and encourage people to seek help. (Chapter 14 discusses campaigns in detail.) There are many examples of such campaigns across many countries, and they can, indeed, have a positive impact. For example, the "Like Minds, Like Mine" media campaign in New Zealand was effective in raising public awareness and improving attitudes toward mental illness (Vaughan & Hansen, 2004). Similarly, *beyondblue*, Australia's national initiative targeting depression, was associated with increased recognition of depression and improvements in the beliefs about the effectiveness of treatments for depression (Jorm, Christensen, & Griffiths, 2005). Our goal as communication researchers is to understand how to apply principles of message design to enhance the positive impact of such campaigns.

MENTAL ILLNESS AND COMMUNICATION IN RELATIONSHIPS

Our understanding of mental illness and communication in relationships can benefit from using a relational theoretical lens. A **relational lens** assumes that human understanding and behavior arise from our interactions with other people, particularly people in close relationships. Researchers from both scientific and interpretive paradigms can adopt a relational lens for understanding mental illness. The scientific paradigm considers the attitudinal and behavioral variables that are correlated with mental illness and the impact of these variables on mentally ill people and their relational partners. The interpretive paradigm strives to uncover and understand the subjective, situated meanings of mental illness and its impact within the context of a relationship. Let's explore the relational approach to studying mental illness more in depth by looking at research on depression.

UNDERSTANDING MENTAL ILLNESS THROUGH A RELATIONAL LENS

Researchers from both scientific and interpretive paradigms can adopt a relational lens for understanding mental illness. The scientific paradigm considers the attitudinal and behavioral variables that are correlated with mental illness and the impact of these variables on mentally ill people and their relational partners. The interpretive paradigm strives to uncover and understand the subjective, situated meanings of mental illness and its impact within the context of a relationship.

James C. Coyne, a professor of psychology in psychiatry, initially advanced the relational approach to understanding mental illness with his interpersonal theory of depression (Coyne, 1976). This theory asserts that devaluation and rejection by relationship partners may exacerbate depressive symptoms. More specifically, Coyne asserts that depressed people are rejected because they induce negative affect in their relationship partners through a process of emotional contagion, and he assumes that it is an irritating, negative experience to interact with depressed people. Because of this negative mood, relational partners would be expected to initially offer non-genuine reassurance and support and then reject and avoid the depressed person.

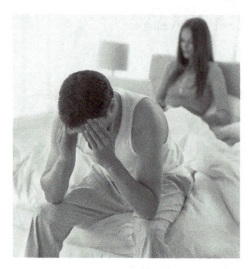

Depressed people appear to be well aware of this rejection, and they internalize further the negative mood state when negative interpersonal feedback occurs (Segrin, 1993). Previous research also suggests that although relationship partners may provide assurance to depressed people through verbal channels, they simultaneously convey devaluation and rejection through nonverbal channels (Coyne, 1976). In response to these subtle signs of rejection, depressed people seek higher levels of reassurance and exhibit higher levels of depressive behaviors, thus intensifying the depressive symptoms over time (Segrin, 1993).

Depressed people engage in more negative and less supportive communication with others and experience rejection from those in their social environment (Segrin, 1993; Segrin & Abramson, 1994). Although rejection is not necessarily the result of a negative mood induction in others (Segrin & Dillard, 1992), depressed people make more negative statements about themselves and their partners, and partners respond in turn with more negative feedback (Vettese & Mongrain, 2000). Similarly, depressed people use more aversive language in conversations (Strack & Coyne, 1983), receive less social support, and experience more problems with intimate members of the social network (e.g., spouses and relatives; Wade & Kendler, 2000) than non-depressed people.

Communication researchers Beth Le Poire and Ashley Duggan have applied a relational lens to explore communication in romantic relationships in which one partner is depressed. Their research is guided by **inconsistent nurturing as control** (INC) theory. This theory, which is based on social exchange and learning theories, describes how non-depressed partners' attempts to help their depressed partners get better may actually backfire and reinforce the very behavior they are trying to curtail (Le Poire, 1995). Previous research in other contexts supports the premise that romantic partners' competing goals of nurturing and controlling serve as a paradox in which controlling the dysfunctional behavior also means risking losing the relationship (Le Poire, 1992).

Guided by INC theory, Duggan and Le Poire (2006) conducted a study to examine the ways non-depressed romantic partners of depressed people changed their influence strategies over the course of the relationship depending on the stage of labeling the problem. They predicted that partners of depressed people would use more negative control strategies before labeling depressive behavior problematic; they would use positive helping and encouraging control strategies following the labeling; and they would revert to a mix of negative control strategies and positive helping or encouraging attempts once they were frustrated that their initial control attempts were not working. These predictions and the statistical methods they later used to analyze their data reflect the scientific paradigmatic perspective guiding this research.

In order to do this study, the researchers recruited 68 couples ($n = 136$ people) that included one depressed person. They screened participants over the phone, using the DSM-IV (the "Diagnostic and Statistical Manual of Mental Disorders," version four), to confirm one (and only one) person experienced depression that interfered with normal functioning and to confirm the couples were living together or married. In face-to-face interviews, the researchers asked background questions about the relationship and asked participants to name the strategies that non-depressed partners used to help with depression. Finally, the researchers categorized the strategies according to the labeling timeframes predicted by the theory.

From these interviews, the researchers examined the types (reinforcement and punishment) and patterns (consistency) of attempts of people seeking to curtail their partner's depression, and they examined the effects of strategy use over time. In line with the INC framework, results suggested that non-depressed partners did change their strategy use over time. Before labeling the depression as problematic, they would use

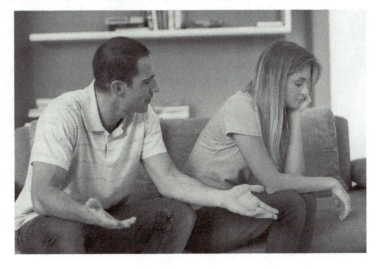

negative strategies such as name calling, making fun of depressive symptoms, and telling their partner to "get over it." After labeling the depression as problematic, however, partners used more positive strategies, including attending counseling with the depressed person, taking the depressed person on vacation, and highlighting positive qualities of the depressed person. At the point that partners became frustrated that their helping and encouraging were not working, they reverted to a mix of negative and positive strategies. This

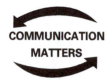

Dear Prudence

Dear Prudence,

I'm a man in his mid-40s who has been happily married for 10 years. I particularly enjoy my wife's dry, some would say sarcastic, sense of humor. Her wit not only attracted me to her as a partner, but it was one of the things that got me through a difficult time in my career, enabling me to see the humor in absurd and uncomfortable situations. About 18 months ago my wife's mother passed away suddenly and my wife began seeing a counselor. After a few appointments, the counselor prescribed an anti-depressant medication, Paxil, and my wife has been taking it ever since. As a result, my wife's personality has changed. Not dramatically, but enough so that she has become a glass-half-full, constantly cheerful type of person. I have no idea if this is common or perhaps if she was always depressed and her dark humor existed for her to deal with it. I'm glad she's happy now but I thought we were happy before and frankly, I miss my old wife! The new rainbows-and-sunshine person I'm living with gives me a headache and I find myself less attracted to her. I feel like a jerk and don't know what to do. Help!

—Dark Side

Dear Dark,

I'll get back to you with an answer in a few weeks, because now that my husband has seen your question I assume he'll start slipping Paxil into my half-empty coffee cup hoping for a similar change in my disposition. I have had many letters from people desperate to get their annoying loved ones on some kind of medication to take the edge off of jagged personalities. But I've never received such a *cri de coeur* from someone who wants the old sarcastic, unmedicated person back. But as an old, sarcastic, unmedicated person myself I appreciate hearing that not everyone wants a partner who has the buoyant outlook of SpongeBob SquarePants. You're right, however, that telling your spouse her new cheerfulness has you wanting to get into bed, alone, and pull the covers over your head, is going to be a difficult, even baffling conversation. It's best if you first broach this in the context of just checking in with her about the grief that propelled her to the therapist's office. If she's feeling more acceptance about her mother's death, you can ask if the therapy has moved on from that to deal with other aspects of her life. This will give you the opportunity to talk about whether she feels the medication is still necessary and why. Depending on how that goes, you can say that you miss the sarcastic take she had on life. Tell her you don't want to interfere with the treatment plan she has arrived at with her thera-pist, but as far as you're concerned, her personality never needed any tweaking.

—Prudie

cycling (change over time) is central to INC theory and has direct implications for couples, as the inconsistent use of strategies that punish and then reinforce and then punish the problematic behavior is likely to *strengthen* depressive tendencies. In other words, the inconsistent behavior from the non-depressed partner can actually reinforce the depressed partner's behavior.

Duggan and Le Poire's (2006) study extended previous research related to interpersonal dynamics within depressed romantic relationships. Findings support the premise that non-depressed partners' competing goals of nurturing and controlling serve as a paradox in which controlling the dysfunctional behavior means losing their ability to control the relationship. People usually think that the goal of treating depression is to relieve it, but the results of this study suggest that partners may actually benefit from some level of depression continuing in the relationship. One explanation is that the nurturing behaviors used during times of crises, or extreme depressive episodes, can help the partner feel nurturing and needed. Similarly, the nurturing during extreme depressive episodes can be rewarding for the depressed person, helping him/her feel loved and cared for. The "Dear Prudence" column we include in this chapter provides an example of the desire for some level of continued depression in a romantic relationship, though for a slightly different reason.

Duggan and Le Poire's (2006) research focused on romantic couples. We also can consider the impact of mental illness on communication in families. What happens in a family when a child is diagnosed with a mental illness? What about a parent? What about a new parent, as in the case of postpartum depression? The impact can be profound.

Johannson and colleagues conducted interviews with mothers and fathers of adult children with serious long-term mental illness, applying an interpretive approach to identify underlying meaning in the data. For the study of mothers (Johansson, Anderzen-Carlsson, Åhlin, & Andershed, 2010), they interviewed 16 women who ranged in age from their 40s to more than 70 years old; their adult children were 13 daughters and three sons, ranging in age from 18 to 49 years and suffering from mental illnesses that included schizophrenia, bipolar disorder, depression, and obsessive-compulsive disorder. The main theme the researchers identified across interviews was "My adult child who is struggling with mental illness is always on my mind" (p. 694). There were three subthemes: "(1) living a life under constant strain, (2) living with an emotional burden, and (3) seeing light in the darkness despite difficulties" (p. 694). For the study of fathers (Johansson, Anderzen-Carlsson, Åhlin, Andershed, & Sköndal, 2012), they interviewed 10 men who ranged in age from their 40s to more than 70 years old; their adult children were six daughters and four sons, ranging in age from 18 to 43 years and suffering from mental illnesses that included schizophrenia, bipolar disorder, depression, and obsessive-compulsive disorder. The main theme the researchers identified across interviews with fathers was "Maintaining a strong façade while balancing on a thin line" (p. 111). There were two subthemes: "(1) A constant struggle and (2) A feeling of powerlessness" (p. 111). It is interesting to note the differences between parental perspectives, with fathers appearing to focus on issues of power and control and mothers appearing to focus on issues of emotion. But the central commonality appears to be the constant strain and struggle of having a child with mental illness.

Another family-focused study out of Sweden considered the experiences of parents, partners, and adult children of people with bipolar disorder. Jönsson, Skärsäter, Wijk, and Danielson (2011) interviewed 17 family members to explore their experiences of living with a family member with bipolar disorder; family members were seven mothers, three fathers, five partners, and two adult children. The researchers used an interpretive analytic approach to allow them to look "behind the text to capture the latent content that yields a meaning and leads to a deeper understanding" (p. 30). They identified two main themes, each with subthemes. The first main theme was family members' views of the bipolar condition, which to them meant "facing change alone," without knowledge or understanding from people on the outside or sometimes even the bipolar family member; "making sense and raising doubts" about the illness; and striving to "maintain normality" in their own lives. The second main theme was family members' views of the future, which included "bearing the burden" of balancing the desire to be helpful and supportive while striving to live their own lives; and "building hope for the future," which meant doing their best to see a positive future with a pleasant life.

TREATMENT OF MENTAL ILLNESS

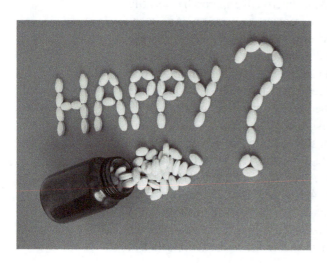

There are different approaches to treating mental illness, depending in part on the diagnosis and severity of the illness. **Medical treatment** from either primary care physicians or psychiatrists is one option. Depression, for example, is commonly managed by primary care physicians. How many times have you seen drugs ads on television that tell you to "talk to your doctor" about depression? Generally speaking, drugs to treat depression assist the body in regulating its own chemistry. Some antidepressant drugs affect neurotransmitters in the brain, such as serotonin, norepinephrine, and dopamine. Scientists have found that these particular chemicals are involved in regulating mood, but they are unsure of the exact ways that they work. The latest information on medications for treating depression and other mental illnesses is available on the U.S. Food and Drug Administration (FDA) website (www.fda.org).

APPROACHES TO TREATING MENTAL ILLNESS

Mental illness can be treated in a variety of ways, including medical or pharmacological, psychotherapy or counseling, self-help or peer-led programs, and Internet-supported interventions.

Not all researchers agree that antidepressant drugs are the best treatment for depression, however, and antidepressant drugs can have serious side effects. Even researchers who suggest and prescribe antidepressant drugs often also suggest and prescribe additional types of treatment, such as counseling or **psychotherapy** ("therapy" for short) from a licensed and trained mental healthcare professional. Such therapy would involve the person with mental illness talking to the therapist to identify and work through the psychological and psychosocial factors that might be causing the illness. Meetings with a therapist also could involve a couple or family or could involve a group setting with people facing similar challenges.

The practice of psychotherapy is a good example of translational research. Let us elaborate by focusing on the treatment of depression as an example. There are several types of psychological treatment for mild to moderate adult depression, and we present the major ones in Table 10.3. Each of these types of treatment is evidence-based and developed from theory.

Amber Hord-Helme, MA LPCC, Nationally Certified Clinical Counselor, Helme Family Counseling, LLC

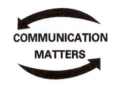

COMMUNICATION MATTERS

As a counselor, I get invited into the most personal and intimate struggles in my clients' lives. They come to counseling because they have tried everything that they know to try to work out the distress in their lives. Clients do what they have learned from their own experiences in their families. It is my job to meet people exactly where they are. They are just looking for other options, for other things to try. Once the pretense is dropped and people honestly identify the patterns of dysfunction in their lives and particularly their relationships, they can clearly identify for themselves other options for change. It is a pleasure to watch people take control of their own personal growth.

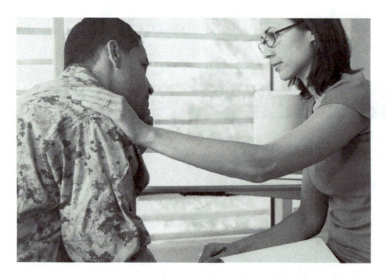

A meta-analysis across 53 studies including all of these types of therapy found only minimal differences in efficacy between the major approaches to psychotherapies for mild to moderate depression, with slightly better effects in interpersonal psychotherapy than the other types (Cuijpers, van Straten, Andersson, & van Oppen, 2008). There was a higher drop-out rate in cognitive-behavior therapy than in the other therapies, and a lower drop-out rate in problem-solving therapy. One important reason to pay attention to drop-out rates is that the therapy can be most effective only if it is completed; depressed people who try a couple of sessions with a therapist and decide "it did not work" might have dropped out without allowing for the process to be effective.

Peer-led and Internet-supported Mental Health Interventions

Alternative approaches to using medication or getting professional counseling for treating mental illness include **self-help** and **peer-led interventions** and interventions available through the Internet. Such alternatives are important to consider because

Table 10.3 Types and Emphases of Therapy for Depression

Type of Therapy	Emphasis
Cognitive-behavior therapy	Focuses on the role of thinking in what we feel
Nondirective supportive treatment	Offers active listening and support
Behavioral activation treatment	Links actions as causing emotions
Psychodynamic treatment	Focuses on unconscious processes as manifest in present behavior
Problem-solving therapy	Focuses on handling stress to improve coping
Interpersonal psychotherapy	Focuses on social roles and interpersonal interactions
Social skills training	Highlights verbal as well as nonverbal behaviors involved in social interactions

they typically are much less expensive and can have greater reach than standard care (Pfeiffer, Heisler, Piette, Rogers, & Valenstein, 2011). They also are popular. A 1995–96 survey determined that an estimated 25 million Americans had participated in a self-help group at some point in their lives (Kessler, Mickelson, & Zhao, 1997). Here we briefly review some of the research on peer-led and Internet-based interventions for treating mental illness.

Peer-led programs to treat mental illness are delivered by people who themselves have mental illness. "The underlying philosophy of these programs is that peers are best equipped to provide the practical information and social support that mental health consumers need to recover and rebuild their lives" (Pickett et al., 2010). A meta-analysis of peer support interventions for treating depression found evidence in favor of the approach (Pfeiffer et al., 2011). Specifically, across seven randomized controlled trials (RCTs) involving 869 participants, peer support interventions were better at reducing depressive symptoms than "usual care." Further, across seven RCTs involving 301 participants, peer support interventions performed as well as group cognitive behavioral therapy. The authors conclude that there is promise in peer support interventions, and they encourage further study to determine the best combinations of program content and approaches to implementation.

An example of a successful peer-led program is the BRIDGES program (Pickett et al., 2010). The curriculum was developed by the Tennessee Mental Health Consumers Association and the Tennessee branch of the National Alliance on Mental Illness. The program is offered over eight weeks in 2.5 hour sessions and serves persons with various diagnoses, including bipolar disorder, depression, and schizophrenia. The topics covered are (a) philosophy of recovery, (b) psychiatric diagnoses, (c) crisis planning and suicide prevention, (d) building social support, (e) medications and mental health treatment, (f) psychiatric rehabilitation and employment, (g) communication and problem management skills, and (h) self-advocacy (Pickett et al., 2010). A clear example of translational research, the BRIDGES program has been implemented in 11 states across the United States and internationally in Canada and England. A large RCT across eight sites in Tennessee found support for the effectiveness of the program in terms of improving perceived self-recovery and hopefulness among participants (Cook et al., 2012).

Internet-based mental health programs represent a second alternative to traditional care. According to a recent survey from the Pew Internet and American Life Project (2010), 79% of American adults now regularly use the Internet, and 66% of them have a broadband Internet connection at home. Another Pew survey (2011) found that 80% of Internet users have searched for health information online, so it's a safe bet that people are seeking information on mental health. But what about seeking treatment for mental health online? The answer to that question is yes.

Barak and Grohol (2011) conducted a comprehensive review of mental health interventions available via the Internet. They found a tremendous number of such interventions and organized them into five categories: (a) online counseling and psychotherapy, (b) psychoeducational websites, (c) interactive, self-guided interventions, (d) online support groups and blogs, and (e) "other types" of online interventions that did not fit the other categories (e.g., mobile applications). The authors reviewed several individual research studies and meta-analyses that evaluated these interventions and found good evidence for their effectiveness. They cautioned, however, that there is still a great deal of work to be done to develop the science of Internet-based mental health interventions. For example, there is need for the research and practice communities to come to terms with the theoretical, ethical, legal, and practical implications of self-help or peer-led interventions and to determine which people are most likely to benefit from Internet-based programs. All in all, though, they concluded that there is great promise in Internet-based or Internet-supported mental health interventions. Indeed, Barak and Grohol suggested that the benefits of online interventions—greater reach, convenience, privacy, anonymity, and potential cost-effectiveness—may result in the people who need treatment but have not yet sought it finally being able to get help. This is an incredible opportunity given that "nearly two-thirds of all people with diagnosable mental disorders do not seek treatment" (p. 156).

CONFLICTING RESULTS

Often, conflicting results in the literature stem from issues related to research design. Perhaps researchers study the wrong population, or perhaps they don't use appropriate statistical analyses. In this section, we briefly review some research on mental illness and social support that highlights these issues.

Depression and anxiety symptoms are predictors of quality-of-life during disease diagnosis and treatment, and social support can minimize the risk of depression and psychological distress (Carpenter, Fowler, Maxwell, & Anderson, 2010). So it's logical to think that social support would be great for everyone who's sick. But is that really true? Segrin, Badger, and Figueredo (2011) had reason to suspect not. These researchers, who represent the disciplines of communication, nursing, and psychology, study men with prostate cancer. They have found evidence of greater psychological distress among men with advanced disease and lower psychological distress among men who are newly diagnosed. They believed, therefore, that the social support needs of these men might also vary with the stage of disease progression. Thus, they designed a study to test the association between social support and depression at different stages of disease progression in men with prostate cancer.

Participants were 71 men diagnosed with prostate cancer and recruited through regional cancer centers, regional Veterans Affairs Health Care Centers, cancer support groups, and research study websites. The men were either in treatment or had completed treatment within past six months. Participants completed baseline assessments of depression, social support, and stage of progression. Next, as part of a larger study, the men participated in one of two randomly assigned health message interventions that lasted eight weeks. Participants completed a second assessment at the end of the intervention and then a third assessment eight weeks after that.

Analyses indicated that social support from family and friends had radically different results in predicting changes in depression in men with prostate cancer depending on the stage of their disease. For men with more advanced prostate cancer, social support was associated with improvements in depression. This finding is consistent with previous research, and it indicates that these men have significant needs related to their illness and the side effects of treatment in ways that social support helps, serving as a buffer between illness (in this case prostate cancer) and depression. For men with an early-stage prostate cancer diagnosis, however, social support was associated with a subsequent *worsening* of depression. Prostate cancer does not necessarily have signs or symptoms in its early stages, so men who are more newly diagnosed might still be processing what it means for them to deal with this disease. Segrin et al. (2011), there-

fore, suggested that these men may not feel the need for assistance from others and may instead prefer to deal with the illness on their own. The researchers also suggested that offers of assistance may indicate that other people now view these men differently (i.e., stigmatized) and that shows of concern can be unwanted reminders of the potentially dire consequences of prostate cancer.

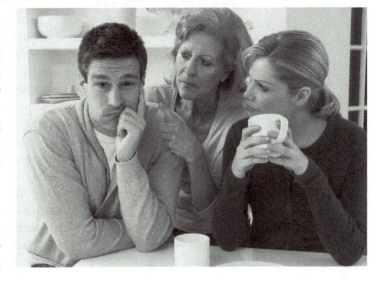

The Segrin et al. (2011) study clearly demonstrated that social support can have different prognostic value for psychological distress among men with prostate cancer depending on the stage of their disease. Had the study sample included only newly diagnosed men, only the negative relationship between social support and depression would have been found; had it included only men who had been diagnosed for some time, a positive relationship would have been found. Had the sample included men along the continuum of diagnosis but the analysis not differentiated between stage of disease, no relationship would have been found. Instead, we now know that social support processes do not work the same ways across all illness contexts and that more social support is not necessarily the goal. Appropriate research design, sampling, and analysis helped to determine this.

DIRECTIONS FOR FUTURE RESEARCH ON MENTAL HEALTH AND ILLNESS

We see a number of directions for future communication research about mental health and illness. Opportunities highlight refining definitional issues, exploring mental health disparities, expanding research on family communication, and exploring different approaches to interventions.

Just as physical health is defined as more than the absence of physical disease, mental health should be defined as more than the absence of mental disorder. In light of that, we believe there needs to be more research on how communication can promote overall good mental health through developing and maintaining positive relationships, supportive social networks, and humorous outlooks on life.

We have to be concerned with mental health disparities. As Fisher et al. (2012) note, ". . . many social and environmental factors affect risk for mental disorders and also influence barriers to receiving mental health care (such as high cost, access, stigma, and mistrust of medical practitioners). People of color, for example, are less likely to receive adequate mental health treatment, in part due to cultural barriers and bias by health providers" (pp. 549–550). As more and more research is being directed at the problem of physical health disparities (Harrington, 2013; Perloff, 2006), we must also be mindful of including the issue of mental health disparities in our efforts.

As we look at the impact of mental illness on communication in family relationships, we must do more to consider the impact on siblings. Oddly enough, there is hardly any research on the experience of brothers and sisters of people with mental illness. Indeed, Jönsson et al. (2011) had no siblings in their study and noted that as one of the study's weaknesses. Growing up with a mentally ill sibling can have profound effects on a person's development, identity, and relationships (Safer, 2002). This is an important gap in the literature.

We also have to consider the opportunities that information communication technologies (ICT) present for reaching those with mental illness and offering new approaches to support and treatment. For example, the Inspire Foundation, an Australian organization established in 1996 to address the escalating rate of youth suicide in that country, uses ICT "to improve and promote mental health and wellbeing for young people aged 14–25" (Stephens-Reicher, Metcalf, Blanchard, Mangan, & Burns, 2011, p. S38). They have reached nearly 400,000 youth

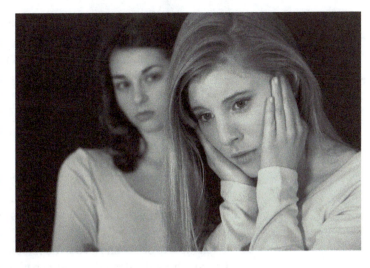

with mental health promotion initiatives. ICT isn't only applicable to a young target audience, either. A survey of 1,592 persons with serious mental illness found that 72% of respondents owned and used a mobile communication device and that both users and current non-users were interested in using mobile devices for things like reminders of appointments or medications, checking in with healthcare providers, and getting information about mental health services (Ben-Zeev, Davis, Kaiser, Krzsos, & Drake, 2013). Clearly, there is opportunity here, and communication researchers have a role to play in understanding how best to use ICT in treating mental illness and promoting mental health.

Finally, we believe there is opportunity in designing interventions targeting friends, family, and co-workers to be the source of persuasive messages encouraging people to seek mental health services (Aldrich, Harrington, & Cerel, 2014; Clark-Hitt, Smith, & Broderick, 2012). Efforts to directly reach people suffering from mental illness and encourage them to seek help are certainly important. There is opportunity, though, in using an "indirect" path by encouraging others to intervene. Theory-based work identifying characteristics of the most credible sources for these messages and then designing messages to persuade those people to intervene is crucial.

CONCLUSION

Our goal for this chapter was to provide you with an overview of communication issues related to mental health and illness. We wanted you to develop an understanding of how mental illness is depicted in the media, how mental disorders can affect communication in relationships, and how mental disorders can be treated through interventions and counseling. Although historically there has been a great deal of stigma associated with mental illness, more and more efforts are being made these days to reduce such stigma and offer hope for treatment and recovery to those suffering from depression, anxiety, and other mental disorders. We hope that if you find yourself or a friend or family member experiencing some form of mental illness, you will not be afraid to seek help.

DISCUSSION QUESTIONS

1. What issues in this chapter are consistent with your expectations about mental health and illness? What issues in this chapter are different from your expectations?
2. What movies or TV shows do you remember seeing that deal with mental illness? Do you think the depiction was negative? Did it seem realistic? Did it influence the way you think about mental illness, or did it influence your response to the film or program?
3. Depression can be considered as a set of symptoms or as an interpersonal/relational concern. What issues arise from considering depression from each perspective? Are there similarities and differences?
4. A dyadic perspective on depression considers the interplay between the depressed individual and other people, such that the depression is manifest as co-constructed between people. For example, depressive symptoms elicit negativity from family members, who respond with more negativity and then contribute to further depressive symptoms. What other health/illness concerns might be considered or explained as dyadic processes? How are these other health/illness issues similar to or different from considering depression from a dyadic perspective?

IN-CLASS ACTIVITIES

1. Students are likely to have either experienced depression or known someone who experienced depression. In small groups, have students describe the degrees of depression, ranging from times when people feel "down" or "sad," all the way to clinical depression. Draw a horizontal line (continuum) on the board. Put "feeling down or sad" at the left end and "clinical depression" on the right end, and illustrate the continuum with examples the students have generated. Discuss the extent to which communication in relationships was affected along the continuum. Remind students that the closer people get to the right end/clinical depression, the more important it is to get help.

2. The following website lists the "Top 5 TV shows that deal with mental health": http://www.theguardian.com/commentisfree/2013/jun/17/top-five-tv-shows-mental-health. Watch an episode from one of these shows and discuss in class how mental illness was portrayed and its impact on interpersonal communication.

RECOMMENDED READINGS

Rasmussen, E., & Ewoldsen, D. R. (2013). *Dr. Phil* and *Psychology Today* as self-help treatments of mental illness: A content analysis of popular psychology programming. *Journal of Health Communication, 18*(5), 610–623.

This study reports a content analysis of episodes of *Dr. Phil* and issues of *Psychology Today*, with a focus on coverage of mental disorders and treatment recommendations.

Knobloch, L. K., Knobloch-Fedders, L., & Durbin, C. E. (2011). Depressive symptoms and relational uncertainty as predictors of reassurance-seeking and negative feedback-seeking in conversation. *Communication Monographs, 78*(4), 437–462.

Based on integrative interpersonal theory, this study explores the interplay of depressive symptoms, relational uncertainty, and communication among 69 romantic couples.

Cook, J. A., Steigman, P., Pickett, S., Diehl, S., Fox, A., Shipley, P., . . . Burke-Miller, J. K. (2012). Randomized controlled trial of peer-led recovery education using Building Recovery of Individual Dreams and Goals through Education and Support (BRIDGES). *Schizophrenia Research, 136*, 36–42.

This article reports the results of a randomized controlled trial of a peer-led mental illness intervention, finding improvements in perceived self-recovery and hopefulness among participants in the treatment group.

Giles, D. C., & Newbold, J. (2011). Self- and other-diagnosis in user-led mental health online communities. *Qualitative Health Research, 21*(3), 419–428.

This article presents a qualitative analysis of three excerpts from discussion forums found in online mental health communities, with a focus on personal identity, informal self-diagnosis, and consultation regarding other-diagnosis.

REFERENCES

Aldrich, R. S., Harrington, N. G., & Cerel, J. (2014). The willingness to intervene against suicide questionnaire. *Death Studies, 38*, 100–108.

Barak, A., & Grohol, J. M. (2011). Current and future trends in Internet-supported mental health interventions. *Journal of Technology in Human Services, 29*, 155–196.

Ben-Zeev, D., Davis, K. E., Kaiser, S., Krzsos, I., & Drake, R. E. (2013). Mobile technologies among people with serious mental illness: Opportunities for future services. *Administration and Policy in Mental Health, 40*, 340–343.

Carpenter, K. M., Fowler, J. M., Maxwell, G. L., & Andersen, B. L. (2010). Direct and buffering effects of social support among gynecologic cancer survivors. *Annals of Behavioral Medicine, 39*, 79–90.

Centers for Disease Control and Prevention. (2013). *CDC report: Mental illness surveillance among adults in the United States.* Retrieved from http://www.cdc.gov/mentalhealth-surveillance/fact_sheet.html

Clark-Hitt, R., Smith, S. W., & Broderick, J. S. (2012). Help a buddy take a knee: Creating persuasive messages for military service members to encourage others to seek mental health help. *Health Communication, 27*(5), 429–438.

Cook, J. A., Steigman, P., Pickett, S., Diehl, S., Fox, A., Shipley, P., . . . Burke-Miller, J. K. (2012). Randomized controlled trial of peer-led recovery education using Building Recovery of Individual Dreams and Goals through Education and Support (BRIDGES). *Schizophrenia Research, 136*, 36–42.

Coyne, J. C. (1976). Toward an interactional description of depression. *Psychiatry, 39*, 28–40.

Cuijpers, P., van Straten, A., Andersson, G., & van Oppen, P. (2008). Psychotherapy for depression in adults: A meta-analysis of comparative outcome studies. *Journal of Consulting and Clinical Psychology, 76*, 909–922.

Duggan, A. P., & Le Poire, B. A. (2006). One down; two involved: An application and extension of inconsistent nurturing as control theory to couples including one depressed individual. *Communication Monographs, 73*(4), 379–405.

Fisher, C. L., Goldsmith, D., Harrison, K., Hoffner, C. A., Segrin, C., Wright, K., & Miller, K. A. (2012). Communication and mental health: A conversation from the CM Café. *Communication Monographs, 79*(4), 539–550.

Goffman, E. (1963). *Stigma: Notes on the management of spoiled identity.* Englewood Cliffs, NJ: Prentice-Hall.

Harrington, N. G. (2013). Introduction to the special issue: Communication strategies to reduce health disparities. *Journal of Communication, 63*(1), 1–7.

Hesley, J. W., & Hesley, J. G. (2001). *Rent two films and let's talk in the morning: Using popular movies in psychotherapy* (2nd ed.). New York: John Wiley and Sons, Inc.

Johansson, A., Anderzen-Carlsson, A., Åhlin, A., & Andershed, B. (2010). Mothers' everyday experiences of having an adult child who suffers from long-term mental illness. *Issues in Mental Health Nursing, 31*, 692–699.

Johansson, A., Anderzen-Carlsson, A., Åhlin, A., Andershed, B., & Sköndal, E. (2012). Fathers' everyday experiences of having an adult child who suffers from long-term mental illness. *Issues in Mental Health Nursing, 33*, 109–117.

Jönsson, P. D., Skärsäter, I., Wijk, H., & Danielson, E. (2011). Experience of living with a family member with bipolar disorder. *International Journal of Mental Health Nursing, 20*, 29–37.

Jorm, A. F., Christensen, H., & Griffiths, K. M. (2005). The impact of *beyondblue: the national depression initiative* on the Australian public's recognition of depression and beliefs about treatments. *Australian & New Zealand Journal of Psychiatry*, *39*, 248–254.

Kessler, R. C., Mickelson, K. D., & Zhao, S. (1997). Patterns and correlates of self-help group membership in the United States. *Social Policy*, *27*(3), 27–46.

Le Poire, B. A. (1992). Does the codependent encourage substance behavior: Paradoxical injunctions in the codependent relationship. *International Journal of the Addictions*, *27*, 1465–1474.

Le Poire, B. A. (1995). Inconsistent nurturing as control theory: Implications for communication-based treatment research and treatment programs. *Journal of Applied Communication Research*, *23*, 60–74.

Perloff, R. M. (2006). Introduction: Communication and health care disparities. *The American Behavioral Scientist*, *49*(6), 755–759.

Pew Internet & American Life Project. (2010). *Home broadband 2010*. Retrieved from http://pewinternet.org/Reports/2010/Home-Broadband-2010.aspx

Pew Internet & American Life Project. (2011). *Health topics*. Retrieved from http://pewinternet.org/Reports/2011/HealthTopics.aspx

Pfeiffer, P. N., Heisler, M., Piette, J. D., Rogers, M. A. M., & Valenstein, M. (2011). Efficacy of peer support interventions for depression: A meta-analysis. *General Hospital Psychiatry*, *33*, 29–36.

Pickett, S. A., Diehl, S., Steigman, P. J., Prater, J. D., Fox, A., & Cook, J. A. (2010). Early outcomes and lessons learned from a study of the Building Recovery of Individual Dreams and Goals through Education and Support (BRIDGES) program in Tennessee. *Psychiatric Rehabilitation Journal*, *34*(2), 96–103.

Pirkis, J., Blood, R. W., Francis, C., & McCallum, K. (2006). On-screen portrayals of mental illness: Extent, nature, and impacts. *Journal of Health Communication*, *11*, 523–541.

Robinson, D. J. (2003). Reel psychiatry: Movie portrayals of psychiatric conditions. Port Huron, MI: Rapid Psychler Press.

Safer, J. (2002). *The normal one: Life with a difficult or damaged sibling*. New York: The Free Press.

Segrin, C. (1993). Social skills deficits and psychosocial problem: Antecedent, concomitant, or consequent? *Journal of Social and Clinical Psychology*, *12*, 336–353.

Segrin, C., & Abramson, L. Y. (1994). Negative reactions to depressive behaviors: A communication theories analysis. *Journal of Abnormal Psychology*, *103*, 655–668.

Segrin, C., Badger, T. A., & Figueredo, A. J. (2011). Stage of disease progression moderates the association between social support and depression in prostate cancer survivors. *Journal of Psychosocial Oncology*, *29*, 552–560.

Segrin, C., & Dillard, J. P. (1992). The interactional theory of depression: A meta-analysis of the research literature. *Journal of Social and Clinical Psychology*, *11*, 43–70.

Shattell, M. M. (2009). Stigmatizing language with unintended meanings: "Persons with mental illness" or "mentally ill persons"? *Issues in Mental Health Nursing*, *30*, 199.

Smith, R. A. (2007). Language of the lost: An explication of stigma communication. *Communication Theory*, *17*, 462–485.

Stephens-Reicher, J., Metcalf, A., Blanchard, M., Mangan, C., & Burns, J. (2011). Reaching the hard-to-reach: How information communication technologies can reach young people at greater risk of mental health difficulties. *Australasian Psychology*, *19*(1), S58–S61.

Strack, S., & Coyne, J. C. (1983). Social confirmation of dysphoria: Shared and private reactions to depression. *Journal of Personality and Social Psychology*, *44*, 798–806.

Stuart, H. (2006). Media portrayal of mental illness and its treatments: What effect does it have on people with mental illness? *CNS Drugs*, *20*, 99–106.

Vaughan, G., & Hansen, C. (2004). "Like Minds, Like Mine": A New Zealand project to counter the stigma and discrimination associated with mental illness. *Australasian Psychiatry*, *12*(2), 113–117.

Vettese, L. C., & Mongrain, M. (2000). Communication about the self and partner in the relationships of dependents and self-critics. *Cognitive Therapy and Research*, *24*, 609–626.

Wade, T. D., & Kendler, K. S. (2000). The relationship between social support and major depression: Cross-sectional, longitudinal, and genetic perspectives. *Journal of Nervous and Mental Disease*, *88*, 251–258.

Watkins, D. C., Hunt, J. B., & Eisenberg, D. (2011). Increased demand for mental health services on college campuses: Perspectives from administrators. *Qualitative Social Work*, *11*(3), 319–337.

World Health Organization. (2001). *The world health report 2001—Mental illness: New understanding, new hope*. Geneva, Switzerland: Author.

CHAPTER

11

Ethical Issues in Health Communication

Allison M. Scott and
Nicholas T. Iannarino

We live in a time when medical technology is advancing at a rapid pace. Many familiar medical procedures are actually relatively new. For instance, did you know that the first surgery to transplant an organ took place just 60 years ago? Now over 25,000 organs are transplanted every year (United Network for Organ Sharing, 2013). Recent technological advances in medicine, such as vaccinations, cardiopulmonary resuscitation (CPR), chemotherapy, and genetic testing, have allowed healthcare providers to prolong many people's lives by many years, but using these kinds of technologies raises complex ethical questions. When should an unconscious patient be put on life support? Can an adolescent refuse to receive a vaccine against her parents' wishes? If an organ donor's liver becomes available, who should get the liver transplant?

The answers to these and many other ethical questions are based on four **ethical principles** of medicine (Beauchamp & Childress, 2001). The first principle is **respect for autonomy**, which involves protecting a person's right to make his or her own decisions when it comes to choosing or refusing medical treatment. The second principle, **nonmaleficence**, means that healthcare providers should "do no harm" to their

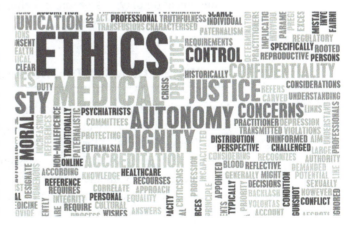

patients. Almost every medical procedure carries some kind of risk, and the principle of nonmaleficence says that these risks should be clearly outweighed by the benefits of treating a patient. The third ethical principle is **beneficence**, which holds that healthcare providers should act in a patient's best interest by working to restore the patient's health or relieve the patient's suffering. Finally, the principle of **justice** mandates the equal distribution of medical benefits and risks, so every person receives the same access to medical treatment and research opportunities, regardless of socioeconomic status, race, or sex.

ETHICAL PRINCIPLES

Medical ethics is based on four ethical principles: respect for autonomy, nonmaleficence, beneficence, and justice.

Ideally, medical practice should uphold all of these ethical principles, and in many cases, it is possible to deliver healthcare in such a way that preserves a patient's autonomy, does not harm but rather serves the best interests of the patient, and does so with fairness. However, in some cases, upholding one ethical principle may come at the expense of another. For example, what if honoring a patient's wishes to give his dying daughter his only good kidney to save her life (respect for autonomy) will ultimately lead to his death (nonmaleficence), which is not in keeping with the patient's own best interest (beneficence) and which also goes outside the legal policies that regulate the fair allocation of organs (justice)?

In this chapter, we examine four instances—informed consent, advance directives, organ donation, and medical mistakes—in which the ethical principles guiding medical practice can potentially compete with each other. In each case, we show how communication plays a key role in helping to resolve some of the tension that arises when ethical principles conflict.

INFORMED CONSENT IN MEDICAL RESEARCH AND PRACTICE

Many medical advances that we benefit from today are the result of systematic medical research seeking to answer all kinds of questions about how to promote health and treat illness. Currently, the gold standard for medical research is the **randomized controlled trial**, a kind of research design that is often used to evaluate the safety or effectiveness of new medications or procedures. The trials are "randomized" because participants are randomly assigned to receive the new treatment or the control treatment (usually standard care or a placebo). When participants are assigned to receive the new or control treatment by chance (like flipping a coin), it ensures that whatever differences are found between the two groups are a result only of the difference in treatment and not something else. The trials are "controlled" because the people who receive the control treatment serve as a baseline point of comparison for the people who receive the new treatment (Torpy, Lynn, & Glass, 2005).

One of the earliest clinical trials recorded in American history was the **Tuskegee Syphilis Experiment**, which began in 1932 in Macon County, Alabama. In this study, which was conducted by the U.S. Public Health Service, researchers documented the natural progression of syphilis by comparing 399 Black men who already had syphilis with 201 Black men who did not have syphilis. The men with syphilis were never told that they had the disease, and they were not given any treatment, even though penicillin was discovered in 1947 to be an effective way to treat syphilis. The study went on for 40 years and only ended in 1972 when the press reported leaked information to the public (Corbie-Smith, 1999). Another notorious example of early medical research is the 1963 **Jewish Chronic Disease Hospital case**. The purpose of this study, which was funded by the U.S. Public Health Service and the American Cancer Society, was to test whether foreign cancer cells would live longer in debilitated non-cancer patients than in debilitated cancer patients. As part of the study, 22 elderly patients who were chronically ill were injected with live human cancer cells without their knowledge. Although public outcry eventually led to the end of the study, the lead researcher was elected president of the American Cancer Society just a few years later (Arras, 2008).

The reason the Tuskegee and Jewish Chronic Disease Hospital studies are infamous is that, in each case, medical research targeted vulnerable populations (violating justice) and put participants at risk of harm (violating nonmaleficence) without any

perceived benefit (violating beneficence) and was conducted without the **informed consent** of participants (violating respect for autonomy). In 1978, prompted by the ethical violations of these research studies and others like them, a national commission released the **Belmont Report**, which became the foundation for establishing ethics committees (called institutional review boards) to oversee medical research at universities, medical centers, and hospitals. One of the main responsibilities of **institutional review boards** is to ensure that a

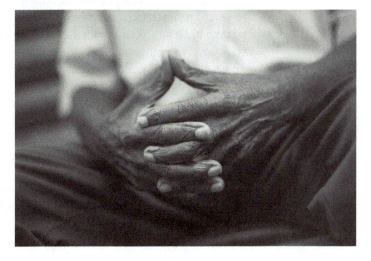

Willowbrook

Willowbrook State School was an institution on Staten Island, New York, that housed and educated predominantly African-American and Puerto Rican children with severe mental handicaps. During the 1950s, Willowbrook director Dr. Saul Krugman conducted groundbreaking hepatitis research studies at the institution, which revealed the existence of two strains of the virus, hepatitis A and B. However, later it was discovered that the researchers came to these conclusions using controversial methods, including feeding new residents live strains of the hepatitis virus that they had collected from the fecal matter of other children. The institution's largely unfurnished and soiled living conditions were also heavily criticized. Dr. Krugman defended his work by stating that, due to overcrowding, the residents would have developed hepatitis regardless of direct exposure from researchers. Dr. Krugman had sent a letter of informed consent to parents with children on the waiting list for admission to Willowbrook, promising immediate enrollment upon their signature. The letter stated that researchers at Willowbrook were attempting to prevent future epidemics of hepatitis and that "no attack or only a mild attack of hepatitis" was expected to occur upon exposure. The researchers also emphasized that participants could develop permanent immunity to hepatitis and asked parents if they would like to give their child "the benefit of this new preventative" (Murphy, 2004, p. 150).

potential participant's decision to participate or not participate in a research study meets the standards for informed consent.

Just like patients must provide informed consent in order to participate in medical research, patients must give informed consent in order to receive certain medical treatment. Before your doctor can operate on a broken arm, put you through a CT scan, or give you certain vaccines, you must sign an informed consent document. Some medical procedures clearly require informed consent, such as surgery and chemotherapy. However, the need for informed consent for other medical treatments is not as obvious. For example, does your doctor need to get informed consent to draw your blood to run tests? To prescribe antibiotics? To conduct a pelvic exam?

Let's consider a specific example. Ladies, let's say that you have been admitted to the hospital to have minor surgery. How would you respond if you found out that after the surgery, while you were still under anesthesia, a medical student performed a gynecological exam on you without your knowledge? This has actually happened to many women. Ubel, Jepson, and Silver-Isenstadt (2003) surveyed 401 medical students at five Philadelphia area medical schools and found that over 90% of students were asked to perform unconsented gynecological exams on anesthetized women for educational purposes. One medical student reported that he conducted unconsented pelvic exams like this four to five times every day during his OBGYN rotation (Barnes, 2012). Is this ethical? (You may be interested to know that, as a result of research studies like Ubel et al. [2003], California, Hawaii, Illinois, and Virginia have all passed legislation requiring specific consent for educational pelvic exams under anesthesia.)

Rooted in the ethical principle of respect for autonomy, the process of informed consent is based on the assumption that an autonomous choice to participate in a clinical research study or receive medical treatment must be based on sound reasoning. Most conceptualizations of informed consent include three criteria: **sufficient information, decision-making competence**, and **voluntariness** (Beauchamp & Childress, 2001). First, the right information must be presented to a person who is considering participating, including the purpose and methods of the study or treatment, as well as the possible risks and benefits of participation. Second, a person must have the capacity to make a reasoned decision. There are a variety of opinions about what counts as decision-making capacity, but most scholars and practitioners agree that a person must have the ability to understand relevant information, appreciate the significance of the information, and rationally manipulate the information to provide reasons for the decision to participate or not participate in the research or treatment (Drane, 1984). This means that someone who is, for instance, very young, very ill, unconscious, or impaired mentally cannot give informed consent (O'Neill, 2003). Finally, a person's decision to participate in research or treatment must be voluntary, which requires that the person's choice to participate or not participate cannot be coerced in any way and that the person can choose to stop participating at any time.

Each of these conditions of sufficient information, decision-making competence, and voluntariness can be difficult to fulfill, making the ideal of truly informed consent rarely possible in practice. Many standard informed consent documents are written at a reading level that is beyond the comprehension of the average educated layperson (Paasche-Orlow, Taylor, & Brancati, 2003), and participants often do not understand the information contained in the informed consent document. For example, in a study from the scientific perspective, which involved a survey of 207 participants from a variety of oncology clinical trials, nearly 30% of

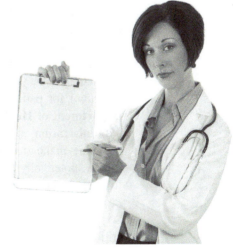

participants believed that the treatment they were receiving as part of the trial had already been proven to be the best treatment for their cancer (Joffe, Cook, Cleary, Clark, & Weeks, 2001). (In that same study, two individuals reported that they did not even know they were enrolled in a clinical trial!) In another study from a more interpretive perspective, analysis of informed consent conversations between physicians and patients revealed that physicians explained the randomization of the assignment to treatment conditions in less than half of the conversations, and in nearly a third of the conversations, physicians made statements that favored either new or control trial treatment (Brown, Butow, Ellis, Boyle, & Tattersall, 2004).

In addition, the information contained in informed consent documents is commonly incomplete. This is especially the case with informed consent for medical research. Informed consent documents often fail to explain the possibility that the clinical trial may not be completed if not enough participants enroll or if a better treatment is introduced in the meantime (Wertheimer, 2013). Even if a trial does reach completion, participants are rarely informed about which, if any, treatment they received as part of the trial (Corrigan, 2003). In fact, the final results of the clinical trial often are not shared with the participants, the medical community, or the public. Half of all completed clinical trials have never been published in an academic journal (Goldacre, 2013), and even though the Food and Drug Administration requires all new clinical trials to submit summaries of results within one year of completion, only 22% of trials comply with this requirement (Prayle, Hurley, & Smyth, 2012). This kind of sporadic reporting can mislead patients, healthcare providers, and the federal government into ill-advised spending on certain medications or procedures.

Although informed consent is designed to facilitate ethical medical research and practice, some researchers have argued that, in certain cases, the process of informed consent actually gets in the way of upholding other ethical principles. For instance, clinical studies on emergency treatments reached a standstill for many years because it was impossible to get informed consent from patients who were (at least temporarily) incapable of giving such consent, and this hampered doctors' ability to learn which treatments yielded the best outcomes (beneficence) and the least harm (nonmaleficence) for patients (Ellenberg, 1997). To address this issue, in 1996 the **U.S. Department of Health and Human Services** in concert with the **Food and Drug Administration** endorsed a waiver of informed consent for research on emergency medicine on the grounds of beneficence, reasoning that it would allow patients access to new, potentially life-saving treatments and that the systematic knowledge gained from clinical trials in emergency medicine would benefit future patients.

So far communication scholars have not been prominently involved in the critical conversation about ethically securing informed consent for clinical trials, but

Informed Consent Around the World

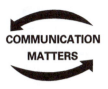

COMMUNICATION
MATTERS

Pfizer is a multinational research and development organization with facilities and experts around the world. Interviews with professionals in three different international geographies highlighted some of the challenges in obtaining informed consent. Below are three illustrative examples.

India

In India, the physician is held in very high esteem, and patients typically proceed with treatment regimens as recommended by their practitioner. This creates two distinct types of issues, one from the point of view of the patient and one from the perspective of the physician. A healthcare professional who practiced in India for more than a decade explained, "in many years of interacting with patients, I never once had someone ask me, 'what are the side effects?' or other such questions about their treatment." Generally, there is an acceptance of disease and its course which may prevent patients from pursuing treatment, or participating in clinical research. Additionally, it creates a sort of quandary for the physician between choosing to guide the patient through the uncertainties new treatments can bring, and maintaining their position as a clinical expert. Because the patient often considers the physician in such high regard, explaining the different options available, or the possible negative effects of a treatment could make it appear as though the physician is not knowledgeable.

Japan

Similar to physicians in India, health practitioners in Japan are held in high esteem by patients and patients are less likely to ask questions about their treatment or treatment options than might be typical in the U.S. Physicians are employed by health institutions that often combine a hospital, a clinic, medical school and research center. Culturally, there is a social obligation from the physician to the institution. As such, if anything happens to a patient being treated that is outside the expectations of the course of their disease or condition, the physician is held personally responsible and would be expected to resign from his or her post. The effect of this high level of trust between a patient and physician can mean explaining to a patient the potential benefits and hazards of research, as recommended by the Declaration of Helsinki might be informative, but perhaps not obtaining "consent." Part of the spirit of informed consent is the weighing of pros and cons by the patient, but if they don't believe there could be any cons, are they giving adequate consent?

Mali

As in many countries in Africa, the informed consent process in Mali is multilayered. The first step for any proposed research effort is to approach the elders of the community in which the study is being considered. If the sponsor is from outside the community, the visit to the community elders would be facilitated by a local host. The second step is for the elders of the tribe or village to assess whether the proposed research effort would be of benefit to the community. If the assessment is positive, the leaders discuss the program with the people living in the village and ask for their assent to participate. After these steps have been taken, perhaps over a series of weeks or months, the local study investigator would then begin to ask patients to participate in the study and engage them in the informed consent process that takes place between a physician and patient.

communication research has the potential to play an important role in the ongoing effort to improve the process of informed consent. How exactly can a communication focus help improve informed consent? One promising line of inquiry involves how people manage information. There is ample evidence in communication scholarship that more information is not always better. Brashers (2001) has argued convincingly that increasing the amount of information given to a person (for instance, on an informed consent document) may not necessarily improve the person's understanding of something (for instance, clinical trials). In fact, it might have the

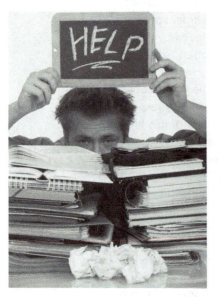

opposite effect. This and other similar lines of research have prompted researchers and practitioners to simplify the language they use in informed consent documents and to present information in a way that is meaningful to potential participants, which means considering not just the kind and amount of information that is provided but also the way in which the information is interpreted (Flory & Emanuel, 2004). Changes such as these help to optimize informed consent for clinical trials, as well as therapeutic practice. Asking potential participants to put key pieces of information into their own words to demonstrate understanding significantly improves their comprehension, while only prolonging the informed consent process by about two-and-a-half minutes (Fink et al., 2010). The value of focusing on how information is presented and interpreted in the informed consent process illustrates how communication can be a valuable means of shoring up the differences between the ideal and the actual practice of informed consent.

INFORMED CONSENT

To conduct medical research and practice ethically, participants must provide informed consent, which is based on the ethical principle of respect for autonomy. For consent to be informed, participants must have sufficient information, decision-making competence, and voluntary choice. Informed consent often falls short of the ideal in practice because participants frequently do not have complete information or do not fully understand the information. Communication research on information management has the potential to improve the process of informed consent.

ADVANCE DIRECTIVES AND SURROGATE DECISION MAKING

Advance directives (also called "living wills") are documents that describe what medical treatments a person does not want to be given in the event that the person loses the ability to make decisions in the future (based on the same criteria for decision-making capacity described above). It is estimated that 70–80% of people will, at some point, be unable to make their own medical choices (American Psychological Association, 2000). This high percentage rate prompted the U.S. Congress to pass the **1991 Patient Self-Determination Act**, which mandates that healthcare institutions must offer all adult patients the opportunity to complete an advance directive whenever they are admitted to a healthcare facility (U.S. P.L. 101–508, 1990). Advance directives focus on specific treatments that a person wants to refuse, such as CPR, mechanical ventilation, tube feeding, artificial hydration, dialysis, or antibiotics.

The primary purpose of advance directives is to preserve respect for a person's autonomy, but advance directives also sustain the ethical principle of beneficence by improving the quality of healthcare a person receives. People who have advance directives report lower levels of depression and anxiety (Pautex, Herrmann, & Zulian, 2008) and are less likely to receive aggressive and medically futile life-sustaining treatments than patients who do not have directives (Teno, Gruneir, Schwartz, Nanda, & Wetle, 2007). But having an advance directive does not always lead to better psychological or physiological outcomes or reduce the use of hospital resources. For instance, Schneiderman, Kronick, Kaplan, Anderson, and Langer (1992) conducted a randomized controlled trial in which patients in the treatment condition were offered the opportunity to complete advance directives, and they found no difference between patients who completed an advance directive and those who did not (control group) in terms of the patient's cognitive functioning, satisfaction, psychological well-being, or health-related quality of life, whether the patient received CPR, mechanical ventilation, artificial nutrition and hydration, or the financial cost of care in the patient's last month of life.

So why don't advance directives necessarily work? One problem is that advance directives are not always practical. For an advance directive to inform medical decision making, obviously it must exist. The good news here is that the number of Americans who have completed an advance directive has doubled in the past 20 years; the bad news is that still fewer than one in three American adults has a directive (Pew Research Center for the People and the Press, 2006). But even when a person has an advance directive, following it can be difficult due to logistical problems, such as misplaced, invalid, or inconsistent documentation (Freeborne, Lynn, & Desbiens, 2000). Some estimates indicate that as much as 86% of the time, doctors are not even aware that their patient has an advance directive (DesHarnais, Carter, Hennessy, Kurent, & Carter, 2007).

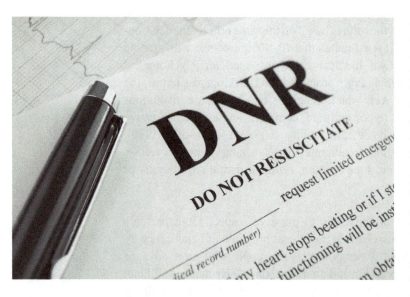

Another problem with advance directives is that they do not always accurately represent a person's wishes about medical treatment. Research comparing what people think they will want and what they actually want when they are ill shows that healthy people tend to do a poor job of predicting their treatment preferences in illness (Jansen, Stiggelbout, Nooij, Noordijk, & Kievit, 2000). This suggests that advance directives may not necessarily be reliable tools for guiding decisions about an individual's medical treatment. People's preferences also are affected by various factors that change over time, such as expected future quality of life, the emotional or financial burden of treatment, how dependent a person is on others, and the level of pain a person experiences (Fagerlin, Ditto, Hawkins, Schneider, & Smucker, 2002). This means that advance directives are never truly up to date because they do not account for changes in a person's preferences between when the directive is written and when a medical decision must be made (Mazur, 2006).

Yet another problem with advance directives is how to interpret them. Some advance directives prompt people to record their general values, such as "take no heroic measures" or "preserve quality of life," but this kind of direction is usually too general and vague to be useful in guiding treatment decisions. Other advance directives are far too specific in documenting treatment preferences, listing detailed instructions like "use oxygen, suction, and manual treatment of airway obstruction as needed for comfort." This degree of specificity is likewise unhelpful because many directions do not apply to a person's actual situation, or a person may face a situation that was not addressed in the advance directive. When researchers have compared what medical treatments people choose in specific real-life scenarios to what they have recorded in advance directives, they have found little to no correlation between a person's actual and documented choices (Winter, Parks, & Diamond, 2010).

The problems surrounding the existence, accuracy, and interpretation of advance directives call into question the ethics of relying on this kind of documentation to guide medical decision making. Consider the famous case of Margo (Dworkin, 1993), a woman in her 50s who, despite having dementia, is very happy. Before Margo developed dementia, she drafted an advance directive in which she says that if she ever has dementia, she wants to refuse any life-sustaining treatment. Margo has contracted pneumonia, which requires an antibiotic treatment. Without the treatment, she will die. Margo, in her demented state, says that she wants to receive the treatment. So should her doctors overrule her advance directive and give her the antibiotics, or should they follow her advance directive and refuse the antibiotic treatment?

Some people argue that dementia fundamentally changes a person, and thus using an advance directive written by Margo when she was of sound mind to make decisions about Margo when she is not of sound mind would be like using any random person's advance directive to make decisions about Margo (which would clearly be unacceptable), so the answer is that competent Margo should not be able to sentence demented Margo to death (Shaw, 2012). But this argument based on nonmalficence goes against the fundamental assumption of advance directives, which is that they are a means of protecting a person's autonomy. Others, however, argue that these two ethical principles do not necessarily contradict one another. They reason that no one could ever have all the information relevant to a medical decision before the circumstances of the decision are known, and thus Margo's decision expressed in her advance directive was necessarily one made in ignorance, which means that it does not meet the standards for informed refusal of treatment and therefore should not be honored (Sokolowski, 2010).

Advance directives can be useful tools for protecting patient autonomy and making medical decisions that are in a patient's best interest, but they are, at best, blunt tools.

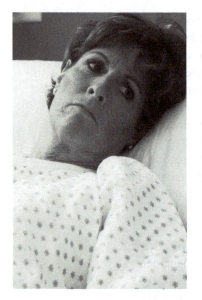

Most research on advance directives has been prompted in direct response to the widely recognized need to improve the quality of medical decision making. This pragmatic focus, however, has yielded a collection of findings about the ethical problems associated with advance directives without any clear guidance for how best to resolve the ethical tensions. In future work, researchers need to use particular perspectives to help focus their research so that we can leverage their findings to improve medical decision making.

In particular, taking a communication perspective holds a lot of promise for informing future research on advance directives. We know that advance directives are not always effective, which raises the question: How helpful is it to rely on advance directives as the basis for making medical decisions? Is there another, more effective basis for making decisions? Communication research suggests that ongoing, informal communication about health decisions may be more helpful in guiding medical decisions. In fact, some scholars have argued that advance directives are only useful to the extent that they promote conversations about health decisions among patients, their families, and physicians (Fagerlin et al., 2002). Tilden, Tolle, Nelson, and Fields (2001) provide empirical support for this argument with their finding that family stress associated with making medical decisions for an ill family member is highest in the absence of any kind of advance directive, lower in the presence of a written advance directive, and lowest when conversations with the patient guided decisions.

Communication with a **surrogate decision maker** about end-of-life decisions is particularly important. A surrogate is someone who takes the responsibility for making choices on someone's behalf when a person's decision-making capacity is impaired. Ethically, the surrogate is supposed to make the same choices the incapacitated person would have made, and most surrogates try to do that. But just how accurate are surrogates in making the same decisions that the ill person would have made? Not very. Many studies have shown that the concordance, or the match, between a person's end-of-life wishes and a surrogate's decisions is no better than chance (Shalowitz, Garrett-Mayer, & Wendler, 2006).

Why don't surrogate decision makers do a better job? There are several possible reasons, such as projection bias (when surrogates project their own preferences onto the ill person) and overtreatment bias (when surrogates overestimate a person's desire for life-sustaining treatment). However, perhaps the most compelling explanation is that, in general, communication between ill individuals and their surrogates is not particularly effective. For instance, Hines et al. (2001) used a scientific approach to

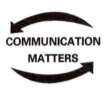

Talking with Your Parents About End-of-life Health Choices

No one wants to talk about end-of-life decisions, but it can be one of the most important conversations you have with your parents. Even though end-of-life healthcare may not even be on your radar right now, it's never too soon to start bringing up the topic. You never know when you might need to know your parents' wishes or they might need to know yours. Plus, if you start talking about these health decisions now, it won't be as awkward or as hard to talk about them later. As you start thinking about having these kinds of conversations with your parents, here are some things to keep in mind that will help make for better discussions:

- Use another person's experience to introduce the topic. If you or your parent knows of someone who has had to make end-of-life choices, start by talking about your impressions of that person's experience and then transition into talking about how you and your parents would like your own experience to be similar to or different from the other person's.
- Talk about general end-of-life values. It is impossible to anticipate every potential end-of-life scenario, so it is especially important to talk about your general end-of-life values. Ask your parents how they define quality of life and what counts as a reasonable chance of recovery, and tell them what you think, too. What you say can provide a useful basis for making choices in the event that you must act on behalf of one another in a health crisis.
- Keep the relationship in mind. Your main goal in having end-of-life conversations is to reach well-reasoned decisions, but it is also important to affirm your parent and your relationship with them. Expressing approval of the other person ("I think your decisions make a lot of sense"), respect for the person's autonomy in making those decisions ("I support whatever choice you make"), and affirming the relationship with your family member ("I'm glad we're close enough to talk about this kind of thing") can make for a more satisfying discussion.
- Start sooner rather than later, and talk often. Starting end-of-life decision making before end-of-life care is necessary allows you to be less stressed and to make more informed choices. So start having these conversations now, and keep the conversations going. Checking in from time to time about your parents' end-of-life preferences will make the conversations easier to have and will keep you more informed.

study family members' conversations about end-of-life care. They conducted face-to-face and telephone surveys with 242 pairs of patients and their surrogates. They found that patients and surrogates who had had at least five conversations about end-of-life decisions still had not talked about issues such as tube feedings or CPR. In another study from a scientific perspective, Libbus and Russell (1995) interviewed 30 pairs of patients and surrogates and found that nearly 40% of the time, end-of-life conversations go so poorly that individuals and their surrogates disagree about whether such a conversation even occurred.

However, recognizing that more communication about end-of-life decisions may not necessarily be translating into better communication, researchers have recently begun to consider how the *quality* of end-of-life conversations between individuals and their surrogates makes a difference in improving end-of-life decision making (Scott & Caughlin, 2012). In a study exemplifying the scientific paradigm, Kirchhoff, Hammes, Kehl, Briggs, and Brown (2010) conducted a randomized controlled trial across six outpatient clinics in Wisconsin. Researchers recruited 313 patient–surrogate pairs to participate in the trial; 153 pairs were randomized to the control group, and 160 pairs were randomized to the intervention group. In the intervention group, a trained facilitator helped patients and their surrogates talk about end-of-life decisions to ensure that the quality of the conversations was high. These conversations specifically focused on the patient's goals for end-of-life care, factors or experiences that have affected the patient's goals for future medical decision making, and the need for engaging in future discussions as situations and preferences change. After engaging in this conversation, the patients and surrogates separately completed a questionnaire, which asked them both about the patient's end-of-life preferences in four different medical situations (e.g., where the patient has low or high chance of survival accompanied by high or low cognitive and functional impairment). The researchers compared the concordance between patients and surrogates in the intervention group with the concordance rates of those in the control group (who received no help with their conversation). They found that in all four situations, surrogates in the intervention group had significantly better understanding of the patient's wishes than surrogates in the control group. In another study that accounted for quality of communication, Lamba, Murphy, McVicker, Smith, and Mosenthal (2012) found that outside ratings of the quality of family conversations about goals of end-of-life care were significantly related to higher rates of "do not resuscitate" orders and life support withdrawal and shorter stays in the intensive care unit. Results such as these show how considering not only the quantity but also the quality of people's conversations about end-of-life decisions can impact important medical outcomes.

ADVANCE DIRECTIVES

Advance directives and conversations with surrogate decision makers provide ways for people to share their preferences about medical treatment in case they ever lose the capacity to make decisions. Advance directives and surrogate decision making are based on the ethical principle of respect for autonomy, and they have the potential to improve the quality of a person's medical care. However, advance directives do not always work well due to logistical, accuracy, and interpretation issues, and surrogate decision makers do not always accurately anticipate an ill person's wishes because of poor communication. Advance directives appear to be most effective when used in concert with informal communication about medical preferences, and surrogate decision making accuracy improves when the quality (not necessarily the quantity) of communication is high.

ORGAN DONATION

Richard and Ronald Herrick were 23-year-old identical twins with one important difference: Richard was dying of kidney disease. Ronald told Richard's physician, Dr. Joseph Murray, that he would gladly give his brother one of his kidneys if it would save his life. Dr. Murray told Ronald that it actually might be possible because the two were identical twins, which significantly diminished the possibility of Richard's body rejecting Ronald's kidney. So on December 23, 1954, in the first successful live organ transplant, Ronald gave his twin brother one of his kidneys, which saved Richard's life.

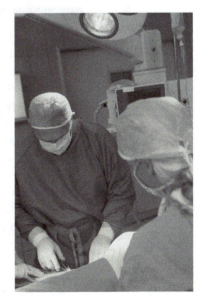

Since then, **organ donation** has come a long way. It is now routine to perform kidney, liver, lung, heart, and pancreas transplants from living and deceased donors. Currently in the United States, there are over 117,000 people who are waiting to receive a donated organ (United Network for Organ Sharing, 2013). In 2012, just over 25,000 people received an organ transplant (United Network for Organ Sharing, 2013). The number of people on the waiting list is growing faster than the number of organ donors, and it is estimated that about half of the people on the waiting list will die while waiting for an organ (Port, Dykstra, Merion, & Wolfe, 2005). Many people consider such deaths to be preventable because an organ transplant can restore many healthful years to a person's life. For this reason, some medical professionals have identified the need for organ donors as a medical crisis.

Nearly 95% of Americans support organ donation, but only about 53% have signed up to be an organ donor (Gallup Organization, 2005). There are a number of ways a person can become an organ donor. You can sign an organ donor card, the back of your driver's license, or an online organ donor registry. In addition, a family member can consent to donating an individual's organs if the person has not documented the decision to become a donor. After a person dies, an organ procurement coordinator presents the person's family with an opportunity to donate the person's organs. Hospitals have the legal authority to continue with organ donation without consent from the deceased person's family if the person has officially expressed the wish to donate. In almost all cases, however, the person's family still makes the final decision about donation (Mesich-Brant & Grossback, 2005).

Communication scholar Susan Morgan and her colleagues developed the **organ donation model** to explain the factors that predict whether someone signs up to become an organ donor (Morgan & Miller, 2001). According to the model, which is rooted in the scientific paradigm, a person's attitudes toward organ donation and perceived social norms about donation give rise to the person's willingness to become an organ donor, which in turn leads the person to sign up to be a donor. Communication research based on the organ donation model has been the basis of a number

---

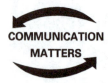

**COMMUNICATION
MATTERS**

Donate Life

Most states give you the option to indicate on your driver's license or state ID card whether you wish to donate your organs and tissue in the event of your death. If you are interested in becoming an organ and tissue donor, there are a number of quick and free ways for you to register. You can sign up with your state's department of motor vehicles (DMV) in person when you update your driver's license or state ID card; many states' DMVs will ask you directly if you would like to become or remain a donor. Or you might find it more convenient to register online with the DMV (dmv. org/organ-donor.php), Donate Life America (donatelife.net/register-now), or the U.S. Department of Health and Human Services (http://organdonor.gov/becomingdonor/stateregistries.html). You can even register through Facebook by clicking on the "Life Event: Health and Wellness" tab on your profile page, which will link you to your state's Donate Life registry. The decision to become an organ and tissue donor is not to be taken lightly, but choosing to donate is as simple as renewing your driver's license or visiting a website.

of federal grant-funded public campaigns to promote organ donation on university campuses, in worksites, and through driver's license bureaus (Morgan & Harrison, 2010). As a result, rates of donor registration have risen. Feeley and Moon (2009) conducted a random-effects meta-analysis of 23 communication campaigns to promote organ donation and found an overall five percent increase in registry signing. This may sound like a modest increase, but this is the average increase across 23 campaigns. (Also, if you consider that one donor can save up to eight lives [U. S. Department of Health and Human Services, 2013], a five percent increase represents significant life-saving potential.) Other investigations report even more dramatic improvements. For instance, a recent intervention promoting organ donation in Michigan increased the number of people who are registered organ donors sevenfold (Harrison et al., in press).

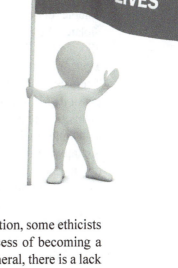

While it is exciting to see the success of intervention efforts, it is important to make sure that the promotion of organ donation does not come at the expense of ethical medical practice. For instance, some ethicists have raised the question about how to tell when a person is dead and thus when the person's organs are available to be transplanted. The **dead donor rule** specifies that organs cannot be harvested unless a person is dead, which upholds the ethical principle of nonmaleficence by preventing one person from being harmed in order to help others (Robertson, 1999). In current medical practice, after consent for donation has been secured from the person or their family, the donor is typically taken to the operating room while they are still alive, medicine that helps preserve the organs is administered, and the patient is taken off life support, and the transplant team waits until the person's heart stops beating. There is no agreement on how long transplant surgeons wait after cardiac death before they start harvesting the organs, and waiting times vary between two and 10 minutes (Joffe et al., 2011). In addition, some ethicists have raised questions about how well the informed consent process of becoming a donor upholds the ethical principle of respect for autonomy. In general, there is a lack of disclosure about the actual process of organ donation on organ procurement organization websites and in online consent documentation, and the information provided to the potential donor by organ procurement coordinators is incomplete at best (Wolen, Rady, Verheijde, & McGregor, 2006). This casts doubt on whether organ donors actually receive and understand the relevant information necessary to make an informed choice about donation.

Another question related to informed consent is whether organ donation should be based on an **opt in** or an **opt out** decision. Currently in the United States, an individual must opt in (by signing up) to be an organ donor. Other countries that have opt in policies include Austria, Great Britain, Israel, and Japan. But some people argue in favor of an opt out system, in which consent to donate is presumed unless a person documents the wish to not be an organ donor. Spain, Germany, Chile, and Brazil currently have opt out policies, and their rate of organ donors is much higher than in countries with opt in formats. One line of reasoning for an opt out policy is pragmatic: Presumed consent provides a way to substantially increase the supply of transplantable organs (Hester, 2006). Other lines of reasoning are more philosophical: Donation should be considered the moral obligation of every person (Saunders, 2011). But others argue that the absence of objection does not meet the standards for informed consent and therefore violates the ethical principle of respect for autonomy (Fabre, 1998). Another option is to use a **mandated choice** system, which requires every person to document their decision for or against donation. Supporters of mandated choice argue that the system preserves the voluntariness of donation and thus the autonomy of donors (Spital, 1996), but opponents argue that it violates a person's autonomy to force a choice to be made at all (Chouhan & Draper, 2003).

Another concern is whether the unsanctioned use of media to promote organ donation violates the ethical principle of justice by interfering with how donated organs are allocated. Policies of organ allocation take into account a variety of factors, including a person's time on the waiting list, immunology, organ size, and geographic location. These policies seek to maximize the best transplant outcomes for the most people possible. Most media promotion of organ donation, such as public service announcements, encourages potential donors to follow these organ allocation policies. However, sometimes individuals use the media to try to circumvent the policies. In 2004, Todd Krampitz, a man with advanced cancer, advertised his need for a liver in the media, online, and on billboards, which led the family of an organ donor to direct the donor's liver to Krampitz (Hopper, 2004). There are many who support the ability of donors or donor families to be able to choose to give transplanted organs to a specific recipient. If a member of your family died, would you want to have some say in who got the person's organs? Many people say you should, citing examples such as families not wanting their loved one's organs being given to people who need an organ because they have abused their bodies in the past, even if they no longer engage in the jeopardizing behavior (such as a former alcoholic who has been sober for 10 years needing a new liver; Richards, 2012). But not everyone agrees. Krampitz had complications with his liver disease that put him at risk for tumors, which is why he was not high on the waiting list to receive an organ. He got the liver transplant (by circumventing the normal allocation system), but he died less than a year after the transplant from a recurrent tumor. This example illustrates the question of whether honoring the wishes of a donor or the donor's family in directing organs bypasses the fair policies of allocation and leads to unnecessary waste (Hanto, 2007).

There are a number of ways that future communication research can help to resolve some of these ethical concerns. First, more work is needed on how organ procurement coordinators talk with families about organ donation. Using a scientific approach, Anker and Feeley (2011) have begun to examine the persuasive strategies that organ procurement coordinators use to gain consent for donation from families, and future research along these lines can assess the extent to which the persuasive strategies are in keeping with the ethical criteria for informed consent. Conversations about organ donation can leave families feeling confused and distressed at a time when grief is already affecting their ability to make decisions. Communication scholars are well positioned to help facilitate more informed consent processes by identifying message strategies that meet the ethical (not just the technical) burden of informed consent.

Second, more work is needed on the quality of family communication about organ donation. One of the reasons that more people do not become organ donors is the high rate of family refusal to allow donation. When family members have discussed organ donation, families are twice as likely to consent to donation than when family members have not discussed the topic (Smith, Kopfman, Lindsey, Yoo, & Morrison, 2004). This has led many researchers to identify the low conversion rate of potential organ donors to actual organ donors as a communication issue. Recent scholarship has recognized the importance of encouraging family discussion of donation as a means of promoting organ donation (Afifi et al., 2006). However, unqualified encouragement to talk about donation with family members can be risky. The assumption inherent in promoting family communication about donation is that families know how to talk ethically about donation, when in fact they may not. Using an interpretive approach, Pitts, Raup-Krieger, Kundrat, and Nussbaum (2009) examined actual family conversations about organ donation and found that families varied in how effectively they used hypothetical ethical scenarios to help establish parameters for circumstances in which a person would or would not donate. Some families talked about hypothetical ethical challenges in which one family member asked about organ procurement and distribution in general (e.g., "What happens if a person on life support never dies?"). Other families talked more specifically using hypothetical family situations in which one member created a "what if" scenario in which a family has to make an organ donation decision concerning another family member (e.g., "Would you pull the plug on Mom if it meant that her kidneys could go to her sister, who has renal disease?"). More research along these lines could assist the developers of organ donation campaigns by providing a means of equipping families to consider the ethical principles of respect for autonomy and justice in conversations about organ donation.

PATIENT SAFETY AND MEDICAL ERRORS

In 2013, a British man who had testicular cancer went into surgery to have his cancerous testicle removed. During the operation, surgeons removed his healthy testicle by mistake—and then sewed it back on 40 minutes later after they realized they had taken the wrong testicle (Smith, 2013). We all know that nobody is perfect, but it may be surprising (and more than a little disturbing) to learn just how common severe mistakes are in the field of medicine.

Medical errors occur when a planned action fails to be executed as intended or when the wrong plan is used to achieve a goal. Mistakes such as missed diagnoses, incorrect treatment implementation, and premature hospital discharge are one of the top 10 causes

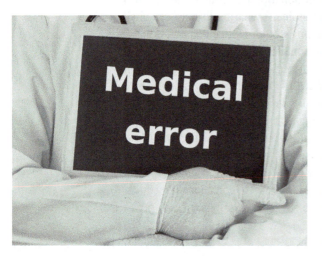

of death in the United States: Between 44,000 and 98,000 patients are believed to die in hospitals each year as a result of preventable medical mistakes. This figure exceeds death rates from motor vehicle accidents, breast cancer, and AIDS (Kohn, Corrigan, & Donaldson, 2000). Errors associated with medication alone cause at least 1.5 million preventable injuries (Aspden, Wolcott, Bootman, & Cronenwett, 2007) and over 7,000 deaths annually (Phillips, Christenfeld, & Glynn, 1998). These harmful and preventable medical errors are estimated to cost between $17 billion and $29 billion in lost income, diminished household production, disability, and additional healthcare (Kohn et al., 2000).

At the root of all this trouble is communication. The **Joint Commission on the Accreditation of Healthcare Organizations** (2002) found that communication problems between patients and providers are the cause of over 80% of all medical errors. For example, a Connecticut woman was readmitted to the hospital with a dangerously low heart rate because she was not informed that she should not mix her old blood pressure medication with a new prescription (Chedekel, 2012). Medical mistakes can also be caused by poor communication between providers. After the hospital staff confused two patients with similar names, a pregnant woman was accidentally given a CT scan of her abdomen, a procedure that could result in cancer or birth defects in an unborn baby (Bonifield & Cohen, 2012). Additionally, a Massachusetts surgeon performed an incorrect operation on a woman's hand after the procedure was moved to a new operating room with different staff members, who inadvertently washed off the marks on the patient's hand and failed to complete a routine pre-surgery site check, which would have likely caught the mistake (Aleccia, 2010). While patients are the obvious victims of medical mistakes, the healthcare provider at fault can be a secondary victim, as they commonly report feelings of self-doubt, self-blame, humiliation, guilt, and fear in the wake of a medical mistake (Newman, 1996).

Despite the ubiquity of medical errors, Americans tend to have an expectation that healthcare providers are above mistakes. We watch television dramas like *House, M.D.* and *Grey's Anatomy*, which reinforce these expectations of perfection by frequently portraying physicians as heroes who rarely make medical mistakes (Foss, 2011). In addition, blame for mistakes is largely placed on the person who committed the error instead of recognizing flaws in the American healthcare system. For example, heavy patient loads, long shifts, burnout, and fragmented care due to specialized medicine likely contribute to most medical mistakes (Kohn et al., 2000). An increasing reliance on a **consumerist approach** to medicine, in which patients evaluate practitioners or healthcare facilities as providers of services that can be bought in the marketplace, could also further diminish the responsibility of healthcare in general for medical mistakes.

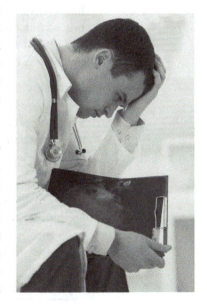

From a critical–cultural perspective, these cases highlight power differences inherent in the media, in patient–provider relationships, and in healthcare as a whole that can serve to control, define, and legitimize the meaning and reality of medical mistakes in society. Medical mistakes violate the ethical principles of beneficence and nonmalficence because they not only fail to work in the patient's best interest but also actually harm patients. They also violate the principle of respect for autonomy because patients obviously do not choose to have medical mistakes happen to them. So what happens when a surgeon accidentally removes a patient's healthy testicle during cancer surgery? What are healthcare providers legally and ethically required to do? If you were the victim of a severe medical mistake, how would you want your medical providers to respond?

Healthcare providers have an ethical obligation to disclose significant errors if the disclosure benefits the patient's physical or emotional well-being (beneficence), prevents further injury or distress (nonmaleficence), affects the patient's future medical decisions (respect for autonomy), or if disclosure would afford the patient the opportunity to be compensated (justice; Wu, Cavanaugh, McPhee, Lo, & Micco, 1997). In many states, healthcare providers also are legally required to apologize or express sympathy to patients or their families after a medical mistake (Kohn et al.,

---

COMMUNICATION MATTERS

Being a Physician Means (Never) Having to Say You're Sorry

Allison Scott, Ph.D. asked her friend Leigh Anne Dageforde, MD, a general surgery resident at Vanderbilt University Medical Center, to discuss apologizing for making a medical mistake. Here's what Dr. Dageforde said:

"Physicians are held to a high standard where society expects that they will not or will very infrequently make a mistake. Some physicians do not know how to admit to an error and instead act defensively when one occurs. When I started training to care for ill and injured people, I rarely considered how each procedure could potentially both help and harm the patient. As I have progressed in my training, the risks of procedures have become more evident as have my own imperfections. Physicians and other care providers cannot be perfect, medications have side-effects, and all procedures have risks.

"Complications and bad outcomes can occur even when everything was done correctly. These events are not only difficult for the patient and their support system but also for the physician who has devoted years of training to care for and help (not hurt) a patient. If the physician or someone on the care team makes a mistake and the patient is harmed, the negative impact influences patients and can emotionally impact physicians.

"Historically, physicians were instructed by administrators and malpractice insurance providers to never apologize to patients or acknowledge mistakes due to concern for liability in court. Recent policies promoted by my institution and others have encouraged physician honesty and appropriate apologies. And as it turns out, physicians face fewer law suits when we apologize than when we don't. But more importantly, these disclosure policies have allowed physicians, patients, and patient supporters to know the truth and to maintain a healthy working relationship."

2000). However, in almost 75% of cases, medical errors are not disclosed to patients or their families, even when severe injury is an outcome (Wu, Folkman, McPhee, & Lo, 1991). Ironically, patients and families usually still realize a mistake occurred even if it is not disclosed (Mazor, Goff, Dodd, & Alper, 2009), and they sometimes sue for malpractice simply to seek answers about their case (Wears & Wu, 2002).

There are several reasons medical errors are not disclosed more often. The main reason is that the laws requiring disclosure do not necessarily provide immunity from medical malpractice litigation, punishment, diminished professional reputation, or rising insurance rates (Carmack, 2010). As a result, healthcare providers are commonly counseled by risk managers and hospital attorneys not to communicate with patients and families after a mistake because an admission of error may be used as legal evidence of liability (Goldberg, Kuhn, Andrew, & Thomas, 2002). Another reason for nondisclosure is that doctors have unrealistic expectations for perfection in their own careers and are not well-trained on how to communicate about errors, which can make it difficult for them to admit responsibility for a mistake (Bonnema, Gonzaga, Bost, & Spagnoletti, 2012).

Even though disclosure of medical errors carries risk, apologizing for mistakes benefits both the patient and provider. Rather than responding with anger, rejection, or possible litigation, patients and their families often express understanding, forgiveness, and appreciation for the healthcare provider's honesty, attention, and concern (Christensen, Levinson, & Dunn, 1992). Patients and their families are more likely to respond positively when their practitioners tell them explicitly that an error occurred, what the error was, why it happened, and how its recurrence will be prevented for future patients, and when they express remorse for the mistake and concern for the patient (Mazor et al., 2009). On the basis of research findings like this, hospitals are increasingly encouraging their healthcare providers to explicitly apologize for mistakes rather than deny responsibility.

While the causes, experience, and disclosure of medical mistakes might seem like an issue that is strongly suited to health communication, this is still a relatively new area of inquiry for communication scholars. Petronio (2006) has used **communication privacy management theory** to investigate through an interpretive lens how healthcare providers' families react when their loved one shares private information about their medical mistake. Although physicians often disclose their mistakes to other physicians on a surface, problem-focused level (Allman, 1998), most providers keep their need for emotional support and reaffirmation of their professional competence private from peers, choosing instead to disclose their mistake on an emotional level to family members. While family members who serve as confidants want to help their loved one cope, they can experience burden in keeping this information necessarily confidential (Petronio, 2006).

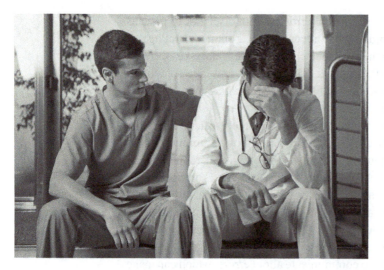

Medical error research stands to gain much more from a communication perspective. For example, communication scholarship on uncertainty and risk management has the potential to inform how providers and patients make sense of medical mistakes. How can healthcare professionals prepare themselves and their patients for the chance that medical errors, which are inevitable, may happen in any given case? There is also a need for communication training in how best to disclose medical mistakes to patients (Bonnema et al., 2012). What kinds of message features make for better or worse outcomes of disclosure? Finally, future research needs to explore the experience of healthcare providers other than physicians (like nurses, lab technicians, and pharmacists), as well as patients who have been victims of medical mistakes.

MEDICAL MISTAKES

Medical mistakes are common and costly. They violate the ethical principles of nonmaleficence, beneficence, and respect for autonomy. Healthcare providers are ethically and legally mandated to disclose medical errors, but they frequently do not do so, even though apologizing for mistakes generally leads to better outcomes than not disclosing error. Communication scholarship on privacy, uncertainty, and risk management would usefully inform future research on medical mistakes. In addition, there is a need for healthcare providers to be better trained in how to disclose errors effectively and appropriately.

FUTURE COMMUNICATION RESEARCH IN MEDICAL ETHICS

Throughout this chapter, we have mentioned several opportunities for future research on ethical issues in health communication. Here, we consider two additional intersections of ethics and communication. First, genetic testing raises many ethical questions about how patients communicate with their families, healthcare providers, and even their insurance companies. For example, who has the right to genetic test results? If your mom finds out that she has the BRCA gene that has been linked to breast cancer, should she tell you? If your boyfriend has Huntington's disease (an inherited neurological degenerative condition that usually leads to death in middle age), should he tell you? If your doctor thinks your newborn baby may have cystic fibrosis but is waiting for test results to know for sure, should she tell you? If your insurance company pays for your genetic testing, should they have access to the results? Questions such as these center around disclosure issues, and while other disciplines have begun to show interest in the who, what, and when of family genetic risk disclosure, communication researchers are well-positioned to look into *how* such disclosure best happens.

Second, the increasingly multi-cultural nature of our country has introduced medical interpreters as part of the healthcare team when a patient and doctor do not speak the same language. (Chapter 6 addresses medical interpreters in more detail.) Interpreters face a number of ethical dilemmas when communicating with a patient. For instance, should they translate exactly what the doctor says, acting purely as a conduit of information? Or should they adapt what the doctor says so that it is more culturally relevant or appropriate? Should 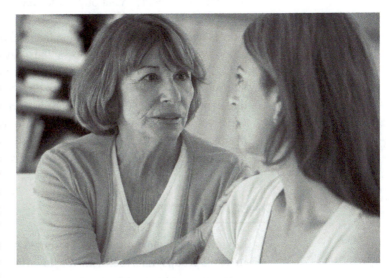 they remain neutral in the interpretation process? Or should they advocate for a patient's needs or desires? Again, taking a communication perspective on these ethical questions has the potential to provide helpful recommendations to practitioners.

CONCLUSION

In summary, medical ethics is based on the four principles of respect for autonomy, nonmaleficence, beneficence, and justice. In this chapter, we reviewed how these four principles are upheld (or not) and how they can potentially work at cross purposes in the context of informed consent, advance directives, organ donation, and medical mistakes. In each of these areas (and in other areas, such as genetic testing and medical interpretation), communication plays a key role in helping to resolve ethical tension.

DISCUSSION QUESTIONS

1. Consider the account of the Willowbrook State School. Which of the ethical principles of justice, nonmaleficence, beneficence, and respect for autonomy did the Willowbrook experiments violate? Do the pioneering results of the study in some way justify the way these discoveries were made? Were the nature and risks of the research disclosed fairly and adequately to parents in the informed consent letter?

2. You are the primary care physician of Margo, the 50-year-old woman who has dementia and has developed pneumonia. Do you overrule her advance directive and give her the antibiotics, or do you follow her advance directive and refuse the antibiotic treatment? What other information would you like to know in order to make this decision?

3. How is organ donation portrayed in the media? (Consider movies like *John Q* and *Seven Pounds* and television shows like *Grey's Anatomy* and *House*.) How do you think this affects people's organ donation behavior? Does Hollywood have an ethical responsibility to portray organ donation in a positive light, or should entertainment media have creative license in portraying organ donation situations?

4. Have you or any of your friends or family experienced a medical error in your healthcare? What happened? How did the healthcare team respond? What would you change about the way the situation was handled?

IN-CLASS ACTIVITIES

1. Review the advance directives presented on this textbook's companion website. In small groups, analyze them for how useful (or not) they would be in various decision-making circumstances.

2. Listed below are four hypothetical scenarios that involve medical mistakes. On your own or in small groups, think of the best (and worst) ways to disclose the error to the patient and/or their family on the basis of the suggestions in the text. How well does your message uphold the four ethical principles discussed at the beginning of this chapter? How does the severity of the mistake affect your disclosure? What are the differences between disclosing to the patient and disclosing to the patient's family? Your instructor may ask you to role play your good and bad disclosures for the rest of the class.

    *   You are a surgeon performing a procedure on a patient who is bleeding heavily somewhere along her digestive tract. You ask your staff for a medication to aid in coagulation to help stop the patient's bleeding. However, the patient is inadvertently treated with a blood thinning medication and dies.

- You are a nursing student rushing to finish your day so that you can make a meeting with your nursing supervisor. Your last task is to remove the urinary catheter in one of your patients. However, instead of double checking the nurse's order, you remove the catheter from the patient next door by mistake. The catheter has to be put back in—a very uncomfortable process.
- You are a radiology technician, and you are preparing a patient for his CT scan by injecting him with contrast dye. However, your co-worker failed to complete the patient's allergy screening form, and the patient breaks out in hives in reaction to the dye.
- You are an emergency room nurse treating a patient with severe pain in her left hand. The patient waited for four hours to be seen in the overcrowded hospital. After taking cultures on the patient's hand, you accidentally label the specimen with another patient's name. As a result, the patient was misdiagnosed with a local infection. Later, doctors were forced to amputate the patient's left arm after discovering that she had flesh eating bacteria that had spread to her forearm.

RECOMMENDED READINGS

Anker, A. E., & Feeley, T. H. (2011). Difficult communication: Compliance-gaining strategies of organ procurement coordinators. *Journal of Health Communication, 16,* 372—392.

In this scientific study, the researchers conducted structured interviews with 102 organ procurement coordinators to see how different ways of asking a patient's family to donate the person's organs can affect whether the family members agree to donation.

Scott, A. M., & Caughlin, J. P. (2012). Managing multiple goals in family discourse about end-of-life health decisions. *Research on Aging, 34,* 670–691.

In this interpretive study, the researchers use discourse analysis to examine actual end-of-life conversations between 242 older adults and their adult children to see how they manage identity and relational goals while making end-of-life decisions.

Ubel, P. A., Jepson, C., & Silver-Isenstadt, A. (2003). Don't ask, don't tell: A change in medical student attitudes after obstetrics/gynecology clerkships toward seeking consent for pelvic examinations on an anesthetized patient. *American Journal of Obstetrics and Gynecology, 188,* 575—579.

In this scientific study, the researchers surveyed 401 medical students to assess their attitude toward conducting unconsented gynecological exams on women who were under anesthesia.

REFERENCES

Afifi, W. A., Morgan, S. E., Stephenson, S. T., Morse, C., Harrison, T., Reichert, T., & Long, S. D. (2006). Examining the decision to talk with family about organ donation: Applying the Theory of Motivation Information Management. *Communication Monographs*, *73*, 188–215.

Aleccia, J. (2010, November 10). Surgery error leads doc to public mea culpa. *Health Care on NBC News*. Retrieved from http://www.nbcnews.com/id/40096673/ns/health-health_care/t/surgery-error-leads-doc-public-mea-culpa/#.UZQjerUsmSo

Allman, J. (1998). Bearing the burden or baring the soul: Physicians' self-disclosure and boundary management regarding medical mistakes. *Health Communication*, *10*, 175–197.

American Psychological Association. (2000). *Report of the APA working group on assisted suicide and end-of-life decisions*. Retrieved from http://www.apa.org/pubs/info/reports/aseol-full.pdf

Anker, A. E., & Feeley, T. H. (2011). Difficult communication: Compliance-gaining strategies of organ procurement coordinators. *Journal of Health Communication*, *16*, 372–392.

Arras, J. D. (2008). The Jewish Chronic Disease Hospital case. In E. J. Emanuel, C. Grady, R. A. Crouch, R. K. Lie, F. G. Miller, & D. Wendler (Eds.) *The Oxford textbook of clinical research ethics* (pp. 73–79). New York: Oxford University Press.

Aspden, P., Wolcott, J. A., Bootman, J. L., & Cronenwett, L. R. (Eds.). (2007). *Preventing medication errors: Quality chasm series*. Washington, DC: National Academies Press.

Barnes, S. S. (2012). Practicing pelvic examinations by medical students on women under anesthesia: Why not ask first? *Obstetrics and Gynecology*, *120*, 941–943.

Beauchamp, T. L., & Childress, J. F. (2001). *Principles of biomedical ethics* (5th ed.). New York: Oxford University Press.

Bonifield, J., & Cohen, E. (2012, November 5). 10 shocking medical mistakes. *CNN Health*. Retrieved from http://www.cnn.com/2012/11/05/health/medical-mistakes-nov

Bonnema, R. A., Gonzaga, A. M. R., Bost, J. E., & Spagnoletti, C. L. (2012). Teaching error disclosure: Advanced communication skills training for residents. *Journal of Communication in Healthcare*, *5*, 51–55.

Brashers, D. E. (2001). Communication and uncertainty management. *Journal of Communication*, *51*, 477–497.

Brown, R. F., Butow, P. N., Ellis, P., Boyle, F., & Tattersall, M. H. N. (2004). Seeking informed consent to cancer clinical trials: Describing current practice. *Social Science & Medicine*, *58*, 2445–2457.

Carmack, H. J. (2010). Bearing witness to the ethics of practice: Storying physicians' medical mistake narratives. *Health Communication*, *25*, 449–458.

Chedekel, L. (2012, December 3). Yale study: Medication errors, confusion common for hospital patients. *New Haven Register*. Retrieved from http://www.nhregister.com/articles/2012/12/03/news/doc50bd213d5f662015750301.txt?viewmode=fullstory

Chouhan, P., & Draper, H. (2003). Modified mandated choice for organ procurement. *Journal of Medical Ethics*, *29*, 157–162.

Christensen, J. F., Levinson, W., & Dunn, P. M. (1992). The heart of darkness: The impact of perceived mistakes on physicians. *Journal of General Internal Medicine*, *7*, 424–431.

Corbie-Smith, G. (1999). The continuing legacy of the Tuskegee Syphilis Study: Considerations for clinical investigation. *American Journal of the Medical Sciences, 317,* 5–8.

Corrigan, O. (2003). Empty ethics: The problem with informed consent. *Sociology of Health and Illness, 25,* 768–792.

DesHarnais, S., Carter, R. E., Hennessy, W., Kurent, J. E., & Carter, C. (2007). Lack of concordance between physician and patient: Reports on end-of-life care discussions. *Journal of Palliative Medicine, 10,* 728–740.

Drane, J. F. (1984). Competency to give an informed consent: A model for making clinical assessments. *Journal of the American Medical Association, 252,* 925–927.

Dworkin, R. (1993). *Life's dominion.* London: Harper Collins.

Ellenberg, S. S. (1997). Informed consent: Protection or obstacle? Some emerging issues. *Controlled Clinical Trials, 18,* 628–636.

Fabre, J. (1998). Organ donation and presumed consent. *Lancet, 352,* 150.

Fagerlin, A., Ditto, P. H., Hawkins, N. A., Schneider, C. E., & Smucker, W. D. (2002). The use of advance directives in end-of-life decision making. *American Behavioral Scientist, 46,* 268–283.

Feeley, T. H., & Moon, S.-I. (2009). A meta-analytic review of communication campaigns to promote organ donation. *Communication Reports, 22,* 63–73.

Fink, A. S., Prochazka, A. V., Henderson, W. G., Bartenfeld, D., Nyirenda, C., Webb, A., . . . Parmelee, P. (2010). Enhancement of surgical informed consent by addition of repeat back: A multicenter, randomized controlled clinical trial. *Annals of Surgery, 252,* 27–36.

Flory, J., & Emanuel, E. (2004). Interventions to improve research participants' understanding in informed consent for research: A systematic review. *Journal of the American Medical Association, 292,* 1593–1601.

Foss, K. A. (2011). "When we make mistakes, people die!": Constructions of responsibility for medical errors in televised medical dramas, 1994–2007. *Communication Quarterly, 59,* 484–506.

Freeborne, N., Lynn, J., & Desbiens, N. A. (2000). Insights about dying from the SUPPORT project. *Journal of the American Geriatric Society, 48,* S199–S205.

Gallup Organization. (2005). National survey of organ and tissue donation attitudes and behaviors. Retrieved from http://www.organdonor.gov/dtcp/publications.html

Goldacre, B. (2013, February 2). Health care's trick coin. *New York Times,* p. A23.

Goldberg, R. M., Kuhn, G., Andrew, L. B., & Thomas, H. A., Jr. (2002). Coping with medical mistakes and errors in judgment. *Annals of Emergency Medicine, 39,* 287–292.

Hanto, D. W. (2007). Ethical challenges posed by the solicitation of deceased and living organ donors. *New England Journal of Medicine, 356,* 1062–1066.

Harrison, T. R., Morgan, S. E., King, A. J., Di Corcia, M. J., Williams, E. A., Ivic, R. K., & Hopeck, P. (in press). Utilizing media priming and design perspectives to promote joining the Michigan Organ Donor Registry: Evaluating the impact of a multi-faceted intervention. *Health Communication.*

Hester, D. M. (2006). Why we must leave our organs to others. *American Journal of Bioethics, 6,* w23.

Hines, S. C., Glover, J. J., Babrow, A. S., Holley, J. L. Badzek, L. A., & Moss, A. H. (2001). Improving advance care planning by accommodating family preferences. *Journal of Palliative Medicine, 4*, 481–489.

Hopper, L. (2004, August 12). Unfair advantage? *Houston Chronicle*, p. B1.

Jansen, S. J. T., Stiggelbout, A. M., Nooij, M. A., Noordijk, E. M., & Kievit, J. (2000). Response shift in quality of life measurement in early-stage breast cancer patients undergoing radiotherapy. *Quality of Life Research, 9*, 603–615.

Joffe, S., Carcillo, J., Anton, N., deCaen, A., Han, Y. Y., Bell, M. J., . . . Garcia-Guerra, G. (2011). Donation after cardiocirculatory death: a call for a moratorium pending full public disclosure and fully informed consent. *Philosophy, Ethics, and Humanities in Medicine, 6*, 17.

Joffe, S., Cook, E. F., Cleary, P. D., Clark, J. W., & Weeks, J. C. (2001). Quality of informed consent in cancer clinical trials: A cross-sectional survey. *Lancet, 358*, 1772–1777.

Joint Commission on the Accreditation of Healthcare Organizations. (2002). *Clinical communication and patient safety*. Retrieved from http://www.jointcommission.org

Kirchhoff, K. T., Hammes, B. J., & Kehl, K. A., Briggs, L. A., & Brown, R. L. (2010). Effect of a disease-specific planning intervention on surrogate understanding of patient goals for future medical treatment. *Journal of the American Geriatrics Society, 58*, 1233–1240.

Kohn L. T., Corrigan, J. M., & Donaldson, M. S. (Eds.). (2000). *To err is human: Building a safer health system.* Washington, DC: National Academies Press.

Lamba, S., Murphy, P., McVicker, S., Smith, J. H., & Mosenthal, A. C. (2012). Changing end-of-life care practice for liver transplant service patients: Structured palliative care intervention in the surgical intensive care unit. *Journal of Pain and Symptom Management, 44*, 508–519.

Libbus, K. M., & Russell, C. (1995). Congruence of decisions between patients and their potential surrogates about life-sustaining therapies. *IMAGE: Journal of Nursing Scholarship, 2*, 135–140.

Mazor, K. M., Goff, S. L., Dodd, K., & Alper, E. J. (2009). Understanding patients' perceptions of medical errors. *Journal of Communication in Healthcare, 2*, 34–46.

Mazur, D. J. (2006). How successful are we at protecting preferences? Consent, informed consent, advance directives, and substituted judgment. *Medical Decision Making, 26*, 106–109.

Mesich-Brant, J. L., & Grossback, L. J. (2005). Assisting altruism: Evaluating legally binding consent in organ donation policy. *Journal of Health Politics, Policy, and Law, 30*, 687–717.

Morgan, S. E., & Harrison, T. R. (2010). The impact of health communication research on organ donation outcomes in the United States. *Health Communication, 25*, 589–592.

Morgan, S. E., & Miller, J. K. (2001). Beyond the organ donor card: The effect of knowledge, attitudes, and values on willingness to communicate about organ donation to family members. *Health Communication, 14*, 121–134.

Murphy, T. F. (2004). *Case studies in biomedical research ethics*. Boston: MIT Press.

Newman, M. C. (1996). The emotional impact of mistakes on family physicians. *Archives of Family Medicine, 5*, 71–75.

O'Neill, O. (2003). Some limits of informed consent. *Journal of Medical Ethics, 29*, 4–7.

Paasche-Orlow, M. K., Taylor, H. A., & Brancati, F. L. (2003). Readability standards for informed-consent forms as compared with actual readability. *New England Journal of Medicine, 348*, 721–726.

Pautex, S., Herrmann, F. R., & Zulian, G. B. (2008). Role of advance directives in palliative care units: A prospective study. *Palliative Medicine, 22*, 835–841.

Petronio, S. (2006). Impact of medical mistakes: Navigating work-family boundaries for physicians and their families. *Communication Monographs, 73*, 462–467.

Pew Research Center for the People and the Press. (2006, January 5). *Strong public support for right to die: More Americans discussing—and planning—end-of-life treatment.* Retrieved from http://people-press.org/reports/display.php3?ReportID=266

Phillips, D. P., Christenfeld, N., & Glynn, L. M. (1998). Increase in U.S. medication-error deaths between 1983 and 1993. *Lancet, 351*, 643–644.

Pitts, M. J., Raup-Krieger, J. L., Kundrat, A. L., & Nussbaum, J. F. (2009). Mapping the processes and patterns of family organ donation discussions: Conversational styles and strategies in live discourse. *Health Communication, 24*, 413–425.

Port, F. K., Dykstra, D. M., Merion, R. M., & Wolfe, R. A. (2005). Trends and results for organ donation and transplantation in the United States, 2004. *American Journal of Transplantation, 5*, 843–849.

Prayle, A. P., Hurley, M. N., & Smyth, A. R. (2012). Compliance with mandatory reporting of clinical trial results on clinicaltrials.gov: Cross sectional study. *British Medical Journal, 344*, d7373.

Richards, J. R. (2012). *The ethics of transplants: Why careless thought costs lives.* New York: Oxford University Press.

Robertson, J. A. (1999). Delimiting the donor: The dead donor rule. *Hasting Centers Report, 29*, 6–14.

Saunders, B. (2011). Normative consent and organ donation: A vindication. *Journal of Medical Ethics, 37*, 362–363.

Schneiderman, L. J., Kronick, R., Kaplan, R. M., Anderson, J. P., & Langer, R. D. (1992). Effects of offering advance directives on medical treatments and costs. *Annals of Internal Medicine, 117*, 599–606.

Scott, A. M., & Caughlin, J. P. (2012). Managing multiple goals in family discourse about end-of-life health decisions. *Research on Aging, 34*, 670–691.

Shalowitz, D. I., Garrett-Mayer, E., & Wendler, D. (2006). The accuracy of surrogate decision makers. *Archives of Internal Medicine, 166*, 493–497.

Shaw, D. (2012). A direct advance on advance directives. *Bioethics, 26*, 267–274.

Smith, R. (2013, February 20). Cancer patient has wrong testicle removed by bungling surgeons. Mirror News. Retrieved from http://www.mirror.co.uk/news/uk-news/cancer-patient-wrong-testicle-removed–1719298

Smith, S. W., Kopfman, J. E., Lindsey, L. L. M., Yoo, J., & Morrison, K. (2004). Encouraging family discussion on the decision to donate organs: The role of the willingness to communicate scale. *Health Communication, 16*, 333–346.

Sokolowski, M. (2010). Advance directives and the problem of informed consent. *Journal of Ethics in Mental Health, 5*, 1–6.

Spital, A. (1996). Mandated choice for organ donation: Time to give it a try. *Annals of Internal Medicine, 125,* 66–69.

Teno, J. M., Gruneir, A., Schwartz, Z., Nanda, A., & Wetle, T. (2007). Association between advance directives and quality of end-of-life care: A national study. *Journal of the American Geriatrics Society, 55,* 189–194.

Tilden, V. P., Tolle, S. W., Nelson, C. A., & Fields, J. (2001). Family decision-making to withdraw life-sustaining treatments from hospitalized patients. *Nursing Research, 50,* 105–115.

Torpy, J. M., Lynn, C., & Glass, R. M. (2005). Randomized controlled trials. *Journal of the American Medical Association, 294,* 2262.

Ubel, P. A., Jepson, C., & Silver-Isenstadt, A. (2003). Don't ask, don't tell: A change in medical student attitudes after obstetrics/gynecology clerkships toward seeking consent for pelvic examinations on an anesthetized patient. *American Journal of Obstetrics and Gynecology, 188,* 575–579.

United Network for Organ Sharing. (2013). *Data.* Retrieved from http://www.unos.org/donation/index.php?topic=data

U. S. Department of Health and Human Services (2013). Retrieved from http://www.organ-donor.gov/index.html

U.S. P.L. 101–508 (1990). *Patient Self-Determination Act.* Washington, DC: US Code.

Wears, R. L., & Wu, A. W. (2002). Dealing with failure: The aftermath of errors and adverse events. *Annals of Emergency Medicine, 39,* 344–346.

Wertheimer, A. (2013). Non-completion and informed consent. *Journal of Medical Ethics.* doi: 10.1136/medethics–2012–101108.

Winter, L., Parks, S. M., & Diamond, J. J. (2010). Ask a different question, get a different answer: Why living wills are poor guides to care preferences at the end of life. *Journal of Palliative Medicine, 13,* 567–572.

Wolen, S., Rady, M. Y., Verheijde, J. L., & McGregor, J. (2006). Organ procurement organizations internet enrollment for organ donation: Abandoning informed consent. *BioMed Central Medical Ethics, 7,* 14.

Wu, A. W., Cavanaugh, T. A., McPhee, S. J., Lo, B., & Micco, G. P. (1997). To tell the truth: Ethical and practical issues in disclosing medical mistakes to patients. *Journal of General Internal Medicine, 12,* 770–775.

Wu, A. W., Folkman, S., McPhee, S. J., & Lo, B. (1991). Do house officers learn from their mistakes? *Journal of the American Medical Association, 265,* 2089–2094.

Technology, Media, and eHealth

12

New Technologies in Health Communication

Nancy Grant Harrington and
Katharine J. Head

"Beam me up, Scotty." In Star Trek, whenever characters find themselves in trouble, a fellow shipmate can simply beam them back to the Enterprise using the transporter. It's kept more than a few Starfleet members from meeting their demise (see opening sequence in *Star Trek into Darkness*, a movie highly recommended by both authors of this chapter!). Wouldn't it be nice if you were sick and a doctor could simply beam you into the clinic and then diagnose and treat you with some Star Trek–like technological wizardry? Well, we aren't quite there yet, but we're working on it (e.g., NASA's working on replicating pizzas). In this chapter, we'll discuss various ways in which new technologies are being used in healthcare in the United States. We'll focus on how information systems promote patient care and how technology promotes information seeking, sharing, and personal health management. We'll also discuss concerns related to the translation and adoption of these technologies, as well as some of the opportunities that these new technologies offer.

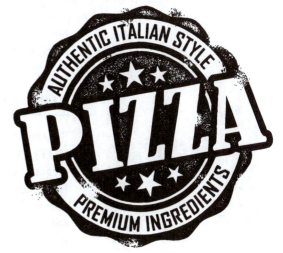

Much of the research on new technologies in healthcare stems from the scientific paradigm, and so you'll see that perspective as you read. However, acknowledging the critical–cultural perspective, we will draw attention to some of the societal implications of these new health communication technologies, as well. Also, we want to point out that the research on technology-based health behavior change interventions is covered in Chapter 15 of this text. This chapter focuses more on the system level and individual use of technology for information management. Now, buckle your seat belts because we are about to hit warp speed!

NEW TECHNOLOGIES IN THE DELIVERY OF HEALTHCARE

To say that the U.S. healthcare system is complex is the understatement of the millennium. To bring the existing system into the twenty-first century by integrating information technology into its operation is the *undertaking* of the millennium. We find it very interesting that a healthcare system that is so in love with technology to support the diagnosis and treatment of disease has been so resistant to technology to manage and exchange information! As Susan Dentzer, editor-in-chief of the journal *Health Affairs*, writes,

> A major anomaly of the Information Age is that a huge sector of the U.S. economy has been so lacking—and for so long—in its use of information technology (IT). As dozens of major industries retooled themselves in the 1980s around new means of conveying, processing, and analyzing information, health care largely sat on the sidelines. We all suffered.
>
> (Dentzer, 2009, p. 320)

Dentzer points out that the "cottage industry" nature of the system, in which most physicians practice in very small groups, is partly responsible for the lack of change. But as U.S. healthcare reform is implemented, along with incentives and mandates for using IT, and as some industry leaders recognize the potential for IT to improve care (and even improve profit), we are seeing IT appearing more and more in the healthcare enterprise.

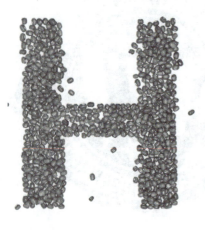

ALPHABET SOUP

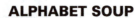

So what's involved exactly in this **health information technology (HIT)** revolution, and what does it do for us? Describing the intricacies and challenges associated with these efforts and everything HIT is capable of is exceedingly complicated and simply beyond the scope of this chapter. So, we're attempting to boil things down to the most pertinent information. If you want to know more detail, we refer you to HealthIT.gov, the website of the **Office of the National**

Coordinator for Health Information Technology (ONC), for a start. For our purposes here, let's consider Table 12.1, which provides you with a list of terms to help you navigate this HIT landscape.

At the heart of HIT efforts are two components: **health information exchange (HIE)** and the **electronic health record (EHR)**. HIE is what it sounds like: the exchange of digital health information. Various initiatives have developed to help manage HIE, addressing issues related to the data that are collected, the computing platforms (software packages, websites) that process and exchange data, and the applications available to utilize the data (e.g., data analysis, decision support). These initiatives come in all shapes and sizes, with differences in funding, governance, and organization, but their ultimate goal is the same: to allow electronic patient healthcare information to be shared within and across healthcare organizations. eHealth Initiative, a national independent, nonprofit organization that promotes research, education, and advocacy related to the use of information technology in healthcare, estimates that there are currently about 300 HIE initiatives in the United States (eHealth Initiative, 2012).

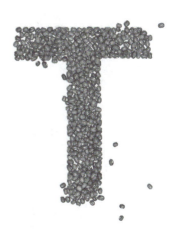

What kind of information is being exchanged, who's exchanging it, and how is it being used? At the organizational level, the information being exchanged is the EHR, which is a digital version of the paper medical records that a doctor or hospital would keep on a patient. With proper use of EHRs, a patient's medical records can be shared by multiple doctors, labs, pharmacies, hospitals, and insurance companies to promote efficient, effective, and safe healthcare. Patient information is available instantly and "follows the patient." At the individual level, depending on the system in place, patients can have access to their EHRs and/or use web-based programs to make appointments, access test results, and communicate with their physicians through email, instant message, or video chat.

HIE/EHR

Health information exchanges (HIE) allow patients and providers to share health information through a digital medium. The most visible example of this type of information exchange in our country today is the electronic health record (EHR), which will soon be a part of most clinics as required by the Patient Protection and Affordable Care Act of 2010.

Table 12.1 List of Important Abbreviations in Health Information Technology

Abbreviation	Full Name	Description
ONC	The Office of the National Coordinator for Health Information Technology	Part of the U.S. Department of Health and Human Services, the ONC is responsible for promoting, coordinating, and supporting the adoption of health information exchange across the United States.
HIT	Health Information Technology	Any computerized technology applied to the comprehensive management of health information, including its secure storage and exchange between patients, providers, and related organizations.
HIE	Health Information Exchange	Electronic sharing of patient health information by healthcare providers, facilitated by HIE initiatives that work toward standardized data meaning, structure, transport, security, and services.
EHR	Electronic Health Record	A digital version of a patient's medical record (e.g., medical history, diagnoses, medications, immunizations, allergies, x-rays, lab and test results) that is maintained by healthcare providers through software systems.
PHR	Personal Health Record	A digital version of patient health information that is maintained by the patient through electronic devices or web-based programs; some PHRs may be linked to EHRs.
HITECH	Health Information Technology for Economic and Clinical Health Act	Legislation designed to improve healthcare delivery and patient care in the United States through health information technology. Provisions of the act provide support and incentives for technical assistance, coordination, connectivity, and training.

As a complement to EHRs, we have PHRs: **personal health records**. PHRs are private, secure software applications that provide patients the opportunity to store, organize, and share their own health information. Estimates are that at least 70 million Americans have some form of a PHR (Kaelber, Jha, Johnston, Middleton, & Bates, 2008). A joint task force convened by the Medical Library Association and National Library of Medicine identified 117 PHRs available through vendors or healthcare providers, employers, or health insurance companies, 91 of which the task force considered "viable" (Jones, Shipman, Plaut, & Selden, 2010). A little more than half were stand-alone programs, approximately one-quarter were integrated with EHRs through a healthcare provider or insurance company, and about a tenth could be either integrated or stand-alone.

Numerous research studies show that EHRs (with or without associated PHRs) have all sorts of positive outcomes, including improved patient safety, more coordinated care, and better healthcare provider adherence to **evidence-based medicine** (e.g., Chaudhry et al., 2006; Kaushal, Shojania, & Bates, 2003). Further, there's evidence to show that most patients want to use information technology to promote healthcare (Deloitte, 2008). There is a question, though, about the impact of these systems on utilization of in-person healthcare resources. You might expect that if patients can access the information and services they need online, then there would be reduced demand for office visits, emergency room visits, hospitalizations, and so on. There is some evidence for this, but there's also evidence of the opposite. Let's take a closer look at this research to learn more about these conflicting results.

Chen, Garrido, Chock, Okawa, and Liang (2009) studied the effects of Kaiser Permanente's (KP) implementation of KP HealthConnect, a "comprehensive health information system" that included an EHR and secure patient–provider email. They focused on the Hawaii region because it was the first to fully implement the program for the physician office setting, and they analyzed data for all patients in the system (approximately 225,000 people). They compared pre- and post-implementation rates for several variables, including total office visits, scheduled telephone visits, and patient–physician emails. Results showed that total office visits declined from 5.01 visits per patient to 3.70 visits per patient. That's a 26% decrease, which is both statistically and clinically significant. Telephone visits and email contact, however, increased. If you consider just the percentages, you'll freak out: Telephone contact increased nearly 900%, and email contact increased nearly 600%. But you have to consider the actual numbers. Telephone visits increased from 0.17 per patient to 1.68 per patient, and email contact increased from 0.03 per patient to 0.23 per patient. The researchers also considered healthcare quality and patient satisfaction data, and they found either no change or trends that looked favorable. What these data suggest is that patients' ability to contact their doctors by telephone or email results in tremendous efficiencies and does not negatively affect health outcomes or patient satisfaction.

A study by Palen, Ross, Powers, and Xu (2012), however, found evidence that patient access to online information and services may actually increase utilization of in-person healthcare resources. These researchers also studied the impact of the KP HealthConnect system, but they were interested in a particular aspect of the system: MyHealthManager (MHM), a component of KP HealthConnect that provides patients access to their health records and lets them manage appointments, refill prescriptions, and email their physicians. The researchers looked at patients enrolled in Kaiser Permanente

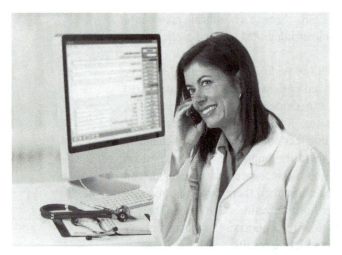

Colorado, an area that serves more than 500,000 members. From the pool of eligible participants (i.e., at least 18 years old, enrolled in the health plan for at least two consecutive years), they selected matched samples of patients who signed up for and used MHM and patients who did not ($n = 44,321$ in each group). Across all of the outcome variables they considered—office visits, calls, after-hour clinic visits, emergency department visits, and inpatient hospitalizations—the MHM users showed an increase in use when compared with MHM non-users.

So what's going on here? Well, as with most things having to do with health information technology, the answer is complicated. First, the study participants were different. Chen et al. (2009) studied all enrollees in the KP Hawaii health plan, whereas Palen et al. (2012) chose a matched subsample of enrollees in the KP Colorado health plan. Second, the time periods of the studies were different. Data for Chen et al. spanned 2004 to 2007, whereas data for Palen et al. spanned 2005 to 2010 (although they just looked at data over a two-year period for any given participant). Perhaps most important, the online technology was different. Participants in Palen et al.'s study had access to MHM, whereas those in Chen et al.'s study almost certainly did not (MHM did not become available until May, 2006). And as Palen et al. point out, patients had to actively sign up to participate in MHM, and this could have introduced several confounding factors that might explain their greater healthcare utilization (e.g., these members were more concerned about their health, they may have discovered additional health concerns through online access).

So, whereas the participants in Chen et al.'s (2009) study seemed to be using online and telephone communication as a substitute for in-person visits, participants in Palen et al.'s (2012) study seemed to be using the more comprehensive MHM system as a prelude to in-person visits. More research is definitely called for here to help us understand the motivation of patients, how they use the various components of these online systems, and ultimately the impact on physician–patient communication and healthcare outcomes.

TELEMEDICINE

Sometimes patients find themselves needing care but they do not have access to a nearby healthcare provider. Or maybe they have access to a nearby healthcare provider, but they really need to see a specialist. One solution to this dilemma is telemedicine.

Telemedicine is the broad term used to describe the many telecommunication technologies used to deliver clinical care across a distance (Turner, 2003). Because the term is so broad, Sood and colleagues (2007) wanted to determine more precisely how people are defining telemedicine. They did a literature search of peer-reviewed articles, they consulted with respected health organizations like the **World Health Organization** and the United Kingdom's **National Health Service**, and they contacted well-known scholars in the field of health and telemedicine. In all, they found 104 different definitions of telemedicine. After reviewing the definitions, though, they figured out that all of them addressed at least one of four contexts: medical (i.e., some mention of the healthcare services being provided), technological (i.e., some description of the technology being used to facilitate the communication), spatial (i.e., some mention of the long distance purpose of telemedicine), and benefits (i.e., some mention of the benefits received from using telemedicine). Strauss's (1998) definition of telemedicine addresses all four contexts: "a means provided by advanced technologies of allowing distant medical resources to meet unfulfilled demands in healthcare services" (p. 111).

Another way to define telemedicine is to classify how it is being used. Building on previous work in this area, Turner (2003) identified six different classifications of telemedicine:

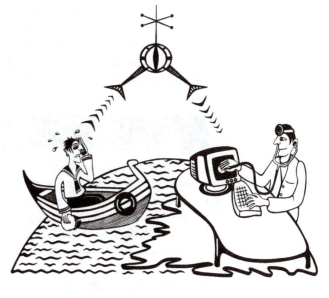

1. Specific disease: using telemedicine to treat a specific condition, like fractures or heart murmurs.
2. Specialty area: using telemedicine in a specific area of medicine, like psychiatry or dermatology.
3. Technology: the type of technology used or the means of transmission, like telephone or interactive videoconferencing; this also addresses the temporal aspect of the technology, like whether it's asynchronous or synchronous communication.
4. Class of clinical problem: using telemedicine at different points in the care continuum, like emergency triage or surgical follow-up.
5. Participants: the responsibilities or roles of the different individuals involved in the telemedicine interaction, like whether the interaction is between a patient and a healthcare provider or between two healthcare providers.

6. History of encounter: the relational aspects of the encounter, like whether it's a one-time visit or a long-term patient–provider relationship.

Matusitz and Breen (2007) explored the effect of telemedicine on health communication, noting that "every individual can benefit from telemedicine, from the patient, to the community, to physicians and other practitioners" (p. 76). They discussed five health communication benefits of telemedicine. The first is transcending geographic boundaries and allowing healthcare services to reach geographically isolated areas. The second is transcending temporal boundaries, meaning that communication can be asynchronous or synchronous. In addition, in most cases it allows for a faster delivery of healthcare because a patient is not waiting for a face-to-face meeting. Third, telemedicine is cost effective and may even help to reduce healthcare costs because people don't need to travel to see a doctor, and it allows for healthcare providers to consult on a case without having to be in the same place. Fourth, telemedicine has the ability to increase patients' comfort, security, and satisfaction, which are very important outcome variables. And fifth, telemedicine can be used to digitize health communication through web-based services. While this last benefit encompasses quite a few ideas (including some of the ones discussed in the HIE section of this chapter), the take away message is that patients can "consult" with online information sites and follow up with a healthcare provider about a possible ailment *before* making an appointment and coming to a clinic or emergency room. As noted by Matusitz and Breen, these benefits of telemedicine "facilitate health communication by eliminating many of the burdens involved in standard health care" (p. 77).

TELEMEDICINE

Telemedicine is a specific kind of HIT in which technology is used to facilitate clinical care when the patients and the providers are separated by a long distance. It is defined as "a means provided by advanced technologies of allowing distant medical resources to meet unfulfilled demands in healthcare services" (Strauss, 1998, p. 111).

But with every benefit, we must also be cognizant of the limitations of telemedicine. Matusitz and Breen (2007) outline four challenges to using telemedicine that directly or indirectly affect health communication. The first is legal issues such as licensing and liability. The healthcare industry is still trying to figure out how telemedicine will work across state and even country lines. The second issue is patient privacy. Legally, healthcare providers are obligated to maintain patient privacy. But with telemedicine, there are more people involved than in standard care (including technicians who assist with the technology), so the possibility increases that confidential patient information may be seen or heard by the wrong person. The third challenge is how health insurance fits into telemedicine. How do consulting physicians get reimbursed? Can a patient only use telemedicine to communicate with an "in network" provider? Such a restriction would severely limit the potential of telemedicine! Finally, there is the challenge of knowledge and expertise with telemedicine. Especially as new telemedicine technologies are developed and become available for use, somebody has to know how to use them. One study of mental healthcare providers at rural VA medical clinics found that about half of the providers reported they were not adequately trained to use the telemedicine equipment at their clinic, that technical problems often interfered with the telemedicine sessions, and that there was not adequate tech support for their telemedicine technology (Jameson, Farmer, Head, Fortney, & Teal, 2011). In sum, telemedicine comes with its

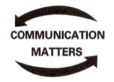

COMMUNICATION MATTERS

The Power of Telemedicine

Imagine you are a young doctor working in a rural clinic with few resources. An older patient who makes his living as a farmer comes in complaining of fatigue and recent weight loss, and although you can find nothing wrong with him, your instincts tell you that something is the matter. You decide to contact the urban university hospital to consult on the case. You send the patient case history along with X-rays. An hour later, a well-respected medical oncologist asks to have a videoconference with you to consult on the patient and lets you know that the X-rays revealed a small carcinoma on the lung. The medical oncologist then asks to speak to the patient about coming to the city for surgery. Although the patient is leery about traveling and leaving his farm, the medical oncologist assures him he will be taken care of and will be able to get back to his farm as soon as possible. The patient travels to the city for the surgery, it is a success, and the patient returns home but continues to use telemedicine for follow-up appointments with the medical oncologist and the young rural doctor.

This care wouldn't have been possible and there might not have been as positive a health outcome if telemedicine weren't being used. And guess what? This is a true story. After his experience with telemedicine, the young doctor said that for the first time in a long time, he didn't feel "so professionally alone," and he felt like "his medical horizon extended all the way back to the city" (Merrell & Doarn, 2013, p. 70). You can see, therefore, that telemedicine not only helps patients but also helps doctors. It's a win-win for everyone.

own unique set of challenges that must be addressed before the full potential of this technology can be realized.

HEALTH 2.0

"Health 2.0" or "Medicine 2.0" refers to the applications, services, and tools that are available via Web 2.0 technology that allow people to seek, share, and manage health information online. Now more than ever, patients and providers alike are empowered

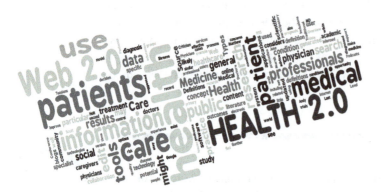

by increased access to information and the increased participation, collaboration, and social networking that information technology affords. The concept of "collective intelligence" or the "wisdom of crowds" means that the whole of knowledge available through socially networked information is greater than the sum of its parts, and that means Health 2.0 is poised to trans-

form healthcare (Sarasohn-Kahn, 2008). In this section, we review research on patient health information seeking, provider and patient information sharing, and patient personal health management in the Health 2.0 environment.

HEALTH 2.0
Health 2.0 is any type of Web 2.0 modality used in the name of healthcare. Health 2.0 technologies can be divided into three major categories based upon the function they serve: information seeking, information sharing, and personal health management.

Information Seeking

It probably comes as no surprise to you that millions of people go online to look up **health information**. In fact, the Pew Research Center determined that 80% of Internet users use the Internet to search for health information (Fox, 2011a). As this online searching behavior becomes more and more popular, it's important that health communication scholars understand what people are searching for online, who is doing this searching, why they are using the Internet to find health information, and where they are searching.

The Basics. As we said a second ago (depending on how fast you read), 80% of people already using the Internet go online to look for health information. But the types of information they seek ranges widely (Fox, 2011a; Fox & Duggan, 2013). According to the Pew Internet & American Life Project (Fox, 2011a), 66% of Internet users go online to look up information about a specific disease or condition; 56% look for information about medical treatments, including medications and procedures; 44% go online to look up information about a particular doctor or other health professional; and 36% look up information about a particular hospital or clinic. People also look for information about health insurance, Medicaid, and Medicare; 25% of Internet users report going online to look up this kind of information (Fox & Duggan, 2013). With healthcare reform (see Chapter 7 for more details on the Affordable Care Act), it is likely that the number will go up as people try to figure out how the new policies affect them.

Just as the health information topics vary, so do the people doing the **information seeking**. Survey research has found that being a younger adult, female, and White, and having a higher income and higher education are all associated with higher levels of online information seeking in the United States (Fox & Duggan, 2013; Koch-Weser, Bradshaw, Gualtieri, & Gallagher, 2010). As Johnson and Case (2012) point out, the Internet has really facilitated people's ability to become active health information seekers instead of passive health information recipients. In their book, *Health Information Seeking*, they review research that explores the reasons that people like to use the Internet to look for information about health and their motivations for doing so. The reasons to use the Internet include "convenience, anonymity, confidentiality, just-in-time decision-making support, and the diversity of information sources" (p. 80). Motivations include "desires for reassurance, for second opinions, for greater understanding of existing information, and to circumvent perceived external barriers to traditional sources (such as a wish not to 'bother' their doctor)" (p. 81).

And just where are people looking on the Internet for their health information? The Internet's a big place (duh). A quick search of the Open Directory Project website uncovers nearly 145,000 open directory sites related to the term "health" (DMOZ, 2013). Thank goodness for search engines that help us find our needle in that haystack. Helpful, too, is knowing where most people tend to look for health information online. The eBusiness Knowledgebase helps us with that, listing the top 15 most popular health websites. Table 12.2 presents the top 10.

Okay, with the who/what/why/where under our belts, let's look at some specific examples of using the Internet to search for health information. In the past decade,

Table 12.2 Top 10 Most Popular Health Websites

Website	URL	Estimated Number of Unique Monthly Visitors
WebMD	http://www.webmd.com	37,000,000
National Institutes of Health	http://www.nih.gov	29,000,000
Yahoo! Health	http://health.yahoo.net	27,500,000
Mayo Clinic	http://www.mayoclinic.com	21,000,000
MedicineNet	http://www.medicinenet.com	12,500,000
Drugs.com	http://www.drugs.com	11,000,000
HealthGrades	http://www.healthgrades.com	10,000,000
Everyday Health	http://www.everydayhealth.com	5,700,000
Health Central	http://healthcentral.com	5,000,000
Health	http://www.health.com	4,000,000

From http://www.ebizmba.com/articles/health-websites, December, 2013.

health communication scholars have studied specific websites both in content characteristics and user characteristics. In this section, we'll examine one particular site (YouTube) and one particular *kind* of site (disease-specific websites) to give you a taste of what's out there. As we go through these examples, think about times you may have used sites like these and what your experience was like.

YouTube. Who knew eight years after Chad Hurley, Steve Chen, and Jawed Karim created YouTube, it would be one of the top visited sites in the world? YouTube reports that more than one billion unique users visit *each month* (YouTube, 2013). They may be looking for cat videos, but they may also be looking for health information. Health communication scholars have approached the study of YouTube by doing content analyses of the specific health topics found on the site.

Researchers have studied a variety of health topics appearing on YouTube, from vaccines (Keelan, Pavri-Garcia, Tomlinson, & Wilson, 2007) to tobacco use (Bromberg, Augustson, & Backinger, 2012; Freeman & Chapman, 2007) to obesity (Yoo & Kim, 2012). Tian (2010) looked at the framing of organ donation videos on YouTube and found that 95.8% of these videos were positively framed and encouraged donation. She also found that over 70% of the videos originated in the United States and the most commonly covered organ was the kidney. Kidneys, of course, can be donated when a person is still alive; 38.3% of the organ donation videos covered this topic. Organs that are transplanted after a person dies were covered less frequently: heart, 24.5%; lung, 18.3%; pancreas, 9.3%. In addition, in terms of *how* videos presented information about organ donation, 29.3% addressed the registration process, 5.4% addressed the transplantation process, and only 2.0% addressed a failed transplantation. Tian concluded that sites like YouTube have great potential for disseminating important health information to a large number of people.

Topical websites. If you find yourself facing a particular health issue, no doubt your search of the Internet will result in at least a few specific websites devoted to the issue. These sites can cover information on the disease, treatments, recent news and research on the disease, and more. Sometimes these sites are hosted by an organization dedicated to this health topic, like the American Diabetes Association website (www.diabetes. org/). Other times, a larger health organization might host a number of websites devoted to diseases. For example, the

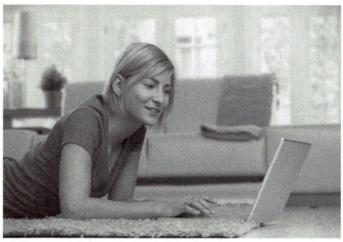

Centers for Disease Control and Prevention has many different websites devoted to specific health topics, from diabetes (www.cdc.gov/diabetes/) to infections from farm animals (www.cdc.gov/healthypets/animals/farm_animals.htm). And then, of course, there are some really interesting sites, such as one that we found that documents how aliens have cured particular illnesses like diabetes, liver diseases, and scoliosis (http://etmedical.com). (*"Paging the Enterprise. Beam me up, Scotty . . ."*)

But returning to Earth, let's take a closer look at one particular topic, HIV/AIDS. Although tremendous advances have been made in treating this disease, it is still frightening, causes patients to have a lot of uncertainty, and comes with a degree of stigma. So in the case of this disease, patients will often rely on searching online for information. Horvath et al. (2010) examined online HIV/AIDS resources by going online and using a variety of keywords in Google to see what popped up. They found 105 unique HIV/AIDS websites. The most common type of website (63%) was what they called an "information clearinghouse," which contained general disease and treatment information, as well as a variety of HIV/AIDS resources. The next most common were sites that gave advice on relationships/dating for those with HIV/AIDS (8%) and AIDS service organizations/community-based organizations (7%). Interestingly, only 33% of these sites contained information specific to persons recently diagnosed with HIV/AIDS, a group with obvious special information needs. The authors concluded that for such a person, the Internet landscape may prove difficult to navigate and that health communication scholars should be aware of this as we continue to study how people with HIV, whether newly diagnosed or not, process the information they find online.

Whoa, Nellie! It's probably time to take a step back and consider the consequences of online information seeking. Much like the website that reports on "alien healings," the Internet is full of lots of information that varies on credibility, accuracy, and more. Related, there is so *much* information out there, knowing which site to pick and which source to believe can feel overwhelming, particularly if you are facing a disease. What are we to do?

Chapter 7 discussed the topic of health literacy, including the more specific health-related media literacy. When considering the vast amount of health information online, health-related media literacy is an essential skill. Called **"eHealth literacy"** by Norman and Skinner (2006), this skill is defined as "the ability to seek, find, understand, and appraise health information from electronic sources and apply the knowledge gained to addressing or solving a health problem" (p. e10). This definition combines aspects of traditional literacy, health literacy, information literacy, media literacy, computer literacy, and scientific literacy. For some of us, we take it for granted that we can go online, search for information, evaluate webpages for credibility, know how to navigate through different websites to find what we are looking for, and be able to think about all that information in terms of how it is similar and different. But for others, it's not so simple.

In discussing some of the recent advancements in webpage formats, compared to several years ago when websites were more simple, Adams (2010) raises this great point:

> [T]he format of [online] information presents new challenges . . . information can no longer be conceptualized as static text with a few hyperlinks, but rather, is a series or blend of audio material, videos, photos, RSS feeds from external sites . . . mixed with reviewed textbook information, subjective information such as opinion and experience, and advertisements.
>
> (p. 396)

This complexity can make information seeking extremely challenging. In Table 12.3, we've listed some of the potential "pitfalls" of going online to search for information, as identified by Metzger and Flanagin (2011). As you read through these challenges, take a second and think about how these apply to you and maybe your last experience looking for health information online.

Table 12.3 Potential Pitfalls of Online Health Information Seeking

	What Does This Mean?	*What to Do?*
Information Accessibility *"Like a Needle in a Haystack"*	There is *so* much information out there, information seekers feel overwhelmed and start to feel like the information they want to find is inaccessible—both in terms of finding the information and comprehending the information.	Satisfice. Scan the information (i.e., list of sites that pop up after you've done a search) that you do find. Don't critically evaluate every source at first, but rather skim over what you find until things start to make sense.
Information Relevance *"Does this pertain to me?"*	Because there is so much information out there, it's likely that much of it won't be a match for what you need, especially if you want very specific, tailored information.	Let the search engine be your guide and always use specific search terms rather than general ones for finding your information.
Information Credibility *"Dr. Feel Good's Website?"* . . . uhhhh, no.	Information should be believable, and it should come from an expert and trustworthy source.	Given the nature of information on the Internet (*anybody* can post *anything*), credibility is crucial. Start with websites that are sponsored by trusted organizations (e.g., the CDC), make sure to look for the HONcode symbol, and follow up with your doctor about any questions you have.

From Metzger and Flanagin (2011).

Beyond following the advice in Table 12.3, there are a couple of other things you can do to more successfully navigate the vast array of health information websites out there. One is to look for the **HONcode** certification symbol on the website. The HON (health on the net) Foundation, established in 1995, is a non-profit, non-governmental organization dedicated to ensuring useful and reliable online health information. According to its website, "HONcode is the oldest and the most used ethical and trustworthy code for medical and health related information available on Internet. It is designed for the general public, health professionals, and web publishers. Currently, the HONcode is used by more than 7,300 certified websites across more than 100 countries." Visit www.healthonnet.org to check it out, and you'll be among the 27,000 people who visit the site daily. Another strategy, although one that's a little more labor intensive, is to apply the DISCERN principles to websites that you visit. DISCERN is a 16-item questionnaire that you fill out to assess the quality of health information that you find on the Internet. Visit www.discern.org.uk for more information.

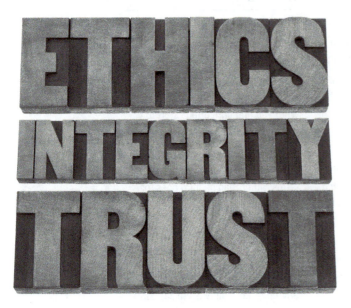

Despite the frequency with which people are searching online for information, one fact remains: *Healthcare providers are still the most trusted source* (Hesse et al., 2005). This is important to remember as health communication scholars because it has implications for patient–provider interaction. In particular, we should be concerned with what happens when patients bring health information they find online to their doctor visits, something that is happening more and more. McMullan (2006) posits this can affect the patient–provider interaction in three ways: (a) the healthcare provider can feel threatened by the patient who brings in information found online, (b) the healthcare provider can assist the patient in evaluating the information he or she found, or (c) the healthcare provider can guide the patient to reliable websites to find information. If doctors remember that they remain the most trusted source of health information, they may be less likely to react defensively. If patients acknowledge that they privilege the expertise of their doctors over sources of information they find on their own, that may help. Have you ever discussed online information with your healthcare provider? How did that go?

In sum, people are going online to search for health information. That isn't changing anytime soon. But in addition to just searching for health information, people are also *sharing* health information online. In the next section, we'll address how people use the Internet to share and exchange health information with family, friends, and other individuals.

Information Sharing

Whether it's through social networking sites, blogs, wikis, health forums, or discussion boards, the Internet is an amazing facilitator of **information sharing**. Because there is so much out there, we've decided to do a highlight reel. First, we'll look at two examples of social networking sites, one for patients and one for physicians. Then we'll look at examples of how patients and physicians blog about health and healthcare.

What will become obvious to you is that what constitutes information *sharing* for one person transforms into an opportunity for information *seeking* for another person. That is the transactional nature of communication, of course.

Social networking sites. Social networking sites (SNS) are any type of online platform where people can connect and interact with other people. The process usually involves people creating user profiles and then building their own network by connecting to others. The Pew Research Center found that 34% of Internet users have gone online to follow someone's health experience, 23% have followed a friend's health experience, and 17% have used a site to memorialize someone who died from a disease (Fox, 2011b). An issue brief from the Deloitte Center for Health Solutions (Keckley & Hoffmann, 2010) on social networking in healthcare reports that 60% of physicians and 65% of nurses are interested in using social networks for professional purposes.

Social networking for patients: PatientsLikeMe.com. PatientsLikeMe.com is a large health-centered social networking site where thousands of patients can connect about a common disease. The site is set up for patients to share information about their illness, their treatments, and their outcomes, along with relevant demographic information. More specifically, the website was created to "provid[e] a better, more effective way for you to share your real-world health experiences in order to help yourself, other patients like you and organizations that focus on your condition" (PatientsLikeMe, 2013, para. 1). And guess what, it works!

Wicks and colleagues (2010) surveyed users of the site and found that these patients believed the site to be helpful in managing their disease. For example, 72% of the users surveyed said they found the symptom information provided by other patients to be moderate to very helpful. In looking at disease-specific benefits, Wicks et al. found that a majority of the HIV patients they surveyed (71%) took more of an interest in their lab values because of the website. In addition, 29% of HIV patients surveyed said the website helped them to decide to take antiretroviral drugs because they were able to learn about other HIV patients' experiences with the treatment. Can you imagine the implications of a site like this, not only in improving patients' health literacy but also in motivating patients and caregivers to take more control over their own health?! As health communication scholars, we get giddy just thinking about it!

Now, you might wonder about the quality of information exchanged on PatientsLikeMe. After all, it's just patients talking about their health issues. But, as noted by Frost and Massagli (2009), given the focus on data reported by each user about their disease, the site provides an opportunity to investigate what evolves when patients "share structured, detailed, and longitudinal medical information with one another and discuss that information online" (p. 229). On the main disease pages, the data presented are at the aggregate level. Therefore, any "outliers" or false reports will often be washed out in the data. On the forum-type pages on PatientsLikeMe where people pose comments, users can (and do) correct false or misleading posts by posting follow-up posts; this is somewhat similar to what happens on Wikipedia, although on that site you can actually correct the post itself. Regardless, as noted by Ancker and colleagues (2009), "a patient community may be more highly motivated to correct information about a disease" in an online environment. While there is decidedly much room for research on this type of medical information sharing, we believe this multi-faceted platform for patients to share health information holds great promise.

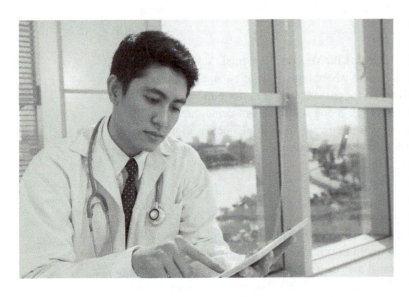

Social networking for physicians: Sermo.com. Sermo.com is the brainchild of Dr. Daniel Palenstrant, a surgeon by training, who is now the company's CEO. Palenstrant noted how so much of the important information doctors shared during grand rounds either took months to make it into medical journals or never made it at all. He created Sermo to be a source for that information. ("Sermo," by the way, is Latin for "conversation.") Since the site became available in October 2007, it has grown to be the largest online community for doctors in the United States. In fact, more than 200,000 MDs and DOs (doctors of osteopathy) representing 68 specialties are members of the network. Doctors sign up by creating a profile; their identity remains anonymous through choice of a username different from their own. After Sermo verifies their credentials, they can "discuss and connect," "collaborate and consult," "stay informed," and even "earn honoraria" by taking surveys and joining physician focus groups. There's even an iPhone app now: iConsult.

Bray, Croxson, Dutton, and Konsynski (2008) conducted an in-depth case study of Sermo. They obtained client observer accounts, which allowed them to log on to the site to see most posts and responses. They also interviewed Sermo leadership, and they reviewed journalistic coverage of Sermo (e.g., press releases, blog posts by critics). The researchers concluded that as a "closed community of experts," Sermo is uniquely positioned to identify and offer "previously unknown solutions to relevant problems" (p. 1). They also observed that Sermo members experience a strong normative sense of community, which can be an important source of social support. The authors did note a few concerns. For example, a crafty non-physician might establish an account with a false identity. Likewise, real physicians may have undisclosed conflicts of interest that may influence their online behavior (e.g., they might try to promote a drug to receive compensation from a pharmaceutical company). Because physicians receive rankings based on their demonstrated expertise within the system, these concerns may be mitigated if users gravitate toward the opinions of higher ranked physicians. Directions for future research include determining the impact of Sermo participation on medical practice and healthcare outcomes.

Blogs. A blog—a combination of the words "web" and "log," as you probably know—is a website where people can make posts and the blog's followers can read the posts and leave comments. While these sites are typically seen as one-way communication, the blogger writes posts with the intention of others reading the posts and often commenting, which suggests these sites are much more interactive and "social" than one would think (Rains & Keating, 2011). Miller and Pole (2010) analyzed some of the most well-known health blogs on the Internet to gain a better understanding of the content and characteristics of blogging about health. They found that most bloggers (63.2%) post at least once a week. Bloggers tended to be female and in their mid–30s, and most were highly educated. Interestingly, half of the bloggers they studied were in a health profession, with 43.3% of them being physicians. In terms of content, the most common focus was on a single disease or health topic, and health blogs tended to not contain audio or video (compared to other, general blogs).

Patient blogs. CaringBridge (CB; www.caringbridge.org) is a specialized blog site dedicated to helping patients and their families share information about a health event. The site was created in 1997 by Sona Mehring, who needed to share a friend's health information with others. The CB site has three purposes: (a) simplify an emotional time by easing communication and encouraging love and support when it matters most, (b) create a safe, personal space where individuals can share as much or as little as they choose on a protected site, and (c) put support in motion by helping individuals tap into their community of support during a health event. Patients and/or their loved ones simply sign up for a site and supply updates whenever they can. Others can follow the site by getting alerts when a new post has been made.

Anderson (2011) studied the use of CB from a **uses and gratifications** theoretical perspective. She wondered about how different people using the site perceived benefits.

First, she found that most CB authors set up the site for their child (50%) or another relative (33%) and less frequently for themselves (13%). Second, she found that the top three gratifications or benefits of using a CB site were sharing information with other people, receiving encouragement from reading comments from others, and enjoying the convenience of the CB site. Third, she found in general that older, female, and more spiritual users tended to rate the benefits of using CB as higher. She concludes that "care pages do not substitute for other media during a health crisis, but become a preferred communication channel, offering users new varieties of social support" (p. 556).

We asked a good friend of ours, Chelsee, to share her experiences using Caring-Bridge. You can read her story below. In all, CB is an excellent resource for those people who may be experiencing a health event and need to share that information with others.

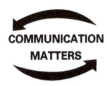

COMMUNICATION MATTERS

Chelsee's Experience

In 2009, I was diagnosed with a rare brain tumor. I decided to start a CaringBridge site where I posted updates on my diagnosis and health for my family and friends. I knew about this site because I had followed a friend's cancer journey on it, and I realized how helpful it was for keeping everyone informed. During my 13-hour brain surgery, my husband was able to continuously update friends and family. Following that, I kept everyone informed as I went through my radiation treatments and eye surgeries. My blog became a source of therapy for me. I've shared many personal details about our life on CaringBridge, such as our struggle with infertility, a miscarriage, and joyous occasions such as the birth of my two daughters.

In 2012, my blog took an unexpected twist. My father was diagnosed with a very rare form of cancer. I told his story on my CaringBridge site, communicating to our loved ones about everything from his surgeries and radiation treatments to taking him to hospice and watching him pass away. I also initiated a fundraiser on CaringBridge to raise money for the exorbitant healthcare costs my parents were faced with. What started as a practical way for me to keep others informed had, over time, turned into so much more. I am thankful that I was able to write about my and my father's health journeys on CaringBridge, not only for me personally but for all of our family and friends.

Provider blogs. As you might imagine, there are a multitude of physician blogs on the Internet. Torrieri (2011) listed nine of them worth checking out. Number one on the list is KevinMD, a blog Torrieri describes as "one of the most beloved health blogs in cyberspace." (That's high praise!) Kevin's blog "takes on some of the biggest healthcare issues affecting patients and the medical community." Other blogs on the list (which are included on this book's companion website) cover medical innovations, cancer research, controversial topics such as medical marijuana, and so on. It's clear that blogs are, indeed, a great way to share information. But did you know that they also may be a way to establish credibility? That's a discovery by Walden (2013), who conducted a qualitative study to explore naturopathic physician blogging behaviors.

Naturopathy is a form of holistic medicine that emphasizes the body's inherent self-healing ability. Naturopathic practitioners go through four years of accredited naturopathic medical school, pass board exams, and earn licenses in states that support them (currently 17 of 50 states). And they face vocal opposition from the American Medical Association. Through conducting interviews with naturopaths and analyzing their blogs, Walden (2013) determined that these healthcare providers use their blogs to promote the credibility of the field. Specifically, naturopath bloggers (a) introduce the public to naturopathic medicine, (b) advance the science and research of naturopathic medicine by sharing peer-reviewed literature, and (c) answer questions and address criticisms, trying in particular to distance themselves from lay naturopaths.

Personal Health Management

In addition to allowing people to seek and share information online, technology offers people many ways to take charge of their own health. We mentioned earlier how PHRs allow people to maintain their own health information as a complement to organizational EHRs. There are also a multitude of apps and websites that allow people to track their health-related behavior. In this section, we describe "the most popular healthy-lifestyle destination on the web," SparkPeople.com, and we present research that evaluates its impact.

SparkPeople.com. Quite possibly the largest online community dedicated to nutrition and fitness is SparkPeople.com. As of October, 2013, the site had 15 million registered members and was attracting 8,000 new members each day (SparkPeople, 2013). People may join for free, although there are additional benefits available with paid membership (e.g., SparkCoach). Members have access to a plethora of nutrition, fitness, and health information through online articles and videos. They can track their food, exercise, weight, and other health goals. They can join numerous teams that focus on seemingly endless health or other interests (e.g., "liberal atheist hippies").

They can post messages to message boards, maintain personal blogs, and gather SparkFriends. They can earn SparkPoints through numerous online activities and use the points to give virtual "goodies" to their friends or themselves. In short, this is an online health behavior management program with a zillion bells and whistles. But does it work?

The answer is a qualified yes. One thing that is abundantly clear in the literature is that there are next to no rigorous scientific evaluations of publicly available weight loss programs; the evidence that does exist indicates some support for such programs' effectiveness (see Collins et al., 2012). Although SparkPeople has not been evaluated in a randomized controlled trial, there is evidence of *how* it works *when* it works. What's interesting about that evidence is that the impact appears to be operating in part through communication among members. Long live social networking!

SparkPeople sent a 64-question email survey to a random sample of its active members and received more than 5,500 responses (Downie, 2009). They then compared "successful members" (people who had met their weight loss goals) with "stuck members" (those who had not met their goals) across goal-setting, nutrition, exercise, and motivation behaviors. They found important differences across all of these categories, including the importance of social support: being surrounded by healthy friends and "tapping into the power of positive people" by interacting on the community pages and reading member success stories. That's all well and good, but has any objective party evaluated SparkPeople? Well, yes.

Hwang et al. (2010) investigated the nature of social support on SparkPeople.com. They conducted a survey of 193 SparkPeople members, did follow-up interviews with 13 of them, and did a content analysis of 1,924 discussion forum messages. The authors identified three major themes of social support: encouragement/motivation, information, and shared experiences. They also determined that members appreciated the anonymity, convenience, and non-judgmental nature of the Internet-mediated social support. Hwang et al. concluded that the **online social support** that members received not only helped them cope with being overweight but also "empowered them to perform behaviors which directly led to weight loss" (p. 11). That's a pretty powerful impact.

TRANSLATION/ADOPTION CONCERNS

In this section, we briefly address a variety of health communication concerns related to the use of technology in healthcare. We consider privacy, motivation to use technology, the rapid pace of technological change, and resources.

Privacy—HIPAA, What?

One of the biggest and probably most important concerns when it comes to using communication technology in healthcare is **patient privacy**. All healthcare providers in the United States are required to comply with the **Health Insurance Portability and Accountability Act**, otherwise known as **HIPAA**. This is a large piece of legislation (what isn't these days?), but what affects patients the most is that HIPAA guarantees that patient health information is safe in the hands of the healthcare providers they visit. You can find out more about HIPAA here: www.hhs.gov/ocr/privacy/index.html.

Unfortunately, given that this act was passed in 1996, there was little guidance in terms of how things like communication technology and social media could be used to talk about health information. Therefore, the federal government clarified the specific guidelines by outlining the Security and Privacy Rules, which concern electronic communication of health information. But there must be a balance between strong safeguarding of information and ease of use, or people may be reticent to actually follow the rules. As noted by Choi, Capitan, Krause, and Streeper (2006), "the struggle to ensure the security of private health information may only be solved by a compromise between ease and efficiency and privacy protection" (p. 63).

Motivating People to Use Technology for Health

"If you build it, they will come" works out great in the movies, but what about in real life? Motivating people to use HIT is crucially important if the potential benefits of such technologies are to be realized. We want to briefly review a study that addresses strategies for motivating people to engage with technology.

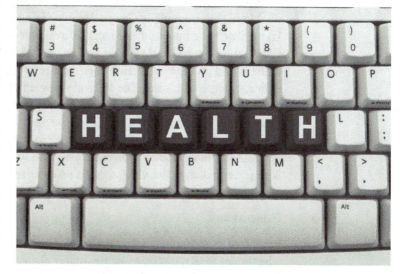

Tripathi, Delano, Lund, and Rudolph (2009) report on the effort of the Massachusetts eHealth Collaborative (MAeHC), a nonprofit, public–private collaborative of more than 30 healthcare delivery organizations in the state, to investigate the costs and benefits of HIE and EHR implementation in three Massachusetts communities.

Importantly (and bravely), the collaborative adopted an "opt-in" approach that required patients to actively consent to their health data being uploaded into the database. A much easier approach would have been "opt-out," in which patient health data would be uploaded unless the patient said no. So MAeHC had to find a way to motivate patients to say yes. They did so by "turning permission into demand," considering patients to be "customers" and trying to find ways to highlight the benefits of the system so that patients would want to participate. Focus groups with patients resulted in five recommendations: (a) show how the new system would address problems that frustrated patients the most (inconvenience and high cost), (b) use healthcare providers to encourage patients to join, (c) emphasize the most important benefits of the system (convenience, safety, ease of information management, patient control), (d) address safeguards related to data security concerns, and (e) make the marketing materials look professional. As students of communication, you will recognize the role of these recommendations in the persuasion process. The good news is that these efforts paid off: Across the three communities, the opt-in rate ranged from 88% to 92%. That's pretty amazing.

Keeping Up with the Kardashians

It's cliché these days to point out how fast technology develops, but that doesn't change the fact that it does. Keeping up with the latest trends, as well as knowing which trends are worth keeping up with, is an information problem of the highest order. Problematic, too, is the disappearance of technologies. Just like our favorite TV shows (poor *Arrested Development* ☹), some technologies lose favor among the public or just don't work out. One example is Google Health. If you use Google for email, you probably know they have many other functions available to users, like Calendars, Blogs, the Cloud, and even a Google Wallet feature. Google is like Leo in Titanic: "I'm the King of the World [Wide Web!]" But when it came to managing personal health information online, Google, um, sunk. The folks at Google note, "our goal was to create a service that would give people access to their personal health information and wellness information," but over a few years, it never caught on with the general public, and so they discontinued the service (Brown, 2011). How we investigate and communicate about these resources when they change so fast—and sometimes disappear before our eyes— is a major challenge for which there is no clear solution.

Resources

Let's face it, technology takes time and money and effort. For example, consider the adoption of EHRs, discussed earlier in this chapter. For an average-sized practice with five physicians, Fleming, Culler, McCorkle, Becker, and Ballard (2011) reported that it would cost more than $230,000 in the first year to implement and maintain the system, that the network and practice implementation teams would need more than

600 hours to prepare and implement the system, and that system users (e.g., physicians, clinic staff) would need more than 130 hours per physician to prepare to use the system. That is a huge investment. From an organizational communication perspective, think of all the challenges associated with making such a change. From a health promotion perspective, though, think of all the opportunities missed if such a change is not made.

CONCERNS IN ADOPTING NEW TECHNOLOGIES AND OPPORTUNITIES FOR ENHANCING HEALTH

New health technologies come with many challenges, but they also present many opportunities for improving health. Some of the challenges include privacy concerns, keeping up with the ever growing number of technologies, and the time and cost associated with adopting a new technology. Some of the benefits and opportunities for improving health include the relative ease for disseminating new technologies given the Internet, the opportunity to address health disparities through these technologies, and the potential to improve health literacy by using these technologies to motivate individuals to learn more about their health and take a more active role in maintaining it.

POTENTIAL OPPORTUNITIES

The benefits of HIT extend beyond improvements in healthcare system efficiency, health information exchange, and patient health outcomes. Indeed, we see promise in at least three areas: dissemination and implementation of healthcare innovations, improvements in health disparities, and assisting low health literacy populations.

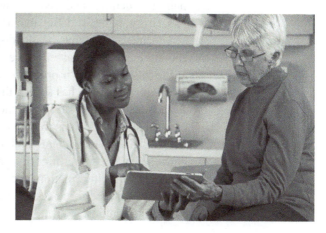

Dissemination and Implementation

One of the points that the authors of the chapters in this textbook have been making is the importance of **translational research**: taking the results of research studies and translating them to practice to improve the health and well-being of society. Unfortunately, translation is very challenging and slow to happen, if it happens at all. Bernhardt, Mays, and Kreuter (2011), however, believe that there is promise in new information technology:

> We believe that the interactivity, deep user engagement and multidirectional information exchange of Web 2.0 information tools can enhance the dissemination of research evidence among intended users and thus facilitate the translation of scientific evidence for effective programs and services into everyday practice.
>
> (p. 34)

Bernhardt et al. (2011) identify four dissemination strategies and associated Web 2.0 techniques: (a) Scientists' dissemination efforts can be increased through online videos, podcasts, blogs, and tweets; (b) inventories of effective programs can be assembled through smart tagging, search engine optimization, and wiki and user-generated content; (c) dissemination partnerships can be built through electronic networks and virtual exchanges; and (d) practitioner demand for evidence-based programs can be increased through social data mining and sharing success stories. We have seen evidence of some of these activities in this chapter. Only time and well-designed evaluations will be able to tell if such strategies effectively promote **dissemination and implementation**.

Health Disparities

As you know from reading Chapters 7 and 8, a perennial problem that has plagued healthcare systems worldwide is **health disparities**. With proper use, HIT is poised to help us identify and reduce these disparities. For example, López, Green, Tan-McGrory, King, and Betancourt (2011) identified health system, provider, and patient factors underlying health disparities and linked them to HIT strategies to ameliorate them. Whereas effectively collecting data on patient race, ethnicity, and language has long been a problem, such data collection can be automated through HIT. Whereas research has shown that physicians can stereotype patients and allow irrelevant demographic characteristics to influence their clinical decision making, HIT can prompt physicians to follow evidence-based guidelines for preventive care, chronic disease management, and drug prescribing regardless of patient demographics. Whereas some minority patients have trouble understanding physicians, patient education information and self-management tools can be culturally and linguistically tailored for access through Web 2.0 technologies. These are incredibly exciting opportunities.

Health Literacy

Attention to the needs of racial and ethnic minority patients to reduce health disparities also can make headway in improving health literacy. As Chapter 7 noted, **health literacy** is defined as "the capacity to obtain, process, and understand basic health information and services needed to make appropriate health decisions" (U.S. Department of Health and Human Services, 2012). As Bickmore and Paasche-Orlow (2012) point out, information technology can be used to assess health literacy and then design health education materials and interventions tailored for low-literate patients. In their own research, which draws on multiple disciplines including computer and information science and medicine, they use "embodied conversational agents" (computer-generated animated characters that mimic human counselors) to educate patients and provide health behavior change interventions. Their research shows that patients respond favorably to these agents regardless of health literacy levels but that low health literate patients find them particularly helpful (Bickmore et al., 2010). This is a perfect example of using information technology to promote health.

TRANSLATIONAL RESEARCH

We find ourselves facing a terrible lack of space for this chapter. There's just too much to cover. Therefore, we direct your attention to other chapters in this book that address translational research in health communication-related technology. See Chapter 1's discussion of David Gustafson's work with CHESS and the section on translational research in Chapter 15.

WHERE NO ONE HAS GONE BEFORE

In their comprehensive review article on current and future trends in Internet-supported mental health interventions, Barak and Grohol (2011) note the tremendous developments in technology in recent years and the profound impact on healthcare: "It would not be an exaggeration to conclude that health- and mental health-related disciplines have gone through dramatic changes in exploiting the Internet, changes that are extensively reflected in many of their operations and activities" (p. 169). The authors conclude that their ability to accurately predict future trends is doubtful. We feel their pain. However, we do want to make a couple of suggestions for future research.

First, we think it's imperative for health communication researchers to seriously explore the impact of technology on patient–provider relationships. Since the dawn of healthcare, that relationship has been central to health and healing. It will continue to be so regardless of what awesome technology we layer upon it. We need to understand how technology may help or hinder that relationship and develop theoretical models to advance research in this respect.

Second, we need to balance ability with responsibility. Just because we can do something doesn't mean we should. With huge advances in EMRs and HIEs, there is tremendous opportunity to track people's health, monitor health behaviors, and predict future disease. For example, specialists can analyze comprehensive EHR databases, identify patients at risk for certain diseases, and reach out to them with tailored messages for treatment instead of relying on primary care physicians for referrals (Chen et al., 2009). Is that okay? Maybe yes, maybe no. What happens, though, when (not if) retailers get in on the act? Remember the big stink about Target's using data to predict which of its female shoppers were pregnant so it could send them baby-related coupons? And Rite Aid's use of data to identify people who filled prescriptions for nicotine patches so it could send them promotional materials on weight loss? Our point is that ability far outpaces responsibility and moves faster than legislators have time to legislate. Be careful out there.

CONCLUSION

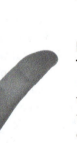

There seems to be almost no limit to people's ingenuity with technology development, and we're getting smarter about applying it in ways that can help us promote our health. As research in this area moves forward, we need to be mindful of the appropriate use of health information technology so that we can improve our lives without compromising values that we hold dear. Whatever happens, we want everyone to live long and prosper. ☺

DISCUSSION QUESTIONS

1.   You just learned about some of the benefits and limitations to using telemedicine. Keeping in mind that telemedicine is often used when a patient would otherwise not have access to a healthcare provider, is there a time when telemedicine would absolutely not be appropriate? If so, why?

2.   Despite the abundance of health information available online, healthcare providers are still identified as the most trusted

source of health information. Why do you think this is true? What are the health communication implications of this finding?

3. On the basis of your own personal experiences and what you learned in this chapter, make a case for what you think is the biggest challenge for adopting new health information technologies in the United States.

IN-CLASS ACTIVITIES

1. Are you currently dealing with a disease or know someone who is? Go to Patients LikeMe.com and look up the disease. (Use the search box in the upper left hand corner; you don't need to be a member.) How useful is the information? Does it seem trustworthy? Would you use this site again for other health issues?
2. Watch the video of members' stories on PatientsLikeMe.com. Have a discussion about the communication and information benefits the members receive from their participation.
3. Go to your favorite search engine (e.g., Google). Type in a common disease (e.g., diabetes, heart disease, breast cancer). How many hits did you get? Randomly pick five of the websites and evaluate them for relevance and credibility using DISCERN (www.discern.org.uk). Repeat this activity with a rare disease (e.g., Dercum's disease, Landau Kleffner syndrome, cyclic vomiting syndrome) and see how your search results differ.

RECOMMENDED READINGS

Mostashari, F., Tripathi, M., & Kendall, M. (2009). A tale of two large community electronic health record extension projects. *Health Affairs, 28*(2), 345–356.

This article reports the experiences of the Massachusetts eHealth Collaborative and the New York City Primary Care Information Project in implementing EHRs in their medical communities, highlighting strategies for overcoming barriers while emphasizing continuity of care (Massachusetts) and preventive care and chronic disease management (New York).

Fortney, J. C., Pyne, J. M., Mouden, S. B., Mittal, D., Hudson, T. J., Schroeder, G. W., . . . Rost, K. M. (2013). Practice-based versus telemedicine-based collaborative care for depression in rural federally qualified health centers: A pragmatic randomized comparative effectiveness trial. *American Journal of Psychiatry, 170*, 414–425.

In this experiment, patients in the telemedicine group saw greater improvements in their depression than patients who saw providers face-to-face for their treatment, suggesting that supplementing mental health care with trained professionals through telemedicine may help in better treating mental illness.

Kim, K., & Kwon, N. (2010). Profile of e-patients: Analysis of their cancer information-seeking from a national survey. *Journal of Health Communication, 15,* 712–733.

This article reports the results of a study of cancer "e-patients" and their online health information seeking behaviors, finding that these patients tended to be older adults and expressed frustration with the online health search for information.

REFERENCES

Adams, S. A. (2010). Revisiting the online health information reliability debate in the wake of "Web 2.0": An inter-disciplinary literature and website review. *International Journal of Medical Informatics, 79,* 391–400.

Ancker, J. S., Carpenter, K. M., Greene, P., Hoffman, R., Kukafka, R., Marlow, L. A. V., Prigerson, J. G., & Quillin, J. M. (2009). Peer-to-peer communication, cancer prevention, and the internet. *Journal of Health Communication, 14,* 38–46.

Anderson, I. K. (2011). The uses and gratifications of online care pages: A study of caring-bridge. *Health Communication, 26,* 546–559.

Barak, A., & Grohol, J. M. (2011). Current and future trends in Internet-supported mental health interventions. *Journal of Technology in Human Sciences, 29,* 155–196.

Bernhardt, J. M., Mays, D., & Kreuter, M. W. (2011). Dissemination 2.0: Closing the gap between knowledge and practice with new media and marketing. *Journal of Health Communication, 16,* 32–44.

Bickmore, T. W., & Paasche-Orlow, M. K. (2012). The role of information technology in health literacy research. *Journal of Health Communication, 17,* 23–29.

Bickmore, T. W., Pfeifer, L. M., Byron, D., Forsythe, S., Henault, L. E., Jack, B. W., . . . Paasche-Orlow, M. K. (2010). Usability of conversational agents by patients with inadequate health literacy: Evidence from two clinical trials. *Journal of Health Communication, 15,* 197–210.

Bray, D., Croxson, K., Dutton, W., & Konsynski, B. (2008). Sermo: A community-based knowledge ecosystem. OII DPSN Working Paper No. 7, Emory University. Retrieved from http://ssrn.com/abstract=1016483

Bromberg, J. E., Augustson, E. M., & Backinger, C. L. (2012). Portrayal of smokeless tobacco on YouTube videos. *Nicotine & Tobacco Research, 14,* 455–462.

Brown, A. (2011). *An update on Google Health and Google PowerMeter.* Retrieved from http://googleblog.blogspot.com/2011/06/update-on-google-health-and-google.html

Chaudhry, B., Wang, J., Wu, S., Maglione, M., Mojika, W., Roth, E., . . . Shekelle, P. G. (2006). Systematic review: Impact of health information technology on quality, efficiency, and costs of medical care. *Annals of Internal Medicine, 144*(10), 742–752.

Chen, C., Garrido, T., Chock, D., Okawa, G., & Liang, L. (2009). The Kaiser Permanente electronic health record: Transforming and streamlining modalities of care. *Health Affairs, 28*(2), 323–333.

Choi, Y. B., Capitan, K. E., Krause, J. S., & Streeper, M. M. (2006). Challenges associated with privacy in health care industry: Implementation of hipaa and the security rules. *Journal of Medical Systems, 30*, 57–64.

Collins, C. E., Morgan, P. J., Jones, P., Fletcher, K., Martin, J., Aguiar, E. J., . . . Callister, R. (2012). A 12-week commercial web-based weight-loss program for overweight and obese adults: Randomized controlled trial comparing basic versus enhanced features. *Journal of Medical Internet Research, 14*(2), e57.

Deloitte. (2008). *2008 survey of health care consumers.* Washington, DC: Author.

Dentzer, S. (2009). Health information technology: On the fast track at last? *Health Affairs, 28*(2), 320–321.

DMOZ. (2013). Open directory project. Retrieved from http://www.dmoz.org/search?q=health

Downie, C. (2009). *The spark: The 28-day breakthrough plan for losing weight, getting fit, and transforming your life.* Carlsbad, CA: Hay House, Inc.

eHealth Initiative (2012). *2012 report on health information exchange: Supporting healthcare reform.* Washington, DC: Author.

Fleming, N. S., Culler, S. D., McCorkle, R., Becker, E. R., & Ballard, D. J. (2011). The financial and nonfinancial costs of implementing electronic health records in primary care practices. *Health Affairs, 30*, 481–489.

Fox, S. (2011a). *Health topics.* Pew Research Center's Internet & American Life Project. Washington, DC: Author.

Fox, S. (2011b). *The social life of health information.* Pew Research Center's Internet & American Life Project. Washington, DC: Author.

Fox, S., & Duggan, M. (2013). Health online 2013. *Pew Research Center Internet & American Life Project.* Washington, DC.

Freeman, B., & Chapman, S. (2007). Is "YouTube" telling or selling you something? Tobacco content on the YouTube video-sharing website. *Tobacco Control, 16*, 207–210.

Frost, J., & Massagli, M. (2009). Patientslikeme: The case for a data-centered patient community and how ALS patients use the community to inform treatment decisions and manage pulmonary health. *Chronic Respiratory Disease, 6*, 225–229.

Hesse, B. W., Nelson, D. E., Kreps, G. L., Croyle, R. T., Arora, N. K., Rimer, B. K., & Viswanath, K. (2005). Trust and sources of health information: The impact of the internet and its implications for health care providers: Findings from the first health information national trends survey. *Archives of Internal Medicine, 165*, 2618–2624.

Horvath, K. J., Harwood, E. M., Courtenay-Quirk, C., McFarlane, M., Fisher, H., Dickenson, T., . . . O'Leary, A. (2010). Online resources for persons recently diagnosed with HIV/AIDS: An analysis of HIV-related webpages. *Journal of Health Communication, 15*, 516–531.

Hwang, K. O., Ottenbacher, A. J., Green, A. P., Cannon-Diehl, M. R., Richardson, O., Bernstam, E. V., & Thomas, E. J. (2010). Social support in an Internet weight loss community. *International Journal of Medical Informatics, 79*, 5–13.

Jameson, J. P., Farmer, M. S., Head, K. J., Fortney, J., & Teal, C. R. (2011). VA community mental health service providers' utilization of and attitudes toward telemental health care: The gatekeeper's perspective. *The Journal of Rural Health, 27,* 425–432.

Johnson, J. D., & Case, D. O. (2012). *Health information seeking.* New York: Peter Lang.

Jones, D. A., Shipman, J. P., Plaut, D. A., & Selden, C. R. (2010). Characteristics of personal health records: Findings of the Medical Library Association/National Library of Medicine joint electronic personal health record task force. *Journal of the Medical Library Association, 98*(3), 243–249.

Kaelber, D. C., Jha, A. K., Johnston, D., Middleton, B., & Bates, D. W. (2008). A research agenda for personal health records (PHRs). *Journal of the Medical Informatics Association, 15*(6), 729–736.

Kaushal, R., Shojania, K. G., & Bates, D. W. (2003). Effects of computerized physician order entry and clinical decision support systems on medication safety: A systematic review. *Archives of Internal Medicine, 163*(12), 1409–1416.

Keckley, P. H., & Hoffmann, M. (2010). *Social networks in health care: Communication, collaboration and insights.* Washington, DC: Deloitte Center for Health Solutions.

Keelan, J., Pavri-Garcia, V., Tomlinson, G., & Wilson, K. (2007). Youtube as a source of information on immunization: A content analysis. *JAMA, 298*(21), 2482–2484.

Koch-Weser, S., Bradshaw, Y. S., Gualtieri, L., & Gallagher, S. S. (2010). The Internet as a health information source: Findings from the 2007 health information national trends survey and implications for health communication. *Journal of Health Communication, 15,* 279–293.

Johnson, J. D., & Case, D. O. (2012). *Health information seeking.* New York: Peter Lang.

López, L., Green, A. R., Tan-McGrory, A., King, R., & Betancourt, J. R. (2011). Bridging the digital divide in health care: The role of health information technology in addressing racial and ethnic disparities. *The Joint Commission Journal on Quality and Patient Safety, 37*(10), 437–445.

Matusitz, J., & Breen, G.-M. (2007). Telemedicine: Its effects on health communication. *Health Communication, 21,* 73–83.

McMullan, M. (2006). Patients using the Internet to obtain health information: How this affects the patient–health professional relationship. *Patient Education and Counseling, 63,* 24–28.

Merrell, R. C., & Doarn, C. R. (2013). Tales of telemedicine. *Telemedicine Journal And E-Health: The Official Journal Of The American Telemedicine Association, 19*(2), 69–70.

Metzger, M. J., & Flanagin, A. J. (2011). Using Web 2.0 technologies to enhance evidence-based medical information. *Journal of Health Communication, 16,* 45–58.

Miller, E. A., & Pole, A. (2010). Diagnosis blog: Checking up on health blogs in the blogosphere. *American Journal of Public Health, 100,* 1514–1519.

Norman, C. D., & Skinner, H. A. (2006). Ehealth literacy: Essential skills for consumer health in a networked world. *Journal of Medical Internet Research, 8,* e9.

Palen, T. E., Ross, C., Powers, J. D., & Xu, S. (2012). Association of online patient access to clinicians and medical records with use of clinical services. *Journal of the American Medical Association, 308*(19), 2012–2019.

PatientsLikeMe. (2013). *About Us.* Retrieved from http://www.patientslikeme.com/about

Rains, S. A., & Keating, D. M. (2011). The social dimension of blogging about health: Health blogging, social support, and well-being. *Communication Monographs, 78*, 511–534.

Sarasohn-Kahn, J. (2008). *The wisdom of patients: Health care meets online social media.* Oakland, CA: California HealthCare Foundation.

Sood, S., Mbarika, V., Jugoo, S., Dookhy, R., Doarn, C. R., Prakash, N., & Merrell, R. C. (2007). What is telemedicine? A collection of 104 peer-reviewed perspectives and theoretical underpinnings. *Telemedicine and e-Health, 13*, 573–590.

SparkPeople. (2013). *Reach your target with SparkPeople.* Retrieved from http://www.sparkpeople.com/advertising-sponsorship.asp

Strauss, A. (1998, May). *Will telemedicine take off?* Paper presented at the IEEE International Conference on Information Technology Applications in Biomedicine, Washington, DC.

Tian, Y. (2010). Organ donation on web 2.0: Content and audience analysis of organ donation videos on YouTube. *Health Communication, 25*, 238–246.

Torrieri, M. (2011, March 24). 9 physician blogs worth checking out. Retrieved from http://www.physicianspractice.com/worklife-balance/9-physician-blogs-worth-checking-out

Tripathi, M., Delano, D., Lund, B., & Rudolph, L. (2009). Engaging patients for health information exchange. *Health Affairs, 28*(2), 435–443.

Turner, J. W. (2003). Telemedicine: expanding health care into virtual environments. In T. L. Thompson, A. M. Dorsey, R. Parrott & K. I. Miller (Eds.), *Handbook of health communication* (pp. 515–535). Mahwah, NJ: Lawrence Erlbaum Associates.

U.S. Department of Health and Human Services. (2012). Health literacy. Retrieved from http://www.health.gov/communication/literacy

Walden, J. (2013). A medical profession in transition: Exploring naturopathic physician blogging behaviors. *Health Communication, 28*, 237–247.

Wicks, P., Massagli, M., Frost, J., Brownstein, C., Okun, S., Vaughan, T., . . . Heywood, J. (2010). Sharing health data for better outcomes on patientslikeme. *Journal of Medical Internet Research, 12*, e19.

Yoo, J. H., & Kim, J. (2012). Obesity in the new media: A content analysis of obesity videos on YouTube. *Health Communication, 27*, 86–97.

YouTube. (2013). Press: Statistics. from http://www.youtube.com/yt/press/statistics.html

Media Effects and Health

*Adam J. Parrish, Sarah C. Vos,
and Elisia L. Cohen*

In a *New York Times* op-ed, Angelina Jolie announces that she's had her breasts removed to avoid cancer, resulting in a media frenzy. On television, commercials promote the use of prescription drugs to supposedly improve our mental and physical well-being. In the medical drama *Grey's Anatomy*, doctors are portrayed as sexy superheroes, making decisions based on gut-instinct and bravado before stealing away to the utility closet for some romance. Each of these examples represents areas in which mass media and health intersect and where media have the potential to influence our knowledge about health, attitudes toward diseases and preventive behaviors, and beliefs about what causes diseases and how to cure them. Media can even influence our beliefs about who is responsible for illness—the individual or society as a whole—and who can make changes that influence health outcomes.

For the purposes of this chapter, we define mass media broadly: newspaper stories, televised sitcoms and dramas, newscasts, websites, commercials, YouTube videos, video games, magazine articles, Twitter feeds, and more. Such a broad definition makes conceptualizing mass media influence difficult, but it also underscores the multiple ways in which media have the potential to converge with health communication.

Scholars who use a scientific perspective to conceptualize media effects on health emphasize mass media's role in transmitting health information and are often concerned with the accuracy of the information being presented. In contrast, communication scholars who use an interpretive perspective focus on the audience's role in understanding that information. Scholars who use a critical–cultural perspective focus on the social structures that shape media coverage and the ways in which public issues and individual health concerns intersect. Each of these perspectives emphasizes different aspects of the relationship between media and health, and each has different underlying assumptions about the agency of individuals and the structural role of media systems in society. These paradigms also illuminate the different pathways through which scholars examine the relationship between media and health.

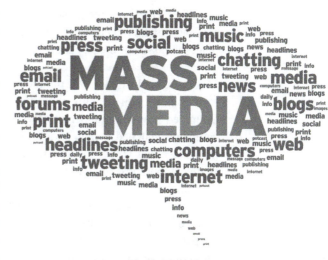

In this chapter, we first discuss some of the most common theoretical perspectives that consider the effects of media on individual and societal health. We then examine in more detail three ways in which media influence health through news reporting, advertising, and entertainment.

THEORETICAL PERSPECTIVES

Scholars from various health-related backgrounds use several prominent communication theories to understand the influence of the news media on health. Some theories stem from the scientific social–psychological tradition of media effects, originally developed to explain the role of media in politics. These theories include agenda setting, priming, and framing. Other theories stemming from the interpretive and critical–cultural traditions examine the social determinants of health. They look at ways social structures such as workplaces, neighborhoods, and schools influence health and the ways that media systems reinforce these structures, ultimately solidifying social and individual understandings of health.

Traditional Theories of Media Effects

Agenda setting. **Agenda setting** focuses on ways media coverage makes certain issues more prominent by covering them more often than others (McCombs & Shaw, 1972). More specifically, according to agenda setting theory, media set the public agenda by covering and drawing attention to certain news stories. Take, for example,

Angelina Jolie's double mastectomy. From an agenda setting perspective, the news coverage of this event raises awareness about genetic testing for breast cancer. It places the issue of breast cancer and its prevention on the public agenda.

McCombs and Shaw (1972) argued that media tell audiences *what* issues to think about but not *how* to think about them. In their seminal 1972 study, the researchers examined how the number of news stories about different political issues during a campaign matched people's views on what issues were most important. The issues that undecided voters thought were most important were also the issues that were written about most often in the newspapers.

This line of research has important implications for health policies and the implementation of healthcare-related legislation. When editors select health-related news stories for publication or broadcast, they are making choices that can affect the relevance and importance of health information for the public. For example, Wang and Gantz (2010) found that local news media frequently broadcast stories about the causes of and treatments for specific physical illnesses (e.g., cancer, heart disease, diabetes) and chose stories about mental illness and aging less often. The researchers also discovered that health news accounted for eight percent of all televised news coverage and stories averaged one minute in length. This type of content analysis highlights the importance of health in local news and reveals the need for further examination of the content of health stories. That is, if a health issue will receive only one minute of coverage on the local news, what information should journalists attempt to include in that minute?

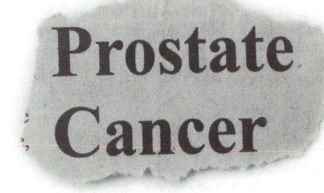

Studies of newspaper coverage of health-related stories also accent the importance of the agenda-setting function of media. Content analyses indicate that cancer is one of the most frequently covered health topics (Wang & Gantz, 2010). Breast cancer is overrepresented in American newspapers when compared to the actual incidence of the disease, whereas more common cancers such as lymphoma, thyroid, and prostate cancer are underreported (Cohen et al., 2008; Jensen, Moriarty, Hurley, & Stryker, 2010). Breast cancer may receive more attention than other cancers because of the political power and media presence of breast cancer nonprofits such as the Susan G. Komen for the Cure© organization. However, Cohen at al. (2008) noted that newspapers targeted to African-American readers might consider health disparities when selecting stories for publication. Black newspaper journalists, for example, may write a story that considers how their readers will understand or evaluate the story from their socio-cultural perspective. African-Americans experience higher rates of breast and prostate cancer mortality and are diagnosed with later stage disease than non-Hispanic Whites, potentially creating a greater need for stories that provide information about prevention, diagnosis, and treatment of illnesses that affect diverse populations disproportionally.

Priming. Priming theory has been used to show how news coverage of health issues influences our knowledge of those issues. Priming may be considered as an extension of agenda setting (Scheufele & Tewksbury, 2007). Like agenda setting, priming focuses on the ways media coverage makes certain issues and ideas more accessible by covering them more often (Weaver, 2007). For example, Stryker, Moriarty, and Jensen (2008) investigated the relationship between what people knew about cancer risks and coverage of those same cancer risks in American newspapers. The study found that the modifiable cancer risks most often covered in the news media were tobacco use and diet, whereas exercise and sun protection were covered less often. Not surprisingly, people who reported reading cancer-related stories in newspapers knew significantly more about tobacco avoidance and healthy eating than they did about exercise and protection from the sun. These findings suggest that media primed consumers to think about certain aspects of cancer prevention (e.g., tobacco and food) rather than others (e.g., exercise and sun protection).

Unlike agenda setting, which focuses on the importance attributed to issues, priming focuses on how mass media content influences the evaluation of issues (Scheufele & Tewksbury, 2007). Priming also considers the short-term effect of media exposure (Roskos-Ewoldsen, Roskos-Ewoldsen, & Carpentier, 2009). As such, much priming research examines how exposure to media violence primes aggressiveness in viewers. Another line of research investigates how media portrayals activate stereotypes, influencing how people perceive others. A related line of health media research examines how representations in media influence public understanding of diseases, including the stigma associated with representations of mental illness in media (also see Chapter 10).

Framing. Framing examines the ways in which issues are presented in media and how those presentations influence the way viewers understand those issues (Scheufele & Tewksbury, 2007). In agenda setting theory, media influence *what* we think about. In framing theory, media influence *how* we think about issues. Entman (1993) argued that frames "diagnose, evaluate, and prescribe" (p. 52). By this, he meant the way an issue is presented makes certain aspects of it more relevant than others and, as a result, the presentation, or frame, influences the way we understand that issue.

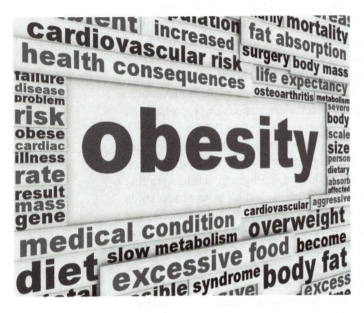

The public debate on obesity provides an opportunity to examine how attributions of blame identify the causes and cures of this epidemic. Lawrence (2004) used a scientific perspective to examine how this issue was framed in news coverage between 1985 and 2003. Setting out to conduct a content analysis, she collected *New York Times* articles about obesity that appeared on the front-page of the paper or in the editorial section. She and a colleague coded the *New York Times* articles deductively. Then they examined news coverage of obesity on television, using abstracts of prime-time news stories. Finally, they searched 10 major newspapers for articles containing key words related to the obesity debate. Before beginning the analysis, Lawrence identified three competing frames for the obesity epidemic from previous studies of the problem: biological, individual, and environmental. In the biological disorder frame, obesity was portrayed as a medical problem that would be cured by a pill, presumably developed and sold by pharmaceutical companies. In the individual behavior frame, obesity was described as an individual problem that would be cured when people individually made choices to eat healthier food and exercise more. In the environmental frame, obesity was presented as resulting from an "unhealthy food and activity environment created by corporate and public policy" (p. 62). After analyzing the data sets, Lawrence found that there was a "vigorous frame contest" going on between the environmental and individual behavioral frames surrounding the obesity epidemic (p. 56). She concluded from her analysis that the obesity epidemic was being reframed from an individual behavioral problem to an environmental problem.

Each frame identifies a different cause of the problem and therefore a different solution. For example, when the obesity epidemic is identified by the news media as a matter of personal responsibility, obese people are responsible for their weight and are at fault if they don't lose weight. The solution is for obese individuals to eat healthier foods and exercise. If they fail, then it is a personal failure. Conversely, if the obesity epidemic is described as an environmental problem, then society is responsible, and policy issues (like subsidies for corn, food advertising, portion sizes, walkable communities, the availability of healthy foods, and physical education in schools) become part of the solution. With a frame emphasizing the social environment, the solution to the obesity problem isn't that people should make personal changes but that policies should be changed to encourage healthier eating and active lifestyles.

What a particular frame leaves out is just as important as what it highlights. Entman (1993) argued that frames often direct attention away from alternative and conflicting explanations of reality. In the example above, the frame of obesity as an individual problem directs attention away from public policies that contribute to obesity. Niederdeppe, Shapiro, and Porticella (2011) have begun to explore how attributions of responsibility for obesity affect public opinion and whether individual differences such as political beliefs influence people's willingness to accept that societal actors (e.g., government and employers) are responsible for addressing the epidemic.

Theories of Media Learning

A second line of research on media and health investigates the ways we learn about health from the media. Cultivation theory and social cognitive theory guide this research and examine how we learn by acquiring and retaining information about health from media. These theories are also rooted in the scientific tradition of communication research.

Cultivation theory. Cultivation theory proposes that the stories told by media, on television in particular, shape the way we view the world (Gerbner, 1990). Much early cultivation research focused on televised portrayals of violence and attempted to measure the cumulative effect of television watching on public perceptions of violence (Shanahan & Morgan, 1999). Essentially, this research demonstrated that people who watched a lot of television perceived the world around them to be more violent than people who did not watch a lot of television. In effect, television exposure was "cultivating" attitudes and beliefs.

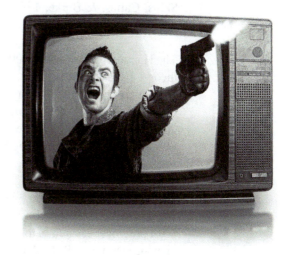

In health communication research, scholars have used this theory to examine how portrayals of health on television affect psychosocial health. For example, Hammermeister, Brock, Winterstein, and Page (2005) examined whether people who watched less than two hours of TV a day (the recommendation of the American Academy of Pediatrics) reported fewer attributes of poor psychosocial health (e.g., loneliness, hopelessness, shyness) than people who watched more than two hours of television per day. Traditionally, scholars engaged in cultivation theory research use a two-step process to understand the effects of television. First, they conduct a content analysis of the television show(s) being examined; second, they survey viewers and non-viewers about television exposure and outcome variables. Hammermeister et al. did not analyze television content first, however. Instead, they assumed that the type of content would not matter; it was the act of television-watching itself that created differences in psychosocial health.

Hammermeister et al. (2005) recruited 430 participants through national media outlets to take an online survey. The majority of participants were White (76%) and were women (75.6%). Participants were asked to report the average number of minutes of television they watched in a day, and they completed several measurement scales to assess their psychosocial health. The researchers then completed a statistical analysis to compare the psychosocial health of people who watched less than two hours of TV a day and those who watched more.

Hammermeister et al.'s (2005) results confirmed that women who watched more than two hours of television had a significantly lower score on the measurements of psychosocial health than women who watched less than two hours of television. However, this relationship was not apparent for men. These results are incongruent with previous studies, which have found that men who were frequent viewers of television were shyer, lonelier, more hopeless, more dissatisfied with their appearance, and had a higher tendency toward eating disorders than did their peers who watched less television (Page, Hammermeister, Scanlan, & Allen, 1996; Williams, Sallis, Calfas, & Burke, 1999). The inconsistency with previous research could be due to the small sample size of men in Hammermeister et al.'s study.

The Hammermeister et al. (2005) study also illustrates a difficult issue for cultivation theory: the issue of causation. The method of analyzing survey research cannot prove that watching more television *causes* psychosocial problems. This method can only show that there is a *correlation*, or relationship, between the two variables. Researchers do not know whether people who are already shy, lonely, depressed, etc., tend to watch more television or whether people who watch more television become more shy, lonely, and depressed.

Whether or not television viewing predisposes people to psychosocial risks or, conversely, whether psychosocial conditions prompt television viewing is uncertain. Most previous research in this area has identified health risks associated with frequent viewing (Dittmar, 1994; McCreary & Sadaca, 1999; Page et al., 1996; Williams et al.,

1999). Researchers also do not know how much television watching might be too much and under what conditions frequent viewing might be harmful. These distinctions need to be made if research is to determine clearly that (a) the time spent with media displaces other time people could spend in more meaningful activities and (b) influential media content shapes individual attitudes and beliefs.

Time spent watching television illustrates another difficulty with cultivation research: How do researchers measure this media exposure variable? In the Hammermeister et al. (2005) study, researchers asked participants to report the number of minutes they spent watching television per day and then divided the sample into two groups, those who watched television for more than two hours a day and those who watched for less than two hours a day. This is traditionally how television viewing is measured in cultivation research (Signorielli & Morgan, 2009): The amount of television watched is measured and then the participants are divided into groups based on their television-watching habits. Researchers often divide the sample into three groups (heavy, medium, light) based on reported television watching. As a result, the amount of time constituting a "large amount" of television watching varies from study to study. This practice is important because how researchers group participants can influence results, as challenges to the cultivation theory have demonstrated (Hirsch, 1980).

The current media landscape also poses difficulties for researchers seeking to measure television watching. When George Gerbner first developed cultivation theory in the late 1960s, television was a different medium than it is today. Gerbner (1990) conceived of television as unique because unlike the other mass media of the day (radio, newspapers, and film), television combined visual and auditory messages and sat in a prominent place in the home; the limited number of channels back then also limited what was available to watch.

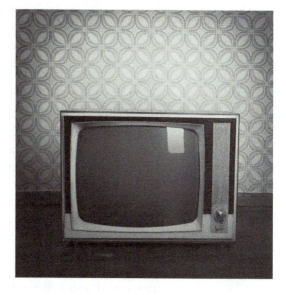

Today television includes a plethora of cable channels and local news. It competes with Internet entertainment and home movie-viewing systems. It also appears online. For the purposes of measurement, these changes raise questions about what watching television actually means. For example, are people watching television while using Netflix to watch old episodes of a particular show? What if they watch YouTube videos of a show on their iPhone? Or, worse yet, what if they watch YouTube videos while watching television?

Should researchers measure that multitasking time twice? Clearly, there are many challenges in this kind of research.

Social cognitive theory. Another theory that conceptualizes the influence of the media through learning is Bandura's **social cognitive theory (SCT)**, a theory that focuses on how we learn by observing others. SCT proposes that media influence our values, thinking, and behavior by modeling behaviors that prompt observational learning (Bandura, 2009). For example, when we watch a sitcom character discuss condom use (or fail to discuss condom use) with a casual sex partner, we acquire information about the role of condoms in casual sex. We might retain that information and remember a useful way to bring up condom use in conversation. Although this type of learning occurs every day in non-mediated interactions, Bandura argued that modeling occurs via media when individuals learn vicariously through the process of identifying with mass media characters. In this way, media portrayals show us what is possible (or what is impossible) and how a task might be accomplished.

SCT is part of the socio-psychological tradition of communication research, and it has a post-positivistic, scientific perspective, meaning it assumes that researchers can observe and measure the world around them. Four constructs critical to understanding SCT are **human agency, human capabilities, vicarious learning**, and **self-efficacy**. SCT assumes that we have agency, which means that we can exercise control over our thoughts, feelings, and actions (Bandura, 1986). Our abilities to symbolize, provide forethought to action, and engage in self-regulation and self-reflection provide the cognitive means by which we act. Additionally, by observing the behavior of others, we can learn vicariously and develop rules to guide our behaviors. Bandura also argued that vicarious learning will not be sufficient to prompt behavior unless we also have self-efficacy. Self-efficacy, essentially, is the belief that you can do something. According to SCT, observing other people who are similar to you can enhance your beliefs about your capacity to engage in a behavior (self-efficacy beliefs).

In this way, SCT is similar to **social comparison theory**, which suggests that we can determine our relative success or failure in any given domain by comparing ourselves to others interpersonally or through media. For example, if you want to gauge your long-distance running abilities, you might enter a marathon. At the end of the race, you will know where you placed in comparison to other competitors (assuming you are still breathing). Knobloch-Westerwick and Romero (2011) noted that upward social comparisons (i.e., comparing yourself to others who are superior in some domain) can have positive or negative effects. When you believe that you can be just as good as or better than other people, you might be more motivated to engage in behaviors that will lead to a higher level of achievement. However, if you believe that the superior goal is unattainable, you might avoid making positive changes. As Vince Vaughn noted in *Dodgeball*: "I found that if you have a goal, that you might not reach it. But if you don't have one, then you are never disappointed. And I gotta tell ya, it feels phenomenal." Mr. Vaughn's advice aside, our point here is that in relation to health, positive upward social comparison can potentially improve health outcomes. So researchers should strive to learn more about that media effect.

Indeed, researchers have investigated the ways in which we use media for vicarious learning and social comparisons in relation to health. Sohn (2009) used a social comparison framework to examine how men and women perceived their own bodies when they compared them to television and magazine representations of idealized body types. Results indicated that women believed their bodies were different from the women they saw on television; men believed that their bodies were similar to the men they saw on television. However, both men and women thought their bodies were different from the images they saw in magazines. Overall, women were more dissatisfied with their bodies after social comparison with media than were men. Sohn noted that differences in these entertainment media might explain the results. For example, television may present more accurate images of men than of women. However, magazines, especially those with a health and wellness focus, often portray idealized images of the human form, thus increasing perceived differences between the real and ideal for both sexes.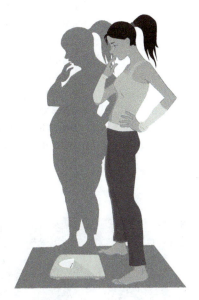

Our existing beliefs about our bodies also can affect the social comparison process. For example, Knobloch-Westerwick and Romero (2011) found that people who reported dissatisfaction with their bodies spent less time reading magazine articles with general interest content that included photographs of ideal body images than they did reading body improvement articles that included similar pictures. This finding indicates that although some images may have negative psychological effects on readers, if the content of the messages accompanying body-ideal images promotes positive and upward social comparison, these effects may be lessened.

Media Power and Inequalities

Several theories argue that mass media reinforce existing power structures that preserve patterns of social inequality. A focus on communication and inequality is important. Research has demonstrated that "differences in health outcomes across social groups result more from social, economic, institutional, and political factors than from access to or quality of medical care or unhealthy decisions by socially disadvantaged groups" (Niederdeppe, Bigman, Gonzales, & Gollust, 2013, p. 9). This means that even more than the individual decisions we make, the environments in which we live influence our health. Another way to think about this is that the environments we live in influence the choices we *have*. Research has shown that people who are poor, discriminated against, or part of marginalized subgroups suffer from higher rates of disease and death than people who are economically secure, not discriminated against, and members of privileged subgroups. Learning how media can make a positive impact on these **social determinants of health** is very important. This type of research may help identify ways that communication can shape public support and collective action to reduce **health disparities**.

Knowledge gap hypothesis. Social inequalities and health disparities can produce differences in the knowledge or information we retain about health-related issues. The **knowledge gap hypothesis** (Tichenor, Donohue, & Olien, 1970) predicts that people with more education and financial means gain and/or retain more from information they encounter in the media. People with less education retain less information, creating a growing gap between the information rich and the information poor. The

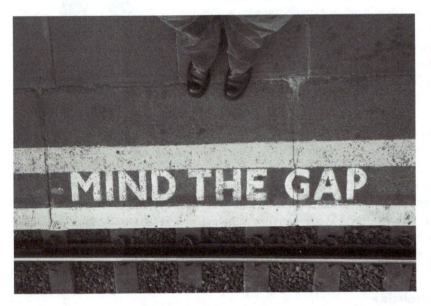

access that we have to news and other health information is shaped by the environments in which we live and the media choices that are available to us. As a result, health communication in the media may contribute to and even expand health disparities, as the knowledge required to positively change health behavior grows among people with more education and means, while it remains the same among people with less education and means.

Communication inequality. Viswanath and Emmons (2006) argued that the same structural factors that contribute to health disparities also contribute to **communication inequality,** or the differences in the ability of social groups to generate, manipulate, and distribute information. For example, empirical studies show that structural factors, such as journalistic practices and values, shape the content and viability of health news stories (Gandy, Kopp, Hands, Frazer, & Phillips, 1997; Hinnant, Oh, Caburnay, & Kreuter, 2011).

Although the media-effects tradition focuses on individual psychological factors to explain differences in our uptake of information, other scholars have taken a more sociological approach. Viswanath and Emmons (2006), for example, called attention to social factors like living conditions, access to a good education, and exposure to environmental factors (e.g., violence) that may affect our ability to obtain and retain information. Beyond information access, these social factors are considered more broadly as social determinants of health.

From a social scientific perspective, communication ecology theory identifies and explains the "array of interpersonal, mediated, and organizational communication options available to an individual to achieve everyday goals" (Katz, Ang, & Suro, 2012, p. 438). In the communication field, this tradition explores how the ecologies in which people live vary by communities and ethnic groups and inform their health communication ecologies (inclusive of both formal and informal communication channels, such as doctors and friendship networks; Katz et al., 2012; Wilkin, Ball-Rokeach, Matsaganis, & Cheong, 2007). From an ecological perspective, Katz et al. have asked whether "a rich set of informal health communica-tion connections—to friends, family, radio, television, Internet, newspapers, magazines, churches, and community organizations—can compensate, even partially for not having access to doctors" (p. 437). The researchers examining responses to the Pew Hispanic Center/Robert Wood Johnson Latino Health Survey found no such compensatory mechanism. However, analysis revealed that "diversified informal health communication ecologies related to health care access (regular doctor visits, uninterrupted health insurance, and regular health care location) and favorable health outcomes (self-ratings of general health, health-related efficacy, and knowledge of diabetes symptoms)" (p. 437). Thus, this line of research confirms that the **communication ecology** in which individuals reside is related to health outcomes.

From a critical paradigmatic perspective, the conceptualization of communication inequality offers a critical lens to examine the relationship between media and health. Such a perspective—one that examines issues of power, social structures, and social class—is rare in the health communication literature. A review of 22 years of scholarship in the field's defining journal, *Health Communication*, found only nine articles (or 1.4% of the total) that employed a critical paradigm (Kim, Park, Yoo, & Shen, 2010). One notable exception is an article that analyzes the symbolic power of an online game designed to promote sugary cereals. Thomson (2011) used a critical semiotic approach to closely examine the marketing rhetoric of Millsberry.com, an online game website created by General Mills to promote its breakfast cereals like Lucky Charms and Trix to children (but not rabbits). A critical semiotic approach meant that Thomson focused on the way in which symbols operated in the game and how those symbols (boxes of cereal, cereal characters) undermined the purported health messages of the site.

To play the Millsberry game, kids created avatars. The avatars earned money by playing games at the arcade and then used this money to buy clothes, decorate houses, and buy food. The object of the game was to keep the avatars healthy in terms of the types of food they ate, the amount of food they ate, and the activities in which they engaged. In order to conduct the study, Thomson created her own avatar, Kidsresearch, and played the game herself for multiple years. Her nine-year-old daughter also played the game, as Jake Spongebob. Thomson's analysis was based on her experiences in the game and her daughter's insights.

Thomson (2011) found that, at a surface level, Millsberry promoted two health messages: (a) Eat from multiple food groups, and (b) eat only until full. However, these messages were undermined by the logic of the game, which encouraged players to eat entire boxes of sugary cereal in one sitting and labeled Fruit Roll-Ups, a product that contains added sugar and food dyes, as fruit. Thomson labeled this type of rhetoric **commodity healthism** (p. 325). Commodity healthism, she explained, "names the way corporations pull a semiotic sleight of hand as they pay lip service to health ideals in order to increase the value of their com-

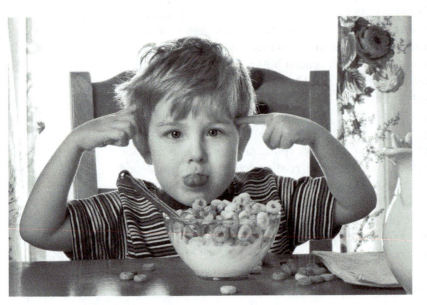

modities, making the brands appear 'healthy' without even having to make specific health claims about their products" (p. 325). Although Thomson's study focused on only one **advergame**, it shows how insidious these messages can be. In effect, the game was encouraging children to eat a cereal that provides more than 25% of its calories from sugar. Thomson's study demonstrates the need to regulate child-targeted food marketing.

PARADIGMATIC PERSPECTIVES ON MEDIA AND HEALTH

Communication theories guide much research about media and health. Scholars from the scientific paradigm often investigate how media messages about health set the public agenda, frame information, prime attitudes, and cultivate perceptions of health. Scholars from the interpretive and critical traditions are more interested in how social determinants of health reinforce inequalities and support institutions that disproportionally affect access to accurate health information, which in turn maintains or increases health disparities.

HEALTH REPORTING IN MEDIA

As we established in the previous section, media representations of health and disease have the potential to exert a substantial influence on health knowledge, attitudes, and even behavior. As a result, researchers and professionals in health communication, journalism, medicine, and public health have dedicated much time to examining how health information is developed and disseminated through media channels. They've paid particular attention to the accuracy of health reporting and how information influences public perceptions and health-related behaviors.

Developing Health-related Stories

How a news story is developed plays a role in what it communicates. Viswanath et al. (2008) noted that media outlets generally follow a **four-step process** in the creation of news. In the first step, journalists decide if a story is interesting, exciting, or unique enough to be told. The second step involves research, which includes selecting sources of accurate and reliable information and translating that information so that it can be understood by laypeople. The third step includes gathering additional information that might make a story appealing, such as personal testimonies and analogies, which leads to the fourth step of news-making: dissemination. Unfortunately, there is not yet a set of rigid journalistic standards that guides this four-step process, and existing standards are not applied uniformly.

National surveys suggest that journalists' education, experience, and the size and type of media organization for which they work influence story selection and development (Viswanath et al., 2008; Wallington, Blake, Tayor-Clark, & Viswanath, 2010). For example, Wallington et al. found that reporters working for national media organizations were more interested in novel and entertaining health news than were

Al Cross, Director, Institute for Rural Journalism and Community Issues, University of Kentucky

There is no "health beat" at most U.S. newspapers, because most are weeklies—small papers that lack the staff, skills, and/or the inclination for aggressive coverage of health problems and disparities. But most readers of these newspapers in rural areas don't read any other newspaper. As larger newspapers have shrunk as a result of the economic recession, their circulation areas—the geographic reach of their newspapers—have also shrunk. This has also meant less coverage.

Helping rural news media pick up that slack, especially on health coverage, is part of the mission of the Institute for Rural Journalism and Community Issues. That's partly because we're based at the University of Kentucky, in a state with chronically low health status. I'm a former state political writer and weekly newspaper editor/manager, and it's clear to me that many rural weeklies' tendency to shy away from "negative news" extends to health coverage. For example, the counties where most Kentucky papers publish stories about their place in the annual County Health Rankings are in the top two quintiles of the rankings. Others avoid, consciously or unconsciously, making the county "look bad."

One of our advisers, cancer specialist Gil Friedell, M.D., says, "If there's a problem in the community, the solution is in the community." To encourage more news coverage that will help communities face up to their health problems and help people make better decisions that affect their health, we have two online publications, one for the state and one for the nation. Kentucky Health News, funded by the Foundation for a Healthy Kentucky, is updated almost daily with excerpts of, and links to, stories about health topics relevant to Kentucky. It's at www.kyhealthnews.blogspot.com. We also do our own stories, because few Kentucky newspapers have a health beat, and we cover health topics extensively on The Rural Blog, a daily digest of events, trends, issues, ideas and journalism from and about rural America. It's at http://irjci.blogspot.com

We sponsor and speak at seminars that help rural journalists cover health topics and post resources for them on our website, www.RuralJournalism.org. We also present research and other presentations at health conferences, to help providers understand how to work with rural journalists.

Our research has found that much rural newspaper health "coverage" is advertorial articles, in which a message promoting a product or service is embedded in what appears to be a news story. We oversaw a project to provide authoritative, independent health articles to rural Appalachian newspapers for use in special health sections and encouraged the papers to use their sample-copy postal powers to send the edition containing the sections to every household in its core area, to reach people with low health literacy. The papers doing that reported a highly positive response.

local reporters, who preferred to focus on health education and decision making for their publics. Furthermore, more educated and experienced journalists cited public education as a priority in story selection, whereas their less-experienced counterparts cited entertainment value as important when selecting stories. In addition, research has demonstrated that newspaper coverage is influenced by the community the paper serves. For example, Pollock and Yulis (2004) found they could accurately predict a paper's position on assisted suicide on the basis of the characteristics (age, education, income, and other factors) of people who read that paper.

Choosing the sources that will inform a story also varies according to education, experience, and type of media organization. Wallington et al. (2010) found that experienced journalists from national organizations were more likely to use information from scientific journals and independent scientists, whereas less-seasoned reporters from smaller organizations were more likely to rely on information from government agencies, local healthcare providers, and press releases when developing stories.

The size and scope of media organizations can also influence journalists' decision-making process regarding story development. Large-scale media outlets may have the financial resources to employ one or more full-time reporters who focus solely on health-related stories (Wallington et al., 2010). These journalists are likely to have more education and expertise in the realms of both health and journalism than are reporters who work for local media outlets. This can affect their abilities to

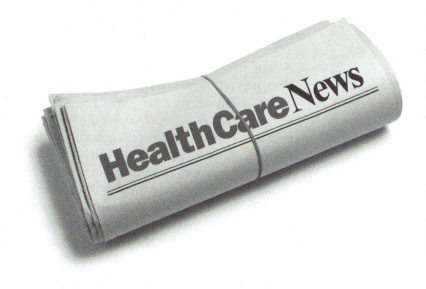

access information from scientific sources, as well as allow for more time and consideration in story development. Local reporters may have to cover a variety of news "beats" and thus have less time to devote to researching and developing health-related news.

The economy has also impacted the quality of health reporting. As a result of the economic downturn that began in 2007 and changing revenue streams, the newspaper industry underwent drastic changes. In the two years following the initial economic crisis, eight major newspaper chains filed for bankruptcy (Kirchhoff, 2010). Major newspapers, like *Rocky Mountain News* in Denver, shut down, and some papers, like the *Seattle Post-Intelligencer*, moved to web-only publications (Westphal, 2009). Thousands of reporters and editors were laid off (Kirchhoff, 2010). According to a survey of health reporters by the **Kaiser Family Foundation** and the **Association for Health Care Journalists** (2009), the financial strain has hurt the quality of health news, as reporters have less time to write in-depth stories and less space to print those stories. In addition, fewer reporters have time to specialize in health coverage (and thus gain expertise), and more experienced reporters have been laid off or moved to other beats.

At the same time that these changes have been occurring in newsrooms, foundations have begun funding projects to fill the gap in reporting (Westphal, 2009). The Kaiser Family Foundation began the Kaiser Health Service Project to provide national reporting on health news. Several other nonprofit projects, like the Center for Investigative Reporting and ProPublica, focus on investigative journalism, and their projects regularly include health-related stories. Whether these nonprofits can fill the gap that has resulted from the structural changes in the news industry is not yet known.

As a result of the economic changes, journalists, especially at smaller news organizations, may rely more often on "information subsidies" packaged by advocacy organizations and industry for story ideas. Len-Rios et al. (2009) noted that public relations (PR) materials (e.g., press releases) often present compact and easily understood information. However, press releases may also contain pre-framed information that is favorable to the entity publishing the release. Therefore, a journalist who uses PR materials as a primary source may not be delivering a story free from bias. Conversely, the ability to translate scientific information varies from reporter to reporter (Forsythe et al., 2012). Wallington et al. (2010) argued that although peer-reviewed journals are considered highly credible and less biased than other potential sources, they contain scientific jargon that can be difficult to render understandable for laypersons.

Reporting Health-related Stories

The way journalists frame news stories can sometimes create inaccurate perceptions of health-related matters. For example, one study found that local television news stories about cancer focused more on the causes of and treatments for cancer than they did on cancer prevention methods (Niederdeppe, Fowler, Goldstein, & Pribble, 2010). The researchers noted that by highlighting many possible causes of cancer and the varying success of treatment options, local TV stories were cultivating fatalistic perceptions concerning viewers' abilities to prevent cancer. That is, if people learn that cancer develops because of genetic, behavioral, and environmental factors, they might think that getting cancer is nearly inevitable and avoid making lifestyle changes that could reduce their risk for cancer. However, if they learn that they can prevent cancer through simple behavioral changes, they may develop healthier attitudes and lifestyle changes.

There are no universal standards that delineate what information should be highlighted in health-related news stories. Some argue that stories in local markets should focus on local sources of information, others call for social justice concerns to guide story and content selection, and still others note that there is illness-specific information that should or should not be included in all mediated health messages (Anhang, Stryker, Wright, & Goldie, 2003; Caburnay et al., 2003; Kim, Kumanyika, Shive, Igweatu & Kim, 2010). However, research indicates that newspapers targeted to minority populations are often primary sources of health information and that locally relevant content can have a powerful impact upon reducing health disparities (Cohen et al., 2008; Len-Rios, Cohen, & Caburnay, 2010). Future research concerning how the roles of national and local media influence health behaviors could provide insight about possible best practices for health journalists.

Media Misinformation

Given the number of factors that can influence how a news story is written and selected for publication, it is no surprise that inaccurate or incomplete health information sometimes reaches large audiences. Journalists, medical professionals, and public health personnel have raised serious concerns regarding the effects of misinformation on public perceptions and health behaviors (Schwitzer et al., 2005).

One notable example of **media misinformation** occurred in 1998 when the British medical journal *The Lancet* reported a link between the measles, mumps, and rubella (MMR) vaccine and autism in children. Before numerous physicians and national and international health organizations could refute the claims made in the report, the damage was done: Media coverage of the report spurred the creation of an organized anti-vaccination movement that is still prevalent today (Gross, 2009). In fact,

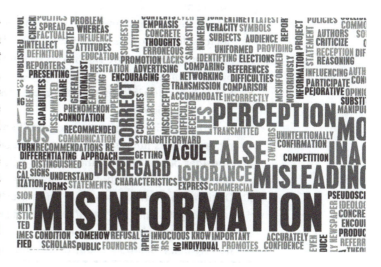

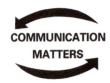
COMMUNICATION
MATTERS

AHCJ Statement of Principles

Statement of Principles of the Association of Health Care Journalists

The Association of Health Care Journalists displays its principles for professionalism, content, and accuracy in health news reporting on its website. The principles are abbreviated here. You can find the full version at http://healthjournalism.org/secondarypage-details.php?id=56

1. **Be vigilant in selecting sources.**
2. **Investigate and report possible links** between sources of information (studies or experts) and those (such as the manufacturers) who promote a new idea or therapy.
3. **Recognize that most stories involve a degree of nuance.**
4. **Understand the process of medical research.**
5. **Preserve journalistic independence** by avoiding the use of video news releases or the use of quotes from printed news releases.
6. **Be judicious in the use of television library or file footage.**
7. **Recognize that gathering and reporting information may cause harm.**
8. **Show respect.** Illness, disability and other health challenges facing individuals must not be exploited merely for dramatic effect.
9. **Remember that some sick people don't like to be called "victims."**
10. **Avoid vague, sensational language** (cure, miracle, breakthrough, promising, dramatic, etc.).
11. **Make sure anecdotes are appropriately chosen** to serve the interests of fairness and balance.
12. **Quantify the magnitude of the benefit or the risk** in the story.
13. **Report the complete risks and benefits of any treatment.**
14. **Clearly identify and explain the meaning of results.** Remember: association is not cause.
15. **Clearly define and communicate areas of doubt and uncertainty.** Explain what doctors don't know as well as what they do know.
16. **Seek out independent experts** to scrutinize claims and evaluate the quality of evidence presented by sources.
17. **Strive to include information about cost and insurance coverage** in any reporting of new ideas in medicine.
18. **Ensure that the total news package (headlines, teases, graphics, promotional material) does not oversimplify or misrepresent.**
19. **Consider public interest the primary criterion when choosing which stories to report.** Follow up on those stories that serve a wider public interest.
20. **Distinguish between advocacy and reporting.** There are many sides in a health care story. It is not the job of the journalist to take sides, but to present an accurate, balanced and complete report.
21. **Be original.** Plagiarism is untruthful and unacceptable.

following a 2011 Republican presidential primary debate, Minnesota Congressperson Michelle Bachmann mistakenly and irresponsibly claimed that the HPV vaccine caused "mental retardation" in a supporter's daughter (Weiner, 2011, para. 6).

Even though the link between vaccines and autism has been widely discredited (10 of the 13 authors of the original *Lancet* article retracted their opinions in 2004), research indicates that MMR vaccination rates decreased significantly in both the United States and England between 1995 and 2004, shortly after this now-discredited research study received media attention (Smith, Ellenberg, Bell, & Rubin, 2007). Given the potentially life-threatening consequences of media misinformation, researchers and ethicists have called for changes in professional and academic standards for health news reporting.

THE CHALLENGE OF MISINFORMATION

Journalists and researchers interested in health reporting face economic and structural obstacles to creating and disseminating accurate health information. These challenges should be addressed systematically by communication scholars and media professionals to develop effective strategies for gathering, interpreting, and reporting on health-related news stories. Future research is needed in this area to avoid the spread of misinformation to the public.

DIRECT-TO-CONSUMER ADVERTISING

So far, we have focused on the influence of news organizations' storytelling practices on health knowledge, attitudes, and behaviors. However, another important source of mediated health information is **direct-to-consumer advertising (DTCA)**. DTCA is the practice of promoting prescription medications to lay audiences through print and electronic media. DTCA began in 1981, when Merck advertised a pneumonia vaccine in the pages of *Reader's Digest*. Today, DTCA spending averages $5 billion a year, making it one of the most prolific and profitable forms of health communication (Lee, 2009; Ventola, 2011). The **Food and Drug Administration (FDA)** provides oversight of the DTCA industry, regulating DTCA to only three forms: "product claim ads," "reminder ads," and "help-seeking ads" (FDA, 2010, para. 13). The FDA requires print ads to provide fine print describing potential drug risks. Televised advertisements must inform potential consumers where they can learn more information about medications.

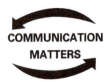

FDA Regulations for DTCA Content

The FDA explicates the three types of DTCA content on its website.

Product Claim Ad	Reminder Ad	Help-Seeking Ad
A product claim ad names a drug, says what condition it treats, and talks about both its benefits and its risks. An ad must present the benefits and risks of a prescription drug in a balanced fashion. Balance depends on both the information in the ad itself and how the information is presented. In this ad, the benefits and risks are presented to give a balanced impression of the drug.	Reminder ads give the drug's name but not the drug's use. The assumption behind reminder ads is that the audience knows what the drug is for and does not need to be told. A reminder ad does not contain risk information about the drug because the ad does not discuss the condition treated or how well the drug works. Reminder ads are not appropriate for drugs whose labeling has a "boxed warning" about certain very serious drug risks.	Help-seeking ads describe a disease or condition but do not recommend or suggest specific drugs. For instance, this ad describes seasonal allergy symptoms, such as runny nose, sneezing, and itchy, watery eyes. People with these symptoms are encouraged to talk to their doctor. Help-seeking ads may include a drug company's name and may also provide a telephone number to call for more information. FDA does not regulate lawful help-seeking ads. They are regulated by the Federal Trade Commission. However, if an apparent help-seeking ad references a particular drug, it is no longer a help-seeking ad, and FDA regulates it.

Quoted from http://www.fda.gov/Drugs/ResourcesForYou/Consumers/PrescriptionDrugAdvertising/default.htm

Although the FDA asserts that its "comprehensive surveillance and enforcement program" attempts to protect consumers from false or misleading advertising, the agency has come under fire from the **Government Accountability Office** for a lack of prompt and thorough reviews of DTCA materials (U.S. GAO, 2006). This is potentially problematic, as some televised advertisements spend more time highlighting a drug's benefits than they do describing potential health risks in an understandable manner (Kaphingst, Dejong, Rudd, & Daltroy, 2009).

Indeed, DTCA is a global controversy. The United States and New Zealand are the only developed nations that allow extensive drug advertising with few regulations; many developed nations have banned the practice ouright (Ventola, 2011). Supporters of DTCA note that it provides patients with important health information that empowers them to initiate communication with their healthcare providers, thus enhancing patient–provider communication. These conversations may in turn promote adherence to medical regimens, leading to improved health. For example, researchers discovered that people with stigmatized illnesses (e.g., social anxiety disorder, erectile dysfunction) felt less embarrassment discussing treatment options with their physicians after being exposed to DTCA for drugs that could treat their symptoms (Khanfar, Polen, & Clausen, 2009; Myers, Royne, & Deitz, 2011).

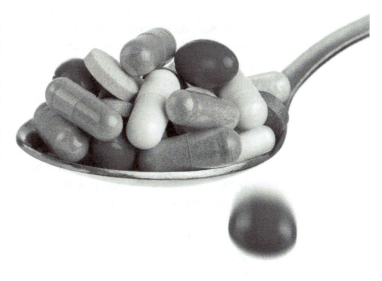

Opponents of DTCA are found mostly in the medical community. Practitioners suggest that the primary purpose of DTCA is to boost corporate profits, which may lead to unethical practices such as using misleading information in ads (Donohue, Cevasco, & Rosenthal, 2007; Frosch, Kreuger, Hornik, Conbolm, & Barg, 2007). This in turn may prompt inaccurate perceptions of illnesses and treatment options, giving patients false hope (An, 2008). In addition, DTCA could increase dissatisfaction with healthcare providers who refuse to grant their patients' requests for advertised medications (Gilbody, Wilson, & Watt, 2005).

Research suggests that DTCA affects patient–provider communication in some interesting ways. For example, Lee (2010) used the two-step flow model to guide a secondary data analysis of a 2002 survey by the FDA. The survey had been administered to 762 U.S. adults and measured participants' information-seeking behaviors relevant to DTCA (e.g., print advertisements, Internet and toll-free phone numbers, and interpersonal communication), influence variables (i.e., asking for drugs from healthcare providers), and response variables (i.e., how healthcare providers responded to requests and how patients reacted to those responses).

The **two-step flow model** suggests that mass media influence people to think about a certain topic (step one) and then seek out more information interpersonally from others whom they deem to be opinion leaders (step two). In this case the first step involves exposure to DTCA from media, and the second step involves talking with healthcare providers as opinion leaders. Statistical analysis of survey data revealed that patients who encountered DTCA most frequently sought more information about prescription drugs from their primary physicians but also consulted pharmacists, nurses, and physicians who were not their primary care providers about specific drugs. Furthermore, patients who consulted pharmacists and other physicians were more likely to receive prescription drugs from their primary care providers after citing other medical personnel as sources of information. This may indicate that primary care providers are more willing to capitulate to patients' requests provided those patients have received endorsement from others within the medical establishment. In other words, the opinion leaders also have opinion leaders! If physicians refused to prescribe pharmacist-endorsed medications, patients reported a desire to switch primary care physicians.

Lee's (2010) study is important for at least two reasons. First, the study supports and adds complexity to the two-step-flow model. DTCA did prompt some participants to ask their providers for advertised medications directly. However, these patients frequently left without the requested medications, feeling dissatisfied with the experience. In contrast, those patients who engaged in interpersonal communication with other medical opinion leaders were the only patients able to sway the prescribing behaviors of their primary care physicians. Second, it seems that both supporters and detractors of DTCA make valid points. DTCA does in fact lead to increased information-seeking behaviors and the initiation of communication with healthcare providers. However, the patient–provider relationship can be affected negatively if these informed consumers do not receive the medications they request. It should be noted that skilled healthcare providers are able to maintain positive relationships with patients even after denying them treatments highlighted in DTCA (Blose & Mack, 2009; Paterniti et al., 2010).

The ultimate effects of DTCA upon physician-prescribing behaviors and patient health outcomes remain unknown. However, given the controversial nature of DTCA, health practitioners have suggested certain reforms to federal policies regarding the industry. For example, Ventola (2011) recommended including quantitative information about drug effectiveness in DTCA and specifically mentioning drug costs in every ad. Only time will tell if these changes become implemented.

DIRECT-TO-CONSUMER ADVERTISING (DTCA)

The United States and New Zealand are the only developed nations that have not banned the controversial practice of direct-to-consumer advertising. Proponents of DTCA believe that it can empower patients, decrease stigma surrounding illness, and increase patient-provider communication. Detractors believe that because DTCA regulations are lax, powerful drug companies misrepresent their products, misinforming patients and affecting the patient-provider relationship negatively. Research about DTCA paints a more complex picture, wherein patients seek out information about advertised drugs from multiple opinion leaders.

ENTERTAINMENT-EDUCATION

Beyond advertisements embedded in broadcast media, a number of entertainment media are relied upon as a vehicle for health education. **Entertainment-education (E-E)** is the process of embedding health-related information into popular media narratives with the goal of changing knowledge, attitudes, and behaviors (Beacom & Newman, 2010; Movius, Cody, Huang, Berkowitz, & Morgan, 2007). E-E occurs when health professionals work with writers and producers to create original storylines for well-known programs and characters.

For example, Movius et al. (2007) discussed consulting writers from the popular crime drama *Numb3rs* in the development of an episode about black-market organ trade in the United States. In truth, there is no market for illegally harvested organs in America; therefore, health communication specialists at **The Norman Lear Center (NLC)** collaborated with writers to include some accurate information in the imaginary tale. Although the fictional organ-harvesting plot drove the drama behind the episode, writers also included facts and statistics concerning the number of people waiting for organs in the United States in various scenes.

Furthermore, the episode included a subplot in which a main character was convinced by others to become an organ donor himself. A follow-up survey conducted by the NLC found that viewers of this episode were more likely than viewers of other dramas featuring storylines about organ donation to think about the importance of organ donation, sign up to become an organ donor, and encourage others to become donors. It seems, then, that presenting medically reliable information

---

The Norman Lear Center

Named after the prolific Hollywood producer and creator of classic television programs such as *All in The Family* and *The Jeffersons*, the University of Southern California Annenberg School of Communication's Norman Lear Center, "probes the meaning of entertainment as a discourse, an industry, and a key component of contemporary life." The Hollywood Health and Society program at the Center has worked with entertainment professionals from popular television shows like *Bones, Law and Order SVU*, and *Grey's Anatomy* to help integrate medically accurate information into fictional storylines and conduct research concerning a host of entertainment and health matters, such as examining representations of disabled individuals in primetime programming, developing effective entertainment-education processes, and promoting national and international diplomacy about health crises. Visit the Center's website for more information: http://hollywoodhealthandsociety.org

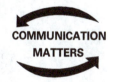

COMMUNICATION MATTERS

through fictional narratives can produce pro-social effects. However, a host of factors might influence whether or not an E-E narrative is educational, entertaining, or both.

Accuracy of health information should be a primary concern for people interested in E-E because media can become powerful sources of information about health-related phenomena for us, especially when we have limited knowledge about certain health issues. For example, Yoo and Tian (2011) noted that people who are uninformed about organ donation can be negatively affected by narratives that portray organ donation as dangerous. Imagine if you tuned in late to *Numb3rs* and saw only the violent black-market organ harvesting scene of the episode discussed above. Would you sign a donor card or tell your friends to become organ donors? It is important, therefore, that messages in E-E provide accurate information and boost self-efficacy to engage in healthy or pro-social behaviors.

Research indicates that accurate information is important in E-E, but so too is the entertainment value of E-E efforts. For example, one study found that adolescents were more interested in theatrical plays with anti-drug messages when those plays contained authentic messages, characters, and plots (Guttman, Gesser-Edelsburg, & Israelashvili, 2008). Teens receive an overwhelming number of health messages from interpersonal and media sources. Guttman et al. warned that because teens are inundated with so much information, stories that do not seem at least potentially relatable could be rejected and perhaps even engender a boomerang effect (i.e., when a persuasive message incites the exact opposite behavior that was advocated). For example, consider the over-the-top emotional tone of the "This is Your Brain on Drugs" PSA, which spawned numerous parodies, or the typical anti-drug educational films shown in high school health classes. The PSA relied on metaphor to convey spurious information (i.e., ANY drug making your brain immediately go all sunny-side up), whereas the films, although

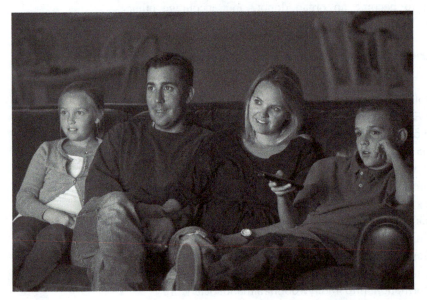

likely more accurate, typically were so poorly acted and produced that they detracted from the overall message.

One interesting line of E-E research considers the effects of repeated exposure to similar messages. For example, researchers found that women who watched analogous breast cancer-related storylines on both *Grey's Anatomy* and *ER* were more likely to have increased knowledge about the topic, more favorable attitudes toward screening, and increased screening-related behaviors than were women who watched only *Grey's Anatomy* or *ER* (Hether, Huang, Beck, Murphy, & Valente, 2008). In other words, repeated exposure to similar E-E messages can positively affect health-related outcomes for populations (e.g., women) who frequently receive similar messages about specific health issues (e.g., breast cancer).

Most researchers seem to agree that learning occurs in E-E because of two similar constructs, involvement and transportation. **Involvement** describes the level of personal identification we have with a specific character in a story. **Transportation** is the degree to which we are engrossed in a general narrative. Moyer-Gusé, Chung, and Jain (2011) found that identification with characters from *Sex in the City* was related positively to self-efficacy and negatively to generating counter-arguments, which led to increased discussion of sexual health with others. Viewers who perceived themselves to be like certain characters from *Sex in the City* were more likely to believe that they could act like their favorite characters and were less likely to question the behaviors of those characters.

Murphy, Frank, Moran, and Patnoe-Woodley (2011) studied the effects of transportation, identification, and emotion on cancer-related knowledge, attitudes, and behaviors among regular viewers of the television show *Desperate Housewives*. For two seasons on the show, Lynette Scavo's storyline depicted her diagnosis, treatment, and recovery from non-Hodgkin's lymphoma. Transportation proved to be the strongest predictor of knowledge, attitudes, and behaviors (e.g., information-seeking and talking about cancer). However, the authors argued that transportation and identification are likely interrelated concepts. That is, people who identified strongly with Lynette may have become more engrossed with the show, or people who were already engrossed in the general narrative of *Desperate Housewives* may have become more involved with Lynette's story. This study seems to reconcile the exposure/ overexposure dilemma. Lynette dealt with cancer for multiple episodes over two seasons. Viewers likely received many messages about cancer. However, because they identified with the character and the show overall, they did not lose interest in the story and the messages did not create a boomerang effect. It seems that the key to E-E is a well-planned mix of science and spectacle.

ENTERTAINMENT-EDUCATION

Entertainment-education is the multidisciplinary process in which health professionals, communication researchers, and entertainers work together to embed health messages in popular entertainment media. Research indicates that accurate information needs to be portrayed in ways that engage audiences so that they connect with characters, stories, and fictional environments. If people are transported into a story and identify with it, they will likely accept health messages and learn new information even upon repeated exposure. However, if the story and characters are not compelling, audiences may have negative reactions to health information.

FUTURE DIRECTIONS

Future studies of mass media and health should focus upon narrowing the theoretical and methodological gaps discussed in the first section of this chapter. Researchers will need to work together to create sophisticated measures and study designs that can more accurately capture how mass media affect our understanding of health.

Journalists and communication researchers should continue to work to overcome structural and economic challenges that affect the development and reporting of health news. Collaborative research among professionals and academics could improve strategies for gathering and interpreting medical information, which might minimize the negative effects of media misinformation.

Considering the controversy surrounding DTCA, more research is necessary to understand how this form of advertising affects patient–provider communication. Similarly, researchers and professionals from the entertainment industry should continue to measure how E-E efforts affect knowledge, attitudes, and behaviors.

Given the ever-changing media landscape, new media such as health-related websites (e.g., WebMD and Yahoo! Health), video games that promote exercise (e.g., *Wii Fit*), YouTube videos demonstrating disease screening processes or offering medical advice, Facebook wellness communities like Healthyshare, and cellphone applications that track weight, food intake, and exercise regimens will become important topics and contexts for future studies of media and health communication.

CONCLUSION

We hope this chapter provided a substantive yet concise discussion of the many ways media affect how we understand health. Tonight you may hear a news broadcast about Michelle Obama's *Let's Move* exercise campaign, watch *The Biggest Loser* as you eat a pint of Ben & Jerry's ice cream, or read a story on *The Huffington Post* about what Amanda Bynes' tweets teach us about mental health. As you encounter these intersections of mass media and health, take a few moments to consider how these messages might affect health knowledge, attitudes, and behaviors at the individual and societal level.

DISCUSSION QUESTIONS

1. How might "new media" (e.g., Twitter, Facebook, Tumblr, etc.) improve or worsen the problems journalists face in the development and reporting of health-related stories?
2. In what ways do you think various types of DTCA (product claim ads, reminder ads, and help-seeking ads) affect patient attitudes toward prescription drugs and communication behaviors with providers?
3. Think about a time you experienced an especially effective example of entertainment education. What features of your example (e.g., messages, characters, drama) made it so effective? How could those features influence future E-E efforts?

IN-CLASS ACTIVITIES

1. Create a health communication media journal for today, making a list of every health communication mediated message you encounter. What messages about health did you encounter from mass media? How would you approach studying them? Develop three research questions guided by theories discussed in this chapter.
2. Visit http://www.fda.gov/Drugs/ResourcesForYou/Consumers/PrescriptionDrug Advertising/default.htm and then click on the examples of correct and incorrect product claim, reminder, and help-seeking ads. Compare and contrast.

RECOMMENDED READINGS

Atkin, C. K., Smith, S. W., McFeters, C., & Ferguson, V. (2008). A comprehensive analysis of breast cancer news coverage in leading media outlets focusing on environmental risks and prevention. *Journal of Health Communication, 13*(1), 3–19.

This study examines media coverage of breast cancer for individual and social determinants of health.

Dens, N., Eagle, L. C., & De Pelsmacker, P. (2008). Attitudes and self-reported behavior of patients, doctors, and pharmacists in New Zealand and Belgium toward direct-to-consumer advertising of medication. *Health Communication, 23*(1), 45–61.

This study examines the effects of DTCA from providers' perspectives in New Zealand (the only other country than the United States to allow DTCA).

Moyer-Gusé, E., Mahood, C., & Brookes, S. (2011). Entertainment-education in the context of humor: Effects on safer sex intentions and risk perceptions. *Health Communication, 26*(8), 765–774.

Although many studies have examined the effects of E-E using televised dramas, this study examines E-E and sitcoms.

REFERENCES

An, S. (2008). Antidepressant direct-to-consumer advertising and social perception of the prevalence of depression: Application of the availability heuristic. *Health Communication, 23*, 499–505.

Anhang, R., Stryker, J. E., Wright Jr., T. C., & Goldie, S. J. (2003). News media coverage of human papillomavirus. *Cancer, 100*(2), 308–314.

Bandura, A. (1986). *Social foundations of thought and action: A social cognitive theory.* Englewood Cliffs, NJ: Prentice-Hall.

Bandura, A. (2009). Social cognitive theory of mass communication. In J. Bryant & M. B. Oliver (Eds.), *Media effects: Advances in theory and research* (3rd ed., pp. 94–124). New York: Routledge.

Beacom, A. M., & Newman, S. J. (2010). Communicating health information to disadvantaged populations. *Family Community Health, 33*(2), 152–162.

Blose, J. E., Mack, R. W., (2009). The impact of denying a direct-to-consumer advertised drug request on the patient/physician relationship. *Health Marketing Quarterly, 26*, 315–332.

Caburnay, C. A., Kreuter, M. W., Luke, D. A., Logan, R. A., Jacobsen, H. A., Reddy, V. C., ... Zayed, H. R. (2003). The news on health behavior: Coverage of diet, activity, and tobacco in local newspapers. *Health Education & Behavior, 30*, 709–722.

Cohen, E. L., Caburnay, C. A., Luke, D. A., Rodgers, S., Cameron, G. T., & Kreuter, M. W. (2008). Cancer coverage in general-audience and black newspapers. *Health Communication, 23*, 427–435.

Dittmar, M. L. (1994). Relationship between depression, gender, and television viewing of college students. *Journal of Social Behavior and Personality, 9*, 317–328.

Donohue, J. M., Cevasco, M., & Rosenthal, M. B. (2007). A decade of direct-to consumer advertising of prescription drugs. *The New England Journal of Medicine, 35*(7), 673–681.

Entman, R. M. (1993). Framing: Toward clarification of a fractured paradigm. *Journal of Communication, 43*(4), 51–58.

Food and Drug Administration. (2010). Keeping watch over direct-to-consumer ads. Retrieved from http://www.fda.gov/ForConsumers/ConsumerUpdates/ucm107170.htm

Forsyth, R., Morrell, B., Lipworth, W., Kerridge, I., Jordens, C. F. C., & Chapman, S. (2012). Health journalists' perceptions of their professional roles and responsibilities for ensuring the veracity of reports of health research. *Journal of Mass Media Ethics, 27*, 130–141.

Frosch, D. L., Kreuger, P. M., Hornik, R. C., Conbolm, P. F., & Barg, F. K. (2007). Creating a demand for prescription drugs: A content-analysis of television direct-to-consumer advertising. *Annals of Family Medicine, 5*(1), 6–13.

Gandy, O. H., Jr., Kopp, K., Hands, T., Frazer, K., & Phillips, D. *(*1997*).* Race and risk: Factors affecting the framing of stories about inequality, discrimination, and just plain bad luck. *Public Opinion Quarterly, 61*, 158–182.

Gerbner, G. (1990). Epilogue: Advancing on the path of righteousness (maybe). In N. Signorielli & M. Morgan (Eds.), *Cultivation analysis: New directions in media effects research* (pp. 249–262). Newbury Park, CA: Sage Publications.

Gilbody, S., Wilson, P., & Watt, I. (2005). Benefits and harms of direct-to-consumer advertising: A systematic review. *Quality and Safety in Health Care, 14*, 246–250.

Gross, L. (2009). A broken trust: Lessons from the vaccine-autism wars. *PLoS Biology, 7*(5), 1–7.

Guttman, N., Gesser-Edelsburg, A., & Israelashvili, M. (2008). The paradox of realism and "authenticity" in entertainment education: A study of adolescents' views about anti-drug abuse dramas. *Health Communication, 23*, 128–141.

Hammermeister, J., Brock, B., Winterstein, D, & Page, R. (2005). Live without TV?: Cultivation theory and psychosocial health characteristics of television-free individuals and their television-viewing counterparts. *Health Communication, 17*(3), 253–264.

Hether, H. J., Huang, G. C., Beck, V., Murphy, S. T., & Valente, T. W. (2008). Entertainment-education in a media-saturated environment: Examining the impact of single and multiple exposures to breast cancer storylines in two popular medical dramas. *Journal of Health Communication, 13*, 808–823.

Hinnant, A., Oh, H. J., Caburnay, C. A., & Kreuter, M. W. *(*2011*).* What makes African American health disparities newsworthy? An experiment among journalists about story framing. *Health Education Research, 26*, 937–47.

Hirsch, P.M. (1980). The "scary world" of the nonviewer and other anomalies: A reanalysis of Gerbner et al.'s findings on cultivation analysis, part I. *Communication Research 7*, 403–456.

Jensen, J. D., Moriarty, C. M., Hurley, R. J., Stryker, J. E. (2010). Making sense of cancer news coverage trends: A comparison of three comprehensive content analyses. *Journal of Health Communication, 15*, 136–141.

Kaiser Family Foundation and the Association of Health Care Journalists. (2009). *Survey of AHCJ Members*. Retrieved from: healthjournalism.org.

Kaphingst, K. A., Dejong, W., Rudd, R. E., & Daltroy, L. H. (2009). A content analysis of direct to consumer television prescription drug advertisements. *Journal of Health Communication, 14*, 451–460.

Katz, V.S., Ang, A., & Suro, R. (2012). An ecological perspective on U.S. Latinos' health communication behaviors, access, and outcomes. *Hispanic Jouranl of Behavioral Sciences, 34,* 437–456.

Khanfar, N. M., Polen, H. H., & Clauson, K. A. (2009). Influence on consumer behavior: The impact of direct-to-consumer advertising on medication requests for gastroesophageal reflux disease and social anxiety disorder. *Journal of Health Communication, 14,* 451–460.

Kirchhoff, S. M. (2010). *The U.S. newspaper indunstry in transition.* (Report No. 7-0658). Retrieved from Congressional Research Service website: www.crs.gov.

Kim, A. E., Kumanyika, S., Shive, D., Igweatu, U., & Kim, S. H. (2010). Coverage and framing of racial and ethnic health disparities in US newspapers 1996–2005. *American Journal of Public Health, 100,* S224–S331.

Kim, J.-N., Park, S.-C., Yoo, S.-W., & Shen, H. (2010). Mapping health communication scholarship: Breadth, depth, and agenda of published research in *Health Communication. Health Communication, 25*(6/7), 487–503.

Knobloch-Westerwick, S., & Romero, J. P. (2011). Body ideals in the media: Perceived attainability and social comparison choices. *Media Psychology, 14,* 27–48.

Lawrence, R. G. (2004). Framing obesity: The evolution on a public health issue. *The International Journal of Press/Politics, 9*(3), 56–75.

Lee, A. L. (2009). Changing effects of direct-to-consumer broadcast drug advertising information sources on prescription drug requests. *Health Communication, 24,* 361–376.

Lee, A. L. (2010) Who are the opinion leaders?: The physicians, pharmacists, patients, and direct-to-consumer prescription drug advertising. *Journal of Health Communication, 15,* 629–655.

Len-Rios, M. E., Cohen, E., & Caburnay, C. (2010). Readers use black newspapers for health/cancer information. *Newspaper Research Journal, 30*(1), 20–35. Retrieved from http://www.ncbi.nlm.nih.gov/pmc/articles/PMC3152198

Len-Rios, M. E., Hinnant, A., Park, S. A., Cameron, G. T., Frisby, C. M., & Lee, Y. (2009). Health news agenda building: Journalists' perceptions of the role of public relations. *Journalism & Mass Communication Quarterly, 86,* 315–331.

McCombs, M. E., & Shaw, D. L. (1972). The agenda-setting function of mass media. *Public Opinion Quarterly, 36,* 176–187.

McCreary, D. R., & Sadaca, S. W. (1999). Television viewing and self-perceived health, weight, and physical fitness: Evidence for the cultivation hypothesis. *Journal of Applied Social Psychology, 29,* 2342–2361.

Movius, L., Cody, M., Huang, G., Berkowitz, M., & Morgan, S. (2007). Motivating television viewers to become organ donors. *Cases in Public Health Communication and Marketing,* 1–20. Retrieved from http://sphhs.gwu.edu/departments/pch/phcm/casesjournal/volume1/peer-reviewed/cases_1_08.cfm

Moyer-Gusé, E., Chung, A. H., & Jain, P. (2011). Identification with characters and discussion of taboo topics after exposure to an entertainment narrative about sexual health. *Journal of Communication, 61,* 387–406.

Murphy, S. T., Frank, L. B., Moran, M. B., & Patnoe-Woodley, P. (2011). Involved, transported, or emotional? Exploring the determinants of change in knowledge, attitudes, and behavior in entertainment-education. *Journal of Communication, 61*(3), 407–431.

Myers, S. D., Royne, M. B., & Deitz, G. D. (2011). Direct-to-consumer advertising: Exposure, behavior, and policy implications. *Journal of Public Policy and Marketing, 30*(1), 110–118.

Niederdeppe, J., Bigman, C. A., Gonzales, A. L., Gollust, S. E. (2013). Communication about health disparities in mass media. *Journal of Communication, 63*(1), 8–30.

Niederdeppe, J., Fowler, E. F., Goldstein, K., & Pribble, J. (2010). Does local television news coverage cultivate fatalistic beliefs about cancer prevention? *Journal of Communication, 60*(2), 230–253.

Niederdeppe, J., Shapiro, M., & Porticella, N. (2011*)*. Attributions of responsibility for obesity: Narrative communication reduces reactive counterarguing among liberals. *Human Communication Research, 37*, 295–323.

Page, R. M., Hammermeister, J. J., Scanlan, A., & Allen, O. (1996). Psychosocial and health related characteristics of adolescent television viewers. *Child Study Journal, 26*, 319–331.

Paterniti, D. A., Fancher, T. L., Cipri, C. S., Timmermans, S., Heritage, J., & Kravitz, R. (2010). Getting to "no": Strategies primary care physicians use to deny patient requests. *Archives of Internal Medicine, 170*(4), 381–388.

Pollock, J. C., & Yulis, S. G. (2004). Nationwide newspaper coverage of physician-assisted suicide: A community structure approach. *Journal of Health Communication, 9*(4), 281–307.

Roskos–Ewoldsen, D., Roskos–Ewoldsen, B., & Carpentier, F. (2009). Media priming: An updated synthesis. In J. Bryant and M. B. Oliver (Ed.), *Media effects: Advances in theory and research* (3rd ed., pp. 74–93). New York: Routledge.

Scheufele, D. A., & Tewksbury, D. (2007). Framing, agenda setting, and priming: The evolution of three media effects models. *Journal of Communication, 57*(1), 9–20.

Schwitzer, G., Mudur, G., Henry, D, Wilson, A., Goozner, M., et al. (2005). What are the roles and responsibilities of the media in disseminating health information? *PLoS Medicine, 2*(7), 576–582.

Shanahan, J., & Morgan, M. (1999) *Television and its viewers: Cultivation theory and research.* Cambridge, United Kingdom: Cambridge University Press.

Signorielli, N. & Morgan, M. (2009). Cultivation analysis: Research and practice. In D.W. Stacks & M.B. Salwen (Eds.), *An integrated approach to communication theory and research* (2nd ed., pp. 106–121). New York: Routledge.

Smith, M. J., Ellenberg, S. S., Bell, L. M., & Rubin, D. M. (2007). Media coverage of the measles-mumps-rubella vaccine and autism controversy and its relationship to MMR immunization rates in the United States. *Pediatrics, 121*(4), 836–843.

Sohn, S. H. (2009). Body image: Impacts of media channels on men's and women's social comparison process, and testing of involvement measurement. *Atlantic Journal of Communication, 17*(1), 19–35.

Stryker, J. E., Moriarty, C. M., & Jensen, J. D. (2008). Effects of newspaper coverage on public knowledge about modifiable cancer risks. *Health Communication, 23*(4), 380–390.

Thomson, D. M. (2011). The mixed health messages of Millsberry: A critical study of online child-targeted food advergaming. *Health Communication, 26*(4), 323–331.

Tichenor, P. J., Donohue, G. A., & Olien, C. N. (1970). Mass media flow and differential growth in knowledge. *The Public Opinion Quarterly, 34*(2), 159–170.

U.S. Government Accountability Office. (2006). *Prescription drugs: Improvements needed in FDA's oversight of direct-to-consumer advertising.* (GAO Publication No. GAO-07-54). Washington, DC. U.S. Government Printing Office.

Ventola, C. L. (2011). Direct-to-consumer pharmaceutical advertising: Therapeutic or toxic? *Pharmacy and Therapeutics, 36*, 669–684. Retrieved from http://www.ncbi.nlm.nih.gov/pmc/articles/PMC3278148

Viswanath, K., Blake, K. D., Meissner, H. I., Gottlieb Sointz, N., Mull, C., Freeman, C. S., ... Croyle, R. T. (2008). Occupational practices and the making of health news: A national survey of U.S. health and medical science journalists. *Journal of Health Communication, 13,* 759–777.

Viswanath, K., & Emmons, K. M. (2006). Message effects and social determinants of health: Its application to cancer disparities. *Journal of Communication, 56,* S238–S264.

Wallington, S. F., Blake, K., Taylor-Clark, K. & Viswanath. (2010). Antecedents to agenda setting and framing in health news: An examination of priority, angle, source, and resource usage from a national survey of U.S. health reporters and editors. *Journal of Health Communication, 15*(1), 76–94.

Wang, Z., & Gantz, W. (2010) Health content in local television news: A current appraisal. *Health Communication, 25,* 230–237.

Weaver, D. H. (2007). Thoughts on agenda setting, framing, and priming. *Journal of Communication, 57*(1), 142–147.

Weiner, R. (2011, September 13). Bachmann claims HPV vaccine might cause 'mental retardation.' *The Washington Post.* Retrieved from http://www.washingtonpost.com blogs/the-fix/post/michele-bachmann-continues-perry-attack-claims-hpv-vaccine-might-cause-mental-retardation/2011/09/13/gIQAbJBcPK_blog.html

Westphal, D. (2009). *Philanthropic foundations: Growing funders of the news.* Retrieved from the University of Southern California, Annenberg School for Communication, Center of Communication Leadership and Policy website: communicationleadership.usc.edu

Wilkin, H. A., Ball-Rokeach, S. J., Matsaganis, M. D., & Cheong, P. (2007). Comparing the communication connections of geo-ethnic communities: How people stay on top of their communities. *Electronic Journal of Communication, 17*(2). Retrieved from http://www.cios.org/EJCPUBLIC/017/1/01711.HTML

Williams, C. D., Sallis, J. F., Calfas, K. J., & Burke, R. (1999). Psychosocial and demographic correlates of television viewing. *American Journal of Health Promotion, 13,* 207–221.

Yoo, J. H., & Tian, Y. (2011). Effects of entertainment (mis)education: Exposure to entertainment television programs and organ donation intention. *Health Communication, 36*(2), 147–158.

14

Campaigns and Interventions

Donald W. Helme,
Matthew W. Savage, and
Rachael A. Record

We are all exposed to health-related campaigns and interventions, both through commercial advertising ("Take this diet pill and lose 20 pounds!") and health behavior change programs designed to prevent us from doing something unhealthy or stupid or to encourage us to do something healthy and less stupid ("Don't Drink and Drive!" "Get the Flu Shot!"). In this chapter, we review three strategies that can be used to influence the health behavior of large groups of people: mass media campaigns, community-based interventions, and school-based interventions. Although we've tried to simplify things by presenting these as separate approaches, in truth there is plenty of overlap between them. The main distinction is in amount of contact with the audience. Whereas a campaign primarily uses some form of mass media to reach a large audience, an intervention—whether community-based or school-based—typically involves practitioners intervening directly in the lives of those they are trying to help. Table 14.1 will help you further compare and contrast campaigns and interventions. Regardless of these differences, the purpose in each case is to improve the health and well-being of people through

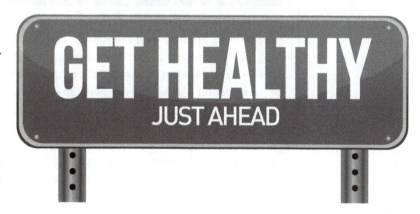

Table 14.1 Characteristics of Campaign Strategies

Campaign/ Intervention Type	Reach	Audience Involvement	Researcher Anonymity	Pace of Information Release	Cost Per Person Reached	Potential Internet Assistance
Mass Media Campaign	High	Low	High	Nonflexible; Pre-determined by Researchers	Low	High
Community-based Intervention	Low	High	Low	Flexible; Influenced by Audience	Medium/ High	High
School-based Intervention	Low to High	High	Low	Flexible; Influenced by Audience	Medium/ High	High

programs designed to prevent disease and to promote general health and healthy behaviors.

In this chapter, we'll explore some of the most common types of health communication campaigns and interventions to provide further insight into what they are and what they can be expected to accomplish. In addition, we'll explain the role of theory in campaigns and interventions, as well as discuss the direction future campaigns and interventions are headed. We hope to illustrate the critical role that mass media campaigns and interventions play in health promotion and risk prevention.

CAMPAIGNS VERSUS INTERVENTIONS

Campaigns and interventions are similar because they both seek to educate people and ultimately lead them to make positive, healthy behavior changes. They differ, however, in that community- and school-based interventions actively "intervene" in the lives of the target audience, whereas campaigns rely on presentation of messages to persuade people.

Before we begin, we do want to point out that the vast majority of the research in mass media campaign and community- and school-based interventions is informed by the scientific paradigm. That is, researchers expect that their campaign and intervention messages will have predictable effects on their target audiences. There is some critical–cultural research that addresses campaigns and interventions and considers the implications of their implementation (e.g., Dutta-Bergman, 2005). In this chapter, however, we focus on research from the scientific perspective. In addition, almost all of the work in this area is interdisciplinary in nature, with research teams having representation from multiple disciplines such as communication, public health, psychology, sociology, nursing, and medicine. In fact, some might argue that in certain areas, the work has reached transdisciplinary status. Prevention research is one example of this, where the area has its own professional organization, conference, and journal (see http://preventionresearch.org).

TYPES OF CAMPAIGNS AND INTERVENTIONS

Mass Media Campaigns

Our daily experiences of watching television, listening to the radio, or using the Internet expose us to mass media messages that promote healthy behaviors and dissuade unhealthy ones. Perhaps you have heard a spot on the radio about being prepared for an emergency or buying food from local and sustainable sources. Or maybe you have seen a **public service announcement (PSA)** on television that presented a frightening portrayal concerning alcohol, tobacco, or substance use. Or you might recall a billboard, poster, or newspaper article that included persuasive messages about managing your health. These are just a few examples of the types of messages that make up what are generally referred to as **mass media campaigns**. When mass media campaigns concern health outcomes, they may be referred to as *public health mass media campaigns* (e.g., Randolph & Viswanath, 2004) or *health mass media campaigns* (e.g., Noar, 2006). While these are umbrella terms that describe strategies using mass communication to change the health-related attitudes or behaviors of individuals, you might come across a specific variation of these efforts known as a *health communication campaign* or a *public communication campaign* (e.g., Atkin & Rice, 2013).

Adding the term *communication* designates that these campaigns include "purposive attempts to inform or influence behaviors in large audiences within a specified time period using an organized set of communication activities and featuring an array of mediated messages in multiple channels generally to produce noncommercial benefits to individuals and society" (Rice & Atkin, 2013, p. 3; see also Rogers & Storey, 1987). This definition implies that not all communication campaigns must involve mass media messages (or mass media messages by themselves) and that sometimes communication campaigns may be smaller in scope and reach a smaller audience than a traditional mass media campaign. In addition, because these efforts are noncommercial, that is, not with the purpose of selling goods or making a profit, health communication campaigns are

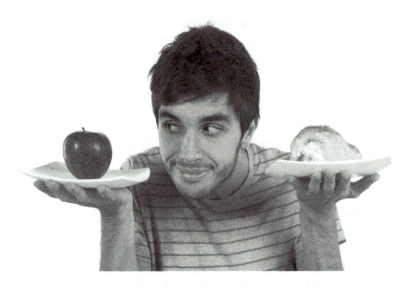

somewhat different from advertising campaigns (Catalán-Matamoros, 2011). Advertising campaigns promote commercial products that may be trivial or superficial, whereas health communication campaigns promote a central, ego-involved, and supremely important topic: one's health (Elliott, 1987). For example, an advertising campaign might market an easily obtainable product that you want (e.g., a delicious cheeseburger), whereas a health communication campaign might advocate for you to avoid negative behaviors that are often enjoyable (e.g., "Put that cheeseburger down!") or to adopt behaviors that involve short-term sacrifice (e.g., checking your cholesterol, exercising for 30 minutes) for the sake of long-term benefits that are not necessarily guaranteed. Although we do not expect health communication campaigns to have the same effects as advertising campaigns, research shows that mass media campaigns have evolved over time in terms of design and achievable expectations to be quite effective at changing attitudes and behaviors among large groups of people (Rice & Atkin, 2013).

The early history of mass media campaigns involved many shortcomings that led to better understandings of how messages affect individuals (see Wartella & Stout, 2002). Zimmerman et al. (2007) pointed out that the potential to reach very large audiences through the media led to an improvement of research methods and a more realistic understanding of campaign expectations. Noar (2006) concluded that we are now in a "*conditional effects era*, in which we have not necessarily discovered new principles of campaign design but rather have seen many of the principles that were formalized in previous eras effectively and creatively put into action" (p. 22). These effective and creative efforts have led to a growing body of research evidence that health mass media campaigns can be effective when properly designed (Hornik, 2002; Randolph & Viswanath, 2004; Rice & Atkin, 2013; Rogers & Storey, 1987). Proper design usually means a trade-off regarding desired effects and the people affected. That is, mass media campaigns can result in *small to moderate* effects among *large to very large* groups of people. These small effects are important when you consider entire populations.

The biggest changes to the design and expectation of mass media campaigns have come from technological advancements. For example, television allowed for the creation of mass-broadcast video messages (including PSAs) to every home with a television. The Internet may be the most important advancement to mass media messages yet, although exactly how to most effectively utilize this ever-changing medium remains to be seen. One of the main benefits of using the Internet as a distribution channel for campaigns is that mass media messages are no longer confined by, say, the traditional 30 seconds of your broadcast television; instead, after seeing the 30 second PSA, you will most likely be directed to check out a website for more information. Websites that accompany mass media campaigns can utilize the full capabilities of the Internet to bring awareness to their purpose, such as webcasts, chat rooms, blogs, and informational videos.

Community-based Health Interventions

The goal of an intervention is to instigate action or bring about some form of change that is beneficial to individuals, families, communities, or all of these groups. Traditionally, **community-based interventions** have focused on engaging with members of the community, organizational representatives (such as local businesses or media outlets), and health experts in all levels of the intervention process. Groups that partner together are able to lend their varied expertise to increase understanding and apply what they know about a given health-related issue. This leads to collective forms of action that will benefit the community and people involved (Israel, Schulz, Parker, & Becker, 1998).

So why would health practitioners choose to do a community-based intervention instead of a mass media campaign? The answer to that depends on the goal. If the goal is to inform a very large group of people about a health risk or persuade many, many people to take some health action, then a campaign to increase awareness or spur self-directed action is ideal. If the goal is to reach a smaller group of people and to work directly with the individuals or groups targeted, then a community-based intervention is probably the way to go. In a community-based intervention, generally only those people in the targeted community or group are exposed to the materials or services that are designed to help them in some measurable or meaningful way. Therefore, an intervention seeks to effect real world change by directly improving the quality of life for the individuals reached, rather than just exposing people to beneficial information and hoping individuals will act on it. In other words, one significant trade-off is that by necessity, community-based interventions tend to be limited in their reach when compared to mass media campaigns, whose reach can be quite broad.

As with mass media campaigns, the Internet has brought community-based health interventions to a new level. There are many different ways the Internet can be utilized to support a community-based intervention. Take, for instance, the hypothetical scenario of

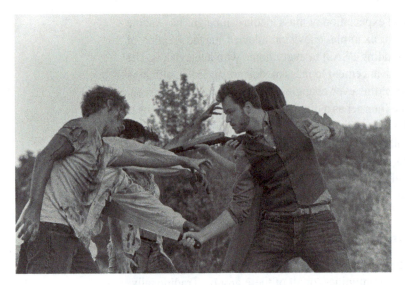

a zombie apocalypse in your community. A state-wide zombie-apocalypse-preparation intervention (led, of course, by the Federal Bureau of Zombie Awareness) may include all of the following community-based components: (a) local self-defense training sessions to teach community members how best to defend against a zombie attack, (b) face-to-face workshops on how a community or neighborhood can build zombie-proof shelters combined with step-by-step directions posted on a website, and (c) coordinated distribution of non-perishable food items to individuals and families who may need to hunker down when a wave of zombies (too large to fight) passes through their community. But the intervention could be supplemented with the following Internet-based components: (a) an online journal to record a history of the struggle in the apocalypse (think *World War Z* the book, not the movie), (b) an Internet chat room to keep track of current zombie locations and offer battle tips, and (c) a website for gardening tips on how to use zombie remains as a non-toxic fertilizer. The purpose of this hypothetical intervention is to encourage members of your community to protect their lives by taking action against zombies; the tools used in the intervention to accomplish these goals are not a cricket bat and a strongly advised double-tap but a combination of direct instruction and training within the community along with critical information distributed via the Internet.

School-based Health Interventions

A **school-based intervention** has many similarities to a community-based intervention with one big exception: As the name suggests, they are conducted in a school or class-room setting (Catalano, Loeber, & McKinney, 1999). So why would you want to conduct research or implement an intervention in a school? Don't the teachers and administrators already have enough to do? Well, yes, they do, and that presents a challenge. However, the primary reason for conducting a health-focused intervention in a school setting is access to the students—who are in essence a captive population (cue the ominous music). There are very few environments or settings that can reliably provide access to that many children or adolescents under one roof where you can be reasonably assured the children will come back day after day (Botvin, 2000). Another reason concerns the educational aspects of many health-based interventions. In a school setting, the environment is already set up for education, and it is not a stretch to include components of a health-related intervention or program in existing classes. Often these interventions or programs can be rolled into existing curricula or can even take the place of existing (and possibly outdated) curricula the school has previously used to meet the same need. Sometimes these interventions meet the requirements of schools that are mandated by local, state, or federal regulations to provide education on certain health-related topics. And often (almost always, really) the intervention or program materials are provided to the schools for free for the duration of the research study, if not longer.

As we just stated, often researchers and practitioners wish to design curricula that can be used by schools to meet the educational requirements for teaching certain health-related components. Implementing and testing the experimental health curriculum in a select group of classrooms or schools provides a real world test of the curriculum before it is rolled out to a larger group or offered for sale to schools for use in their classrooms (Wagner, Tubman, & Gil, 2004). School-based interventions allow researchers to investigate an experimental curriculum because classrooms, schools, and even school districts can be randomly assigned to conditions and compared in experimental designs.

The Internet has also advanced the capabilities of school-based interventions. Indeed, one of the biggest changes that the Internet affords is the ability to connect with students without intervention staff having to walk in the classroom. Twenty years ago if a health organization wanted to improve the health of a group of students with an intervention in classrooms, people would have had to be available to bring materials to the classroom (either getting the messages to the teacher or giving them directly to students). Now, however, the Internet can be used as the middle-man for school-based interventions. For example, a research group may want to conduct an intervention to increase drug awareness in junior high schools. Instead of having a person come to the schools every week to present information, the researchers could create a webcast for all classrooms to view online.

CAMPAIGN AND INTERVENTION STRATEGIES

There are a variety of campaign and intervention strategies that can be used to promote healthy behavior change, such as mass media-, community-, or school-based strategies. All of these strategies can be supplemented with Internet-based support, and sometimes these strategies are entirely Internet based.

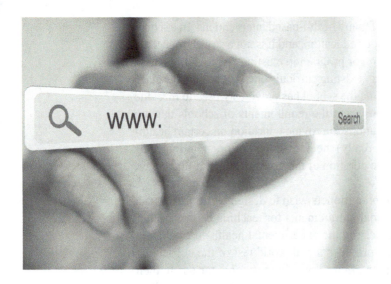

Take a Breath

If we are explaining this right, you should be getting the idea that a long line of research has consistently demonstrated that there is a place for the use of mass media, community-, and school-based approaches to promote health behavior change; that success is more likely under certain circumstances; and that many if not most interventions combine one or more of the approaches in order to meet the needs of the population targeted. Further, a now common strategy is to add an Internet component to otherwise traditional campaigns and interventions, making them what's known as **Internet-inclusive**. In fact, adding an Internet component is becoming so common that mass media campaigns and community- and school-based interventions that do not include an Internet component appear to be more the exception than the norm.

THEORETICAL CONSIDERATIONS FOR ALL CAMPAIGNS AND INTERVENTIONS

While there is considerable overlap in terms of theoretical and methodological considerations across campaigns and interventions, each approach does have its own issues that must be taken into consideration. The best way to guide the decision-making process of selecting a strategy is to draw upon communication theory to inform choices and strategies. Rice and Atkin (2013), Glanz, Rimer, and Viswanath (2008), and Noar and Zimmerman (2005) all do an excellent job of thoroughly covering the most common and useful theories specific to health behavior change interventions and mass media campaigns. In Table 14.2 we present some of the theoretical frameworks and models that these scholars discuss, focusing specifically on the different variables and goal of each framework.

Communication theories can also be used to determine the extent to which **target audiences** have attempted to change their behavior. For instance, the transtheoretical model (Prochaska & Velicer, 1997) is a stage-of-progression model that describes

Table 14.2 Theoretical Frameworks and Models for Campaigns/Interventions

Theory/Model	Citation	Key Variables	Theory/model determines . . .
Activation Model of Information Exposure	Donohew, Palmgreen, & Duncan, 1980	– Need for Sensation – Argument Strength	. . . amount of sensation value required to hold attention to a message.
Elaboration Likelihood Model	Petty & Cacioppo, 1986	– Message-processing Ability – Personal Motivation – Response Efficacy	. . . how people will process messages.
Extended Parallel Process Model	Witte, 1992	– Self-efficacy – Severity – Susceptibility – Benefits to Health – Barriers to Behavior	. . . likelihood of performing a behavior to avoid a health threat.
Health Belief Model	Becker, 1974	– Cues to Action – Severity – Susceptibility	. . . if action will be taken to prevent, screen for, and/or control illness.
Integrative Theory of Behavior Change	Cappella, Fishbein, Hornik, Ahern, & Sayeed, 2001	– Attitude – Behavioral Intention – Environmental Constraints – Personal Skills – Self-efficacy – Social Norms	. . . likelihood of performing a behavior.
Social Cognitive Theory	Bandura, 1997	– Personal Goals – Outcome Expectancy – Self-efficacy	. . . how people learn behaviors from observing others.
Theory of Planned Behavior	Ajzen, 1991	– Attitude – Behavioral Control – Social Norms	. . . intention to perform a behavior.

how to determine where the target audience is in their progress toward behavior change for a specific health behavior. The stages range from precontemplation (not even thinking about a change), to contemplation (starting to think about it), to preparation (getting ready to change), to action (changing), to maintenance (sticking with the change). Determining where most of your audience is helps you figure out what the content of your campaign messages should be. For example, an anti-tobacco campaign designer would want to determine if the target audience even views tobacco use as a problem (precontemplation) or has tried to quit in the past (they've taken action but haven't maintained the change). This knowledge can help campaigners and public health practitioners design their approach to persuade the audience on the basis of their readiness to attempt, adopt, or sustain a recommended behavior. This framework helps us appreciate how target audiences who don't know they have a problem probably won't listen to persuasive messages designed for supporting people who have tried to change their behavior multiple times.

In addition to these theories that describe behavior change, some theories are specific to designing certain types of messages within the campaign or intervention. For example, the extended parallel process model (Witte, 1992) is specific to designing effective fear appeals, and prospect theory (O'Keefe & Jensen, 2007) focuses on how messages are constructed in terms of gains (emphasizing good things that will happen if you follow message advice) or losses (emphasizing bad things that will happen if you don't follow message advice). Collectively, these are just some of the most cited theories that can be used to inform the design of mass media campaigns and health interventions alike.

THE ROLE OF THEORY IN CAMPAIGNS AND INTERVENTIONS

Selecting a health promotion strategy, creating motivational messages, and assessing campaign and intervention effectiveness should all be driven by theory. There are a variety of theories that can be used to guide campaign and intervention research. Some, like the activation model of information exposure or the elaboration likelihood model, focus on how audience members cognitively process persuasive messages. Others, like the health belief model or social cognitive theory, focus on health behavior change processes and the variables that have to be influenced to lead to behavior change.

At this point, we are going to delve deeper into some of the specific methodological and practical considerations for each of these approaches. We'll also take a look at exemplar studies. Let's begin with mass media campaigns.

MASS MEDIA CAMPAIGNS

Special Considerations

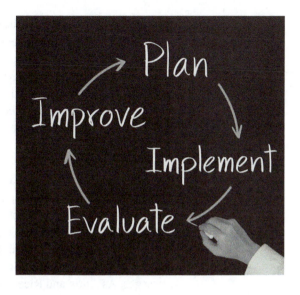

Catalán-Matamoros (2011) offers a useful summary of when to use mass media campaigns for health promotion. He suggests that campaigns are most appropriate when (a) wide exposure is desired, (b) the timeframe is urgent, (c) public discussion is likely to facilitate change, (d) awareness is a main goal, (e) media authorities (e.g., journalists, editors, producers, stations) are on your side, (f) other program components support change, (g) long-term release of information is feasible, (h) a generous budget exists, (i) the behavioral change is simple, and (j) the agenda includes public relations to increase wide-ranging exposure. Additionally, Noar (2006) concluded that health communication campaign success is more likely when campaign designers (a) conduct **formative research**, (b) use theory as a foundation for the campaign, (c) **segment** the audience (i.e., split it up based on relevant characteristics), (d) use a targeted message design focus (i.e., design messages based on the relevant targeting characteristics), (e) place messages in strategic communication channels, (f) conduct a **process evaluation**, and (g) use a sensitive **outcome evaluation** that will generate causal arguments about the campaign's influence on attitudes and behaviors. Noar's suggestions for success can be accomplished through careful design, implementation, and evaluation of mass media campaigns.

Design. Let's explore campaign design. While much of what is discussed here can also apply to interventions, we will use campaigns as our context for illustration. To begin, perhaps the most cited model for considering the development of all the parts of a mass media campaign is **McGuire's communication–persuasion matrix**, or input–output model (see McGuire, 2013). This model provides a framework for what goes into and what comes out of a campaign. You might think of it like a recipe for a campaign, where you get to change the ingredients based on your goals. The input variables are source, message, channel, and audience, terms you have probably heard quite repetitively if you are a communication major! Outcomes of the campaign are the result of two processes: audience exposure to and processing of campaign stimuli. The outcomes of the mass media campaign are described at different levels, including learning, yielding, and actual behavior. Learning is the outcome made up of information gain, new knowledge, and skill development. Yielding is the outcome described by changes or developments in attitudes, values, and beliefs. Behavior is the outcome that is usually of most interest, as it represents whether people in your audience adopted the behavior change recommended in the mass media campaign. As you can see, there are many decisions to be made about all the parts of a campaign.

Implementation. After campaign design comes a transition to implementation. Atkin and Rice (2013) say that campaigners must forward "a coherent set of strategies and implement the campaign by creating informational and persuasive messages that are disseminated via traditional mass media, new technologies, and interpersonal networks" (p. 3). To that end, an audience's exposure and processing (recall McGuire's matrix) depend on the campaign messages and the media placement choices for these messages. As Atkin and Rice summarize, campaign messages might focus on prevention of a harmful behavior or the promotion of a beneficial one. Messages should also promote awareness but ultimately be persuasive and influential.

Further, how the messages are disseminated and to whom they are targeted are of the utmost importance—recall Noar's (2006) conclusion that effective campaigns segment the audience, use a targeted message design focus, and place messages in strategic communication channels. This process of targeting, which we also mentioned earlier in the chapter, refers to directing campaign messages at segments of the population who might benefit from the campaign because of their risk or need for help. For example, messages targeting women's heart health probably should not be broadcast on Spike TV. Campaigners will achieve greater effects when they find means for getting persuasive messages to targeted groups, as opposed to disseminating messages among larger audiences who aren't as likely to be persuaded. The key to this endeavor is determining who needs the campaign and where or when they are likely to pay attention to campaign messages. With advents in technology, campaigns can be improved by finding ways to interact with audience members through the use of social media.

Evaluation. Three types of campaign evaluation happen at different points in time to serve different purposes. Initially, formative evaluation is conducted to inform the design of a campaign before it launches. Atkin and Freimuth (2013) provide an in-depth overview of formative research, which entails preproduction research and message pretesting. Preproduction research involves learning as much as possible about the target audience, including their current cognitions, skills, and behaviors related to the campaign topic. In addition, focus groups, survey research, and ratings data about media exposure can help to determine which forms of media would best reach target audience members.

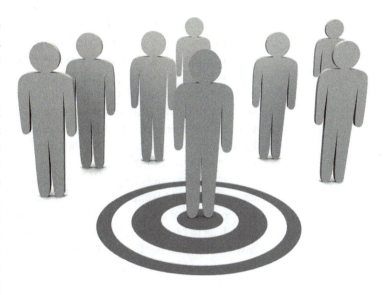

Once messages begin to be constructed and refined, message pretesting can begin. Your goal here is to gauge audience reactions to preliminary versions of messages and to refine the messages before final production. Once the campaign messages are designed and campaign implementation is under way, a process evaluation should be conducted to assess the extent to which the campaign is being implemented as it was designed. Monitoring exposure and attention to campaign messages is useful for determining the success of campaign management and identifying any obstacles to campaign effectiveness.

Last, an outcome evaluation takes place at the end of a mass media campaign to assess the success of the effort. Valente and Kwan (2013) give a detailed overview of the research methods used to determine the effects of the campaign. For the most part, these include cross-sectional or longitudinal field experiments that allow for causal arguments about the relationship between campaign exposure and attitude or behavior change. Some qualitative research is conducted from this perspective, too, such as focus groups and interviews. These forms of inquiry can also provide additional perspectives on the impact of the campaign. Although it may sound like you would do each type of evaluation one after the other, in practice there is quite a bit of overlap between the process and outcome evaluation efforts. To that end, it is incredibly important to have all aspects of the evaluation planned before the start of the campaign.

Mass Media Campaign Exemplar

Now that you have a primer in mass media campaigns, let's explore the development, implementation, and evaluation of one notable traditional exemplar mass media campaign known as the ONDCP *Marijuana Initiative* and the *Two Cities Study*.

Development. The **Office of National Drug Control Policy (ONDCP)** is the federal agency in charge of the efforts dedicated to regulate and control drug abuse in the

United States. In 1998, the ONDCP launched the five-year *National Youth Anti-Drug Media Campaign*, the largest national anti-drug media campaign in U.S. history. The campaign was very well funded (approximately $1 billion dollars!), had very high exposure as measured by gross rating points, and was designed to target at-risk nonusers and occasional users. Also, the campaign messages were produced in several languages to reach multiple audiences. Sadly, the first four years of the campaign were found to be ineffective: Adolescent marijuana use had peaked in 1997 (one year before the campaign began) and remained essentially flat during the campaign's first four years. Why did the campaign not work? Arguably, because the target audience was not appropriately segmented. Therefore, the ONDCP revamped the campaign for the final year and launched the *Marijuana Initiative*, which strategically targeted high sensation seekers. High sensation seekers are known to be at greater risk for drug use, as well as to respond well to messages that are high in sensation value, such as those that elicit strong sensory, emotional, and arousal responses (Palmgreen et al., 1991; Zuckerman, 1990; also see Chapter 9).

Implementation. The *Marijuana Initiative* was directed toward at-risk adolescents 14–16 years old and used several "hard-hitting" ads appearing mostly on television but also on the radio. The messages featured several negative consequences of marijuana use in dramatic and novel fashion (Palmgreen, Lorch, Stephenson, Hoyle, & Donohew, 2007). The *Marijuana Initiative* ads also were seen much more than the ads in the previous *National Youth Anti-Drug Media Campaign*. For example, only one or two television ads with corresponding radio ads were run in a one- to three-month timeframe in the original campaign, but the *Marijuana Initiative* ran four new television ads and corresponding radio ads each quarter (every three months), providing more varied content, which is preferred by high sensation seekers. Considered together, the shorter yet more intensive nature of the *Marijuana Initiative* made it a very different campaign from the original.

Evaluation. Palmgreen et al. (2007) examined the effectiveness of the *Marijuana Initiative* on high sensation seeking youths, comparing youth in Kentucky who would have seen the ads to those in Tennessee who had not seen the ads. The results showed the campaign to be effective. Specifically, it reversed upward developmental trends in 30-day marijuana use among high sensation seeking adolescents and significantly reduced their positive marijuana attitudes and beliefs. Results also indicated that the campaign's dramatic depiction of negative consequences was responsible for its effects on high sensation seeking youths. This research suggested that substance use prevention campaigns using an approach that includes dramatic negative-consequence messages targeted to high sensation seekers can be effective.

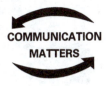

COMMUNICATION
MATTERS

Philip C. Palmgreen, Ph.D., Professor Emeritus, University of Kentucky

My interest in campaigns research grew from a project funded by the National Institute on Drug Abuse (NIDA) that I worked on 25 years ago with Lewis Donohew. The study focused on developing televised anti-drug PSAs that would be more effective in reaching and persuading high sensation seeking youth. High sensation seekers (HSS) are much more likely to engage in risky behaviors such as drug use. Through formative research and two experiments, we found that high sensation value (HSV) messages, which elicit strong sensory, affective and arousal responses, are much more effective with HSS youth.

This led us to a series of campaign studies also funded by NIDA to test the effectiveness of our approach called SENTAR, which stresses the importance of employing HSV messages targeting HSS in campaigns to reduce risky behaviors like drug use. Probably the most influential (and my favorite) of these studies we termed the Two Cities Study. Televised anti-drug campaigns targeting HSS teens were carried out in Lexington, KY (two campaigns) and Knoxville, TN (one campaign) and evaluated using a sophisticated controlled interrupted time-series design. Results revealed that all three 4-month campaigns were successful in reducing teens' 30-day marijuana use for several months after each campaign. At the conclusion of this study, I was a member of a scientific panel charged with overseeing the design and implementation of the Office of National Drug Control Policy's multi-billion dollar anti-drug campaign (1998–present), the largest such federally-funded initiative in history.

The reason I termed the Two-Cities Study "influential" is that its findings persuaded ONDCP to adopt the SENTAR approach as a primary scientific basis for its campaign. It also influenced the design of a number of other prevention efforts including a campaign I was a part of that reduced risky sexual attitudes and behavior of HSS young adults.

COMMUNITY-BASED INTERVENTIONS

Special Considerations

Interventions can be (and often are) conducted as stand-alone activities. More and more often, however, interventions are being used in conjunction with some form of campaign (be it large or small) to inform, persuade, or motivate the intended audience to either participate in the intervention or take advantage of the services offered. Essentially, campaign messages draw attention to the intervention and make

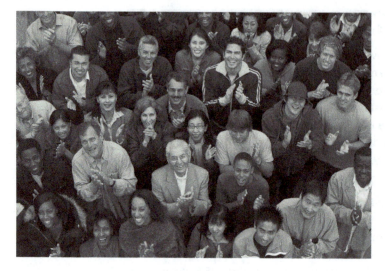

community members aware that the intervention is taking place in their community. Because campaign messages add additional costs to the intervention, they are only used when interventions have adequate funds available. Still, getting the word out somehow is critical: Just because you build it, doesn't mean they'll come.

So what can a community-based intervention do for you that a campaign cannot? Well, as we've been saying all along, a community-based intervention gives health experts an opportunity to work directly with the people of the community. Never underestimate the value and benefits of working one-on-one with someone whom you want to help. Think about it in your own lives: What has had the most effect on you in the past? A commercial or PSA you saw on television? Or your doctor or similar trusted health professional telling you face-to-face that you need to do (or not to do) something? Face-to-face direct intervention will almost always have a greater impact than viewing or listening to a mediated message (all things being equal, of course).

Given this admission, why not ditch campaigns altogether and just have community-based or some other kind of face-to-face intervention? Well, for starters there is cost. Interventions require a lot of staff—staff in the form of paid, volunteered, or donated time. Then there are the materials necessary for the intervention (such as medical supplies or testing equipment). These things cost money, and that can add up. Then there are the facilities needed to conduct the intervention and permission or cooperation from local agencies or organizations to even conduct the intervention in the area, not to mention advertising the intervention even exists (as well as many other issues not mentioned here). While potentially very effective, community-based interventions are by necessity much more difficult (and expensive) to implement.

There are important elements that need to be considered when planning an intervention. Some of these are obvious, such as being aware of exactly who you are trying to help and whether they need the type of help you want to offer (e.g., are these services already available and just not being utilized appropriately?). Some elements require a bit more nuanced consideration, such as making sure whatever type of intervention you plan is appropriate for the culture, ethnic background, geography, and socioeconomic status of the people and area in which they live. How so, you may wonder? Consider the following somewhat hypothetical scenario.

Let's say a group of investigators would like to test an intervention designed to increase physical activity of children in order to reduce obesity and increase health in a very rural, lower socioeconomic status, mountainous area of Appalachia. As part of their overall intervention strategy, they challenge students to exercise in exchange for money for their school. Specifically, every week the students are encouraged to participate in particular exercise activities, such as swimming, riding a bicycle, playing a sport with friends, and walking; each student who performs an activity for six straight weeks will earn their school a set amount of money. This all sounds good, right? Potentially, yes, as long as all the children have access to relatively flat, paved areas on which they can ride bikes, convenient locations that have space and equipment for playing sports, and safe, clean bodies of water or swimming pools that can be accessed. Not all children in Appalachia have access to such facilities or equipment (or even paved roads) that would be necessary to engage in the activities required for this project. For many of the children, attempting the intervention would basically be pointless, potentially frustrating, and could undermine the credibility of the intervention and its promoters.

How could this sort of disaster be prevented? The designers of the study could conduct formative research to identify the barriers to physical activity for children in the area. They could also identify viable physical activities for the area and recommend those instead of ones not readily accessible to children of the area. They also could identify "positive deviants," or people who tend to come up with creative solutions on their own for engaging in physical activity and staying healthy. Knowledge about the barriers could prevent the mistake of setting unachievable participation goals.

Community-Based Intervention Exemplar

Now that you have an idea of some of the peaks and valleys you might encounter when engaging in community-based research, we'll give you a brief look at an exemplar study. Note the integration of both community- and Internet-based approaches in the project, *Web-based Support for Community Tobacco Control Coalitions*.

Development. The *Web-based Support for Community Tobacco Control Coalitions* (Buller et al., 2011) project ran from November 2002 through April 2004 and was

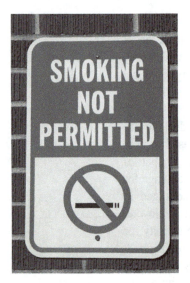

funded by the **National Cancer Institute**. The main purpose of the intervention was to improve public health in Colorado by assisting local coalitions with increasing tobacco control regulations and policies. The research team decided on an Internet-based intervention combined with a community-based approach for two key reasons. First, it would more effectively reach people in rural areas where government budget cuts were affecting public health initiatives, and second, the website would be an easy way to provide participants with lots of different information.

Implementation. The coalition's intervention had a text-based website for control participants and an interactive website for intervention participants. The intervention website was designed to give tobacco control workers access to information and tools that they would need for improving tobacco-control policy in their communities. The interactive features on the website included a calendar; a bulletin board forum, which allowed participants to discuss, share, and interact with each other; and webcasts, which provided educational sessions that participants could watch live or later as an archived recording. The website also provided the latest tobacco control news, gave community profiles of the participating communities, distributed a newsletter, gave tips of the day, and had a learning center that focused on coalition building and intervention strategies. One of the most notable decisions made by the research team was to "market" the website in order to keep participants interacting on the webpage. The marketing strategy included mailing messages to the coalition members (letting them know about the website and its features) and e-mailing participants reminders about the website and its capabilities.

Evaluation. The intervention results found that the communities using the interactive website either maintained or improved their tobacco control efforts, whereas the comparison communities had a reduction in tobacco control efforts (Buller et al., 2011; Young, Montgomery, Nycum, Burns-Martin, & Buller, 2006). These findings demonstrate the overall success of the interactive website with marketing in comparison to the text-based website. Although the program was generally effective, there were some common weaknesses experienced by this and similar Internet-inclusive interventions of the time that shed light on challenges that come with relying on Internet components in community-based intervention approaches. First, despite the purpose of using the Internet to better reach the rural communities, some of the participants reported not knowing how to use the Internet and, therefore, were not used to using it for finding information. Given the geographic dispersal of the coalition participants, this was not a problem the designers were effectively able to overcome. Second, maintaining website participation was a challenge; this was most likely due to intervention fatigue (that is, not remembering to check the website or no longer being interested in checking the website). This weakness was addressed by keeping much of the content fresh on the website (rotating news stories and adding new journal articles) and by encouraging participation with the interactive components offered.

Although the intervention experienced some of these common weaknesses, it also demonstrated many strengths. Specifically, aside from some of the rural communities that struggled with using an Internet-based information source, many rural communities embraced the strategy and took full advantage of the website; therefore, the intervention did improve on the reach of previous campaigns. In addition, the website utilized both interactive (e.g., chatroom) and non-interactive features to appeal to different participants' preferences. For example, participants who did not want to interact in the discussion forum could read journal articles or news stories to receive information.

David Buller, Ph.D., Research Director, Klein Buendel

In addition to being involved in tobacco prevention research, David Buller is involved in sun safety research. This is the story of the genesis of the *Go Sun Smart* program.

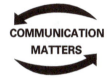

COMMUNICATION MATTERS

In the late 1980s, I was an Assistant Professor of Communication at the University of Arizona. My spouse, Mary, was a program manager at the Arizona Cancer Center, administering clinical trials and community education on skin cancer prevention. Intrigued by her work, we initiated a 25-year research program aimed at developing effective health communication strategies to increase sun safety by children and adults. One of my most compelling studies was on *Go Sun Smart*, a health communication program designed to improve sun safety by outdoor workers. Working with a team of communication and health researchers, Barbara Walkosz, Peter Andersen, Michael Scott, Gary Cutter, and Mark Dignan, we created *Go Sun Smart* based on principles of diffusion of innovations theory, persuasive message research, and feedback from managers and employees. It contained signage, printed materials, articles, a training program, and a website.

Starting in 2000, my research team conducted three community-based studies evaluating *Go Sun Smart* with employees in the North American ski industry. In a first randomized trial, we assigned 13 ski areas to use *Go Sun Smart* and another 13 to be untreated controls. Employees at *Go Sun Smart* ski areas reported fewer sunburns during the ski season and fewer sunburns and more sun protection behaviors in the following summer than those at control ski areas. Next, the National Ski Areas

Association decided to distribute *Go Sun Smart* to its membership of over 300 ski areas throughout North America and allowed us to study this dissemination. In a second randomized trial, we recruited 68 ski areas and assigned half to an enhanced dissemination strategy, using personal contact and printed and online communication to convince managers to use the program, again based on diffusion of innovations theory. The enhanced ski areas used more of the *Go Sun Smart* program than ski areas that just received it from NSAA. Further, employees reported practicing more sun protection at ski areas that used nine or more program messages. In a third study, we returned to these 68 ski areas up to seven years later and discovered that while use of *Go Sun Smart* declined as expected, employees still took more precautions at ski areas with continued high use of *Go Sun Smart*. Currently, we have combined the health communication from *Go Sun Smart* with messages advocating that workplaces adopt formal policies on occupational sun protection. We are testing this enlarged program in a randomized trial with 98 local governments with outdoor workers in public works, public safety, and/or parks and recreation. In the *Go Sun Smart* research, we identified health communication strategies that changed both individual and organizational behavior in ways that improved the safety of workers in a major U.S. recreation industry.

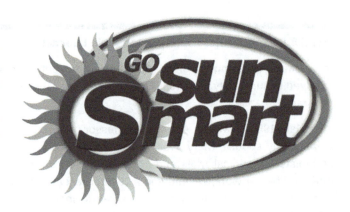

SCHOOL-BASED INTERVENTIONS

Special Considerations

School-based interventions need to take into account many if not all of the theoretical and methodological considerations we've discussed so far for mass media, community, and Internet-based or inclusive approaches. That is, there certainly can be campaign messages that are included as part of a school-based intervention. Schools do exist in community settings. And more and more curricula now include an Internet component. In addition, however, the unique educational setting of the class-room and administrative structure of schools present their own unique set of challenges that must be addressed.

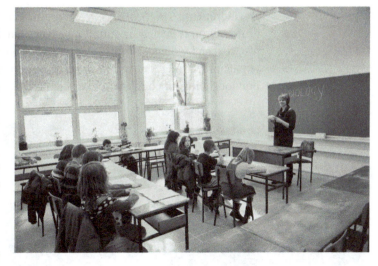

As we previously alluded to, schools already have a lot to do, not a lot of money to do it with, and increasing responsibilities in regard to testing and evaluating student outcomes with already existing curricular requirements. Because of these existing requirements and stresses on the educational system, getting schools to cooperate can be a difficult, if not daunting, task. When schools do agree to cooperate, the intervention will need to operate within the existing structure and schedule of the school (Botvin, 2000). Some-times this means conducting the intervention during class time, but other times it means conducting it after school with students who agree (and whose parents agree) to stay after. Conducting the intervention during class time can be challenging since it requires fitting within whatever time periods the schools use. Many schools use a standard 50-minute window, but some use shorter or longer periods or have unusual meeting patterns. No matter the length or schedule of a class, you need to factor in the time it takes to get the students in their seats, settled down, and focused on the task at hand. If the intervention takes longer than a single class period (and most do), it needs to be broken down into segments that can be delivered over a series of class periods. On top of everything else, schools also have holidays that need to be accounted for and things such as fire safety drills, not to mention that a certain number of kids will always be absent due to illness or other reasons. Any experimental design to evaluate the effectiveness of a school-based intervention will need to be flexible to account for these unavoidable and often random occurrences.

School-based Intervention Exemplar

As before, now that we've discussed the do's and don'ts, as well as the risks and rewards, of conducting health-based interventions in school settings, let's take a brief look at one notable example known as *All Stars*.

Development: *All Stars* is a theory-driven, school-based intervention focused primarily on reducing or curtailing several adolescent risk behaviors—namely drug use, sex, and violence (Harrington, Giles, Hoyle, Feeney, & Yungbluth, 2001). Based on social learning theory, *All Stars* strives to enhance four key mediating variables previously identified in the social scientific literature as having a protective effect on

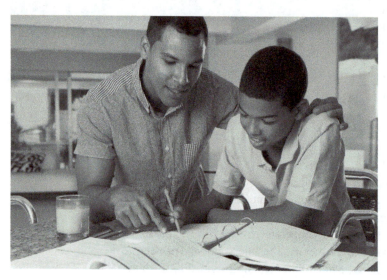

keeping youth from engaging in risky behaviors: (a) help students identify their ideal desired life-style and then influence their perceptions that drug use, sex, and violence can interfere with that lifestyle; (b) increase students' beliefs about peer norms in relation to abstinence from drugs, sex, and violence; (c) have students make a personal commitment to avoid drugs, sex, and violent behavior; and (d) have students develop stronger feelings of attachment and acceptance at their school (Harrington et al., 2001, p. 535). The activities and lessons in the curriculum are designed to create positive normative beliefs about risky behavior, demonstrate how it is incongruent with students' lifestyles, and make students feel like an accepted part of the school community. The curriculum involves a combination of in-class exercises, a series of one-on-one meetings between instructors and students, and a concerted effort to involve parents in the program, primarily through homework assignments.

Implementation: The *All Stars* experimental curriculum consisted of 22 sessions: 14 during class time, four outside of class with small groups of students selected to be assistants or serve as peer leaders, and four outside of class in one-on-one sessions between instructors and students. Apart from the homework assignments to involve parents, the classroom activities include interactive elements such as debates, games, and discussion about the problems with using substances, engaging in sexual activities, or being violent. In the initial study, schools were assigned to one of three conditions: (a) to have the program delivered by specialists from outside the school, (b) to have it delivered by regular classroom teachers, or (c) to receive whatever regular health education classes the school usually used (i.e., the comparison group). Students were surveyed both before and after the program to assess whether the program had any effect on student risky behaviors.

Evaluation. Results from the independent evaluation conducted by Harrington et al. (2001) found that *All Stars* had a modest effect on reducing the onset of student substance abuse. Most interesting was that the results showed that teachers were the most effective persons to deliver the intervention in school. Unlike the outside specialists, teachers were more involved and integrated into the school, and so they probably were better able to influence some of the important mediator variables of the study, namely normative perceptions and student integration (or bonding) with the school community. Results also showed that perception of lifestyle incongruence, making personal and public commitments to not use drugs, and correcting or creating drug-free normative beliefs were three of the most important predictors to program effectiveness and subsequent reductions in student risky behaviors (McNeal, Hansen, Harrington, & Giles, 2004).

William B. Hansen, Ph.D., President, Tanglewood Research

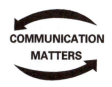

COMMUNICATION
MATTERS

As a graduate student in 1975, I was part of the first federally funded research project on preventing cigarette smoking in adolescents. The project was strictly a research project designed to try to see what impact a variety of approaches might have on deterring the onset of cigarette use among 7th and 8th grade students. At the time, there were no well-formulated theories about how to prevent tobacco, alcohol, or other drug use. Participating on the project proved influential on the direction of my career.

After graduate school, I spent 10 years at UCLA and USC developing and testing various alcohol, tobacco, and drug prevention programs. In all, there were about 40 versions of programs that were tested in randomized control trials, some of which showed promise, others of which did not. However, it wasn't until I moved to North Carolina that the key insight came. I called it "the law of maximum expected effect." Essentially, epidemiologic research I conducted on 6th through 12th grade students allowed me to understand that in order to have a preventive effect on substance use, programs must target mediating variables that had very strong predictive relationships with those outcomes. In the North Carolina study, we tested 12 mediators that prior research had included in school-based programs. Of these, only three showed promise as mediators—normative beliefs, commitment to avoid substance use, and a perception that substance use did not fit with desired lifestyle.

I designed *All Stars* to specifically address these topics. When teachers are able to change these mediators, the program has its intended effects, meaningfully deterring the onset of risky behaviors.

DO RESEARCH RESULTS CONFLICT?

In the history of campaign and intervention research, we find that sometimes our efforts work, sometimes they don't, and sometimes they can actually backfire. One thing is certain, however, and that is that we've learned enough over the years to have solid theory-based principles for campaign and intervention development, implementation, and evaluation. And if we follow those principles, we have a much better chance at success. As we mentioned earlier, we are now in what Noar (2006) calls a **conditional effects era**. This simply means that campaigns and interventions can be effective "on the condition" that we follow the principles of campaign and intervention design.

We also mentioned that campaigns, in particular, tend to have small to medium effects. This means that only a percentage of the target audience is affected by the campaign. However, if your campaign is large enough (e.g., nationwide), small effects can have big impacts, affecting thousands and thousands of people. More intensive community- and school-based campaigns are poised to have larger effects, but the tradeoff typically comes with smaller reach. Knowing precisely what your goals are and whom you want to reach will help guide your decisions in which campaign or intervention strategy to use.

No matter what, researchers and practitioners must always be vigilant for unintended consequences, such as boomerang effects. We're reminded of the story of a teacher who tried to convince his students of the dangers of alcohol by showing them a bottle of tequila "con gusano" (with the worm in the bottle). He wanted to make the point that alcohol can be deadly. He held up the bottle and asked his students, "What do you think this means?" One student replied simply, "If you drink tequila, you won't get worms." Yeah, wrong message. Fortunately, theory and proper formative research will help us avoid a great deal of such trouble—but only if we put our principles into practice.

APPLICATION TO REAL WORLD SETTINGS

A lot of campaigns and interventions that are conducted for the purpose of research start and stop with the research study. That is sad but typical. However, there are some shining examples of campaigns and interventions that have had lasting impact because they have been translated into practice. A great example of translational campaign research is the *Marijuana Initiative* evaluation we discussed earlier. Research on audience targeting and high sensation value message design influenced national policy for substance abuse prevention campaigns. That's a pretty big impact!

More examples of translational research come in the form of school-based interventions. The *All Stars* program we profiled is a clear example. Two other examples of successful school-based interventions are *LifeSkills Training*, a program designed for elementary, middle, and high school students targeting alcohol, tobacco, marijuana, and violence prevention, and *keepin' it R.E.A.L.*, a narrative and performance-based multicultural substance abuse prevention program for students ages 12–14. All three of these programs are used extensively across the nation, and all are listed on the **Substance Abuse and Mental Health Services Administration (SAMHSA)** national registry of evidence-based programs and practices (http://www.nrepp.samhsa.gov).

FUTURE DIRECTIONS OF CAMPAIGNS AND INTERVENTIONS

So, what does the future hold for mass media campaigns and interventions? Research across the field of health communication suggests that interest will continue to grow for understanding the role of technology in health decision making and behavior. The impact of technology on health communication research and practice is tremendous, particularly for campaigns and interventions. As we mentioned earlier, mass media campaigns now can be supplemented by Internet-based components, and community- and school-based interventions no longer have to be confined to a particular physical location—they can be conducted partially (or entirely) in cyberspace. So future research needs to address this technology revolution head-on. Some potential research questions include the following:

1. How can the smartphone be used effectively to deliver interventions previously delivered via desktop computer or web-only?
2. Does the incorporation of specialized social media sites (such as Facebook pages) increase attention to and adoption of health promotion recommendations?
3. Is there an optimal balance between traditional and new media components of a campaign, and what variables may moderate that balance?

In addition, media campaign and intervention research needs to consider the role of interpersonal communication in influencing program effects. Programs are not implemented in a vacuum. How people talk about what they see on television or hear in community- or school-based interventions may have an important impact (van den

Putte, Yzer, Southwell, de Bruijn, & Willemsen, 2011). If we are truly to understand effects, we cannot ignore this fact.

ally assist share
help
Partner
sustain →support
cooperate collaborate
participate

Although we cannot fully predict the future for campaigns and interventions, we are pretty confident that future efforts will continue to come from interdisciplinary or even transdisciplinary teams and the results of these efforts will be expected to be translational in nature. As the **Coalition for Health Communication** (2013) advocates, the notion of transdisciplinary research proposes that by working with those who have different backgrounds and training, we can achieve "a sense of synergy where advocates, social scientists, and hard scientists as well as other stakeholders work in coalition with each other to work on basic and applied research for the public good" (p. 1). Further, campaigners and interventionists will be expected to find ways to translate their research findings to those who work with targeted audiences, to those who make health policy decisions, and to the public at large. Collectively, the future of health communication work promises to involve partnerships between health communication experts, other social and behavioral scientists, health practitioners, community stakeholders, and policy makers. These partnerships should result in robust research that is shared broadly.

CONCLUSION

In the beginning of this chapter, we asked you to think about all of the advertisements and persuasive attempts you are exposed to on a daily basis. At this point, we hope that you see how health communication messages fit into these attempts. Mass media campaigns and community-, school-, or Internet-based interventions are the primary mechanisms to get health-related messages to intended audiences. The exemplars we shared with you throughout the chapter suggest that novel approaches that take into account relevant audience factors lead to the largest changes in attitudes and behaviors. Indeed, health communication practitioners will continue to try to secure the limited attention of an already media-saturated population through increasingly innovative and creative means—so don't expect your friendly neighborhood PSA or community-based health promotion event to go away any time soon. But do expect them to become more exciting (or at least more interesting) as we seek to help guide you toward making better and healthier lifestyle choices. We hope (famous last words)!

DISCUSSION QUESTIONS

1. Campaign researchers are looking to Internet-based technologies as the future of campaigns and interventions. Ten years from now, how do you expect the Internet will be utilized in campaign and intervention projects?

2. Think about your favorite campaign/intervention. After reading this chapter, critically analyze the campaign. What type was it? What features were utilized? What made it your favorite campaign/intervention? How could it have been improved?

3. What health-related issue do you perceive as the most in need of awareness? What type of campaign/intervention style would you use to increase awareness? Why would your strategy be effective?

IN-CLASS ACTIVITIES

1. Campaigns and interventions are all around us. To demonstrate this, have the students list all the campaigns/interventions they know of and document them on the board. Select a few examples and ask students to tell you what they know about them. For example, what was the purpose, what health behavior was targeted, did there appear to be a particular target audience?

2. Split the class into groups of four to six students and assign each group a health behavior. For example, the behaviors could be smoking, exercise, alcohol, bullying, cancer screening, etc. Have each group create a campaign/intervention plan. Their plan should include (a) whether it is a campaign or an intervention, (b) what theory will guide their work, (c) what channels will be used, (d) who the target audience is, and (e) how the Internet could be utilized to enhance the plan.

3. Awareness ribbons are one of the most recognized and well-known campaign strategies. On the textbook's companion website, you will find two files for Chapter 14: *Awareness Ribbons—Questions* and *Awareness Ribbons—Answers*. Have the class try to identify as many of the ribbon colors as possible. Note that some ribbon colors do represent more than one awareness. However, the answers page presents the most well-known awareness for each color.

RECOMMENDED READINGS

Crawford, N. D., Amesty, S., Rivera, A. V., Harripersaud, K., Turner, A., & Fuller, C. M. (2013). Randomized, community-based pharmacy intervention to expand services beyond sale of sterile syringes to injection drug users in pharmacies in New York City. *American Journal of Public Health, 103,* 1579–1582.

This article reports the effectiveness of a community-based intervention designed to reduce racial/ethnic disparities in HIV transmission by involving pharmacies in delivering HIV risk reduction information as part of an existing nonprescription syringe access program for injection drug users.

Porto, M. P. (2007). Fighting AIDS among adolescent women: Effects of a public communication campaign in Brazil. *Journal of Health Communication, 12,* 121–132.

This study reports the results of a nationwide television and radio campaign targeting 13–19-year-old Brazilian women to encourage them to participate in the purchase and use of condoms.

Schneider, M., DeBar, L., Calingo, A., Hall, W., Hindes, K., Sleigh, A., . . . Steckler, A. (2013). The effect of a communications campaign on middle school students' nutrition and physical activity: Results of the HEALTHY Study. *Journal of Health Communication, 18*(6), 649–667.

The HEALTHY Study involved the implementation and evaluation of a three-year school-based intervention that included a communication campaign component; this article investigates and reports on campaign implementation across intervention schools and the relationship between student exposure to campaign materials and behavior change.

REFERENCES

*References marked with an asterisk indicate studies included only in Table 14.2.

*Ajzen, I. (1991). The theory of planned behavior. *Organizational Behavior and Human Decision Processes, 50*(2), 179–211.

Atkin, C. K., & Freimuth, V. (2013). Guidelines for formative evaluation research in campaign design. In R. E. Rice & C. K. Atkin (Eds.), *Public communication campaigns* (4th ed., pp. 53–68). Thousand Oaks: Sage.

Atkin, C. K., & Rice, R. E. (2013). Theory and principles of public communication campaigns. In R. E. Rice & C. K. Atkin (Eds.), *Public communication campaigns* (4th ed., pp. 3–19). Thousand Oaks: Sage.

*Bandura, A. (1997). *Self-efficacy: The exercise of control.* New York: Freeman.

*Becker, M. H. (1974). The health belief model and personal health behavior. *Health Education Monographs, 2*, 324–508.

Botvin, G. (2000). Preventing drug abuse in schools: Social and competence enhancement approaches targeting individual-level etiologic factors. *Addictive Behaviors, 25*(6), 887–897.

Buller, D. B., Young, W. F., Bettinghaus, E. P., Borland, R., Walther, J. B., Helme, D., . . . & Maloy, J. A. (2011). Continued benefits of a technical assistance web site to local tobacco control coalitions during a state budget shortfall. *Journal of Public Health Management & Practice, 17*(2), e10–e19.

*Cappella, J. N., Fishbein, M., Hornik, R., Ahern, R. K., & Sayeed, S. (2001). Using theory to select messages in antidrug media campaigns: Reasoned action and media priming. In R. E. Rice & C. K. Atkin (Eds.), *Public communication campaigns* (3rd ed., pp. 214–230). Thousand Oaks: Sage.

Catalán-Matamoros, D. (2011). The role of mass media communication in public health. In K. Smigorski (Ed.), *Health management: Different approaches and solutions* (pp. 399–414). Rijeka, Croatia: InTech.

Catalano, R. F., Loeber, R., & McKinney, K. C. (1999). *School and community interventions to prevent serious and violent offending* (Juvenile Justice Bulletin). Washington, DC: U.S. Department of Justice.

Coalition for Health Communication. (2013). *Future directions of health communication.* Retrieved from http://www.healthcommunication.net/CHC/research/future.htm

*Donohew, L., Palmgreen, P., & Duncan, J. (1980). An activation model of information exposure. *Communication Monographs, 47*(4), 295–303.

Dutta-Bergman, M. J. (2005). Theory and practice in health communication campaigns: A critical interrogation. *Health Communication, 18*(2), 103–122.

Elliott, B. J. (1987). *Effective mass communication campaigns: A source book of guidelines: Conception, design, development, implementation, control and assessment of mass media social marketing campaigns.* Transportation Research Board of the National Academies: Victoria, Australia.

Glanz, K., Rimer, B., & Viswanath, K. (2008). *Health behavior and health education: Theory, research, and practice.* Jossey-Bass: New York.

Harrington, N. G., Giles, S. M., Hoyle, R. H., Feeney, G. J., & Yungbluth, S. C. (2001). Evaluation of the All Stars character education and problem behavior prevention program: Effects on mediator and outcome variables for middle school students. *Health Education & Behavior, 28*, 533–545.

Hornik, R. C. (2002). *Public health communication: Evidence for behavior change.* Mahwah, NJ: Lawrence Erlbaum Associates.

Israel, B. A., Schulz, A. J., Parker, E. A., & Becker, A. B. (1998). Review of community-based research: Assessing partnership approaches to improve public health. *Annual Review of Public Health, 19*, 173–202.

McGuire, W. J. (2013). McGuire's classic input-output framework for constructing persuasive messages. In R. E. Rice & C. K. Atkin (Eds.), *Public communication campaigns* (4th ed., pp. 133–146). Thousand Oaks: Sage.

McNeal, R. B., Hansen, W. B., Harrington, N. G., & Giles, S. M. (2004). How All Stars works: An examination of program effects on mediating variables. *Health Education & Behavior*, *31*(2), 165–178.

Noar, S. (2006). A 10-year retrospective of research in health mass media campaigns: Where do we go from here? *Journal of Health Communication*, *11*(1), 21–42.

Noar, S. M., & Zimmerman, R. S. (2005). Health behavior theory and cumulative knowledge regarding health behaviors: Are we moving in the right direction? *Health Education Research*, *20*(3), 275–290.

O'Keefe, D. J., & Jensen, J. D. (2007). The relative persuasiveness of gain-framed loss-framed messages for encouraging disease prevention behaviors: A meta-analytic review. *Journal of Health Communication*, *12*(7), 623–644.

Palmgreen, P., Donohew, L., Lorch, E. P., Rogus, M., Helm, D., & Grant, N. (1991). Sensation seeking, message sensation value, and drug use as mediators of PSA effectiveness. *Health Communication*, *3*(4), 217–227.

Palmgreen, P., Lorch, E. P., Stephenson, M. T., Hoyle, R. H., & Donohew, L. (2007). Effects of the office of national drug control policy's marijuana initiative campaign on high-sensation-seeking adolescents. *American Journal of Public Health*, *97*(9), 1644–1649.

*Petty, R. E., & Cacioppo, J. T. (1986). The elaboration likelihood model of persuasion. *Advances in Experimental Social Psychology*, *19*, 123–181.

Prochaska, J. O., & Velicer, W. F. (1997). The transtheoretical model of health behavior. *American Journal of Health Promotion*, *12*(1), 38–48.

Randolph, W., & Viswanath, K. (2004). Lessons learned from public health mass media campaigns: Marketing health in a crowded media world. *Annual Review of Public Health*, *25*, 419–437.

Rice, R. E., & Atkin, C. K. (2013). Theory and principles of public communication campaigns. In R. E. Rice & C. K. Atkin (Eds.), *Public communication campaigns* (4th ed., pp. 3–20). Thousand Oaks: Sage.

Rogers, E. M., & Storey, J. D. (1987). Communication campaigns. In C. R. Berger & S. H. Chaffee (Eds.), *Handbook of communication* (pp. 817–846). Thousand Oaks: Sage.

Valente, T. W., & Kwan, P. P. (2013). Evaluating communication campaigns. In R. E. Rice & C. K. Atkin (Eds.), *Public communication campaigns* (4th ed., pp. 83–98). Thousand Oaks: Sage.

van den Putte, B., Yzer, M., Southwell, B. G., de Bruijn, G-J., & Willemsen, M. C. (2011). Interpersonal communication as an indirect pathway for the effect of antismoking media content on smoking cessation. *Journal of Health Communication*, *16,* 470–485.

Wagner, E. F., Tubman, J. G., & Gil, A. G. (2004). Implementing school-based substance abuse interventions: Methodological dilemmas and recommended solutions. *Addiction*, *99*(2), 106–119.

Wartella, E. A., & Stout, P. A. (2002). The evolution of mass media and health persuasion models. In W. D. Crano & M. Burgoon (Eds.), *Mass media and drug prevention: Classic and contemporary theories and research* (pp. 19–34). Mahwah, NJ: Lawrence Erlbaum.

Witte, K. (1992). Putting the fear back into fear appeals: The extended parallel process model. *Communication Monographs*, *59*(4), 330–349.

Young, W. F., Montgomery, D., Nycum, C., Burns-Martin, L., & Buller, D. B. (2006). Web-based technical assistance and training to promote community tobacco control policy change. *Health Promotion Practice*, *7*(1), 78–85.

Zimmerman, R. S., Palmgreen, P. C., Noar, S. M., Lustria, M. L. A., Lu, H., & Horosewski, M. L. (2007). Effects of a televised two-city safer sex mass media campaign targeting high-sensation-seeking and impulsive-decision-making young adults. *Health Education and Behavior*, *34*, 810–826.

Zuckerman, M. (1990). The psychophysiology of sensation seeking. *Journal of Personality*, *58*, 313–345.

15

Internet and eHealth

Seth M. Noar

The emergence of computer technology, which advanced from personal computers to the Internet to fully functional mobile computers (i.e., smartphones), has brought with it immense opportunities for health communication. Consider the following statistics: 79% of American adults now regularly use the Internet, and 66% of American adults have a broadband Internet connection at home (Pew Internet & American Life Project, 2010a). While the digital divide was an early concern, the gap in home broadband access among racial groups is closing, with 56% of African Americans now having such access compared to 67% of Whites (Pew Internet & American Life Project, 2010a). The number of people using social media sites (e.g., Facebook) doubled between 2008 and 2011, such that 59% of adult Internet users now use social media (Pew Internet & American Life Project, 2011b). Nearly three-fourths of adolescents and young adults use social media sites (Pew Internet & American Life Project, 2010b), with a majority of young people interacting with social media every day or nearly every day (Whiteley et al., 2011).

In addition, computer technologies and Internet access are now widely available "on the go." Eighty-eight percent of Americans own cell phones, with young people tending to get their first cell phone at age 12 or 13 (Pew Internet & American Life Project, 2010c). Three-fourths of adolescents (aged 12–17) have cell phones, and 88% of those adolescents use text messaging, up from 51% in 2006 (a 42% increase). Half of teens using text-messaging send 50 or more text messages per day, and one in three send more than 100 text messages per day (Pew Internet & American Life Project,

2010c). Interestingly, while the use of texting has been increasing over time, the use of other cell phone functions, such as voice calling, email, and instant messaging, has remained stable during that same period of time (Pew Internet & American Life Project, 2010c).

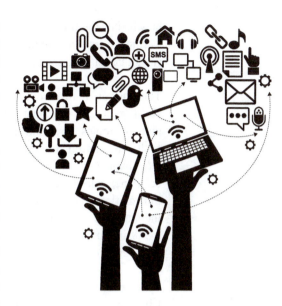

These statistics, which continue to increase over time, attest to the fact that we have seen a communications revolution over the past two decades (Viswanath, 2005). Health communicators would be remiss if we did not consider the host of opportunities that these technologies create for effective health messaging. Indeed, the current chapter will demonstrate that health communicators from a variety of disciplines have been investing much time and effort in this area, and this investment has quickly led to an emerging, interdisciplinary field—the field of eHealth. In fact, the eHealth field is a true example of *transdisciplinarity* (discussed in Chapter 1), where knowledge from multiple discplines comes together to create an innovative, new field. The purpose of this chapter is to discuss (a) what the eHealth field is, what we know from extant research, and how we know it, (b) different types of eHealth applications and some exemplar studies from this field, (c) conflicting results in the field, (d) applications in real world settings, and (e) gaps and future directions for research in eHealth.

WHAT IS eHEALTH?

eHealth has been defined as "the use of emerging information and communication technology, especially the Internet, to improve or enable health and health care" (Eng, 2001, p. 1). Although this emerging, interdisciplinary field is relatively new, it is developing at a rapid pace. Indeed, the evidence base for a whole range of eHealth applications and interventions is quickly growing (Noar & Harrington, 2012c). Before discussing

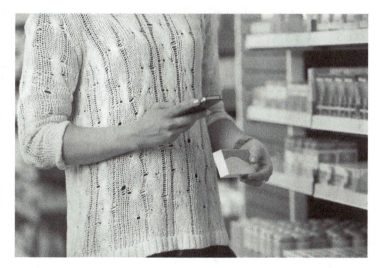

how health communicators are harnessing eHealth, I must first take a step back and ask a critical question: Are people, on their own, using the technologies discussed above in ways that relate to their health?

The answer, it turns out, is a resounding *yes*, and studies on **health information seeking** clearly demonstrate this. Indeed, health information is one of the most popular topics searched for online, with 80% of Internet users having sought such information. In fact, more people use the Internet to seek health information than bank (61%), book travel (65%), or even shop (71%) online (Pew Internet & American Life Project, 2011a). Interestingly, while people trust health information from their doctors much more than information found online, when they have a question, people are much more likely to go to the Internet first (49% in one study) versus going to their doctor (11% in the same study; Hesse et al., 2005).

When people go online, what are they searching for? The Pew Internet & American Life Project (2011a) reports that multiple studies have shown that the most common health-related search topic involves looking for information about a specific disease or medical problem. Thus, it appears that the most common motivation for health information seeking is when a person, friend, or family member is having some type of health issue, and more information and/or a remedy is sought. The next most common search topic is information about medical treatments or procedures. It is perhaps not surprising that such searching is common, as needed medical treatments can bring with them a great deal of uncertainty (see Chapters 2 and 7), and information about a treatment may serve to reduce that uncertainty. Still other relatively common searches are for information about particular doctors or health professionals, hospitals or other medical facilities, and public or private health insurance programs.

The kinds of data above have led experts in the eHealth field to make the following declaration: "The question now is not whether the public is ready for eHealth information, but whether eHealth information is ready to meet the public's expectations" (Goldberg et al., 2011, p. S187). Not only that, but because studies show that simply having particular health knowledge often does *not* lead to healthy lifestyles or health behavior change (Cook & Bellis, 2001), the focus of many health fields, including eHealth, is on strategies (e.g., changing beliefs, engendering skills) that effectively help people to modify their behaviors to promote health or manage/treat disease (Noar & Harrington, 2012b). Thus, I next discuss applications and interventions that can help people improve their health and manage chronic conditions.

THE NEW FIELD OF eHEALTH

This chapter introduces what can really be seen as a new field—the field of eHealth. The eHealth field is *transdisciplinary*. That is, knowledge from multiple disciplines has come together to create an innovative field that did not exist before. Think about how an almost endless number of disciplines can and do contribute to eHealth—computer science, medicine, communication, journalism, public health, business, advertising, marketing, psychology, sociology, nursing, and so forth. The bringing together of these various perspectives and expertise into a cohesive, new field is what makes eHealth a transdisciplinary field.

Before I discuss these applications, though, I raise a question: Why have we invested so many resources in this area already, and why is there so much excitement about eHealth? The answer is the following: Creating health communication programs that are both efficacious (that work) *and* that reach large proportions of the intended audience has been elusive. In fact, communication researchers have long noted that while interpersonal communication approaches are the most persuasive (but have the lowest reach), mass communication approaches achieve the greatest reach (but have lower

Lynn Miller, Ph.D., Professor, University of Southern California and John Christensen, Ph.D., Assistant Professor, University of Connecticut

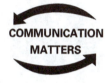

COMMUNICATION MATTERS

Everyday, people get "carried away" by the situation and their emotions, and before they know it, or understand what's happening, they do something they later regret. Interventions to enable individuals to have better emotional self-regulation in such situations were nearly impossible before eHealth. eHealth affords "just in time" interventions that interrupt risky choices when people are actually making them. Our approach, SOLVE (Socially Optimized Learning in Virtual Environments), uses virtual environments/games to recreate scenarios/choices in people's lives. Users' virtual choices actually predict their real-life choices. *If* users make virtually risky choices, these are interrupted with messages designed to change behavior. The goal is to make the risky choices less automatic, addressing the affective and motivational issues that led to those unhealthy decisions. In our latest game, agents are "intelligent": A given agent's goals/beliefs affect agent reactions. Imagine interacting with different virtual romantic partners and seeing how things unfold differently! We also record users' brain patterns while playing games to examine if our "model" of the user's psychology predicts user's brain patterns and behavior. It's exciting and tremendously rewarding to develop and do research on these eHealth interventions and to know we've kept some people from contracting diseases, like HIV.

efficacy; Rimal & Adkins, 2003). eHealth technologies have the potential to achieve both high **efficacy** and high **reach**, which to date has been unprecedented in the history of the health communication field.

For instance, eHealth applications can be persuasive, most notably through the use of interactive features (Cassell, Jackson, & Cheuvront, 1998). Indeed, while interactive interventions were previously the sole territory of the interpersonal domain, computer technologies introduce the opportunity for **interactivity** in the absence of human interaction. Websites, mobile phones, and social media all offer numerous opportunities for interactivity. While scholars debate the exact definition and nature of interactivity (Bucy & Tao, 2007), one useful definition is provided by Kiousis (2002):

> Interactivity can be defined as the degree to which a communication technology can create a mediated environment in which participants can communicate (one-to-one, one-to-many, and many-to-many), both synchronously and asynchronously, and participate in reciprocal message exchanges ... it additionally refers to their ability to perceive the experience as a simulation of interpersonal communication. (p. 372)

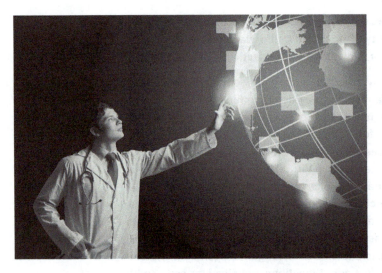

This definition makes clear that interactivity takes place using communication technology, it involves an exchange of messages and/or information, and it mimics the experience of interpersonal communication. In addition, there is both theoretical (Cassell et al., 1998) and empirical (Hawkins et al., 2010) literature to suggest that interactivity plays a significant role in eHealth efficacy and health behavior change. While many studies focus on *medium interactivity*, or cases where we interact with a computer (e.g., interactive website, health video game, health app; Hawkins et al., 2010), studies also offer support for the efficacy of *human interactivity* (Tate, Jackvony, & Wing, 2006), where we interact with other people through media (e.g., chat room, social media, text messaging). Combining the interactive properties of eHealth applications with the global reach of the Internet as a delivery system makes for a potent set of tools for health communication.

Beyond these two powerful features of eHealth applications (interactivity and Internet as delivery system), such applications offer additional advantages (Noar & Harrington, 2012b). These are summarized in Table 15.1. As we can see, eHealth applications offer a number of attractive features. For example, while face-to-face counselors may be expensive, only available at particular times, and may (verbally or nonverbally) judge a patient, eHealth applications can be low cost, available on demand 24/7, and used in an anonymous and non-judgmental fashion. Similarly, while printed health education materials tend to be generic, unappealing, and offer only one-way communication, eHealth applications can be tailored to the individual, use multimedia, games, and other appealing features, and offer two-way communication. Different applications will offer different sets of advantages, of course, and each is discussed more below.

Table 15.1 Advantages of eHealth Applications

Characteristic	*Description*
Anonymity	Programs can be used in an anonymous fashion, which may lead to increased reporting of sensitive behaviors and increased engagement with health communication programs
Automated data collection	Collection of data is built into the program and takes place effortlessly
Appeal	Particular applications (e.g., video games) hold appeal among certain audiences (e.g., youth), which may increase engagement in programs
Convenience/support on demand	Users can interact with programs whenever the need exists
Flexibility/modifiability	Ability to change and adapt the program; relative ease of updating the program, particularly with those programs that are online
Increased access to information	Particularly with online programs, opportunity for the user to access vast amounts of health information
Interactivity	Technological attributes of mediated environments that enable reciprocal communication or information exchange
Internet-driven delivery system	Use of the Internet as an intervention delivery system allows for broad access via desktop, laptop, tablet computers, and mobile devices
Low cost	Ability to use standalone programs or programs as adjuncts to other kinds of health efforts (e.g., interpersonal, mass media) can reduce costs; cost to deliver likely to be low once development is complete

(Continued)

Table 15.1 Continued

Characteristic	Description
Multimedia platform	Ability to use multiple forms of media, such as still images, video graphics, and sound files
Networkability	Programs online can be networked and can allow for connections with others, including other users, health educators, etc.
Simulated environment	Opportunity to role-play risky situations in a simulated environment without the possibility of harm
Tailoring potential	Ability of the program to customize content to the individual, based on an assessment of the individual

Table 15.2 lists several types of eHealth applications, along with descriptions, key advantages, applications available, effects to date, and some cautions. It is important to note that the eHealth field tends to take a scientific paradigmatic perspective. There has been little work in this field from an interpretive or critical–cultural perspective. In fact, eHealth applications are typically tested using quantitative research, most notably randomized controlled trials (RCTs). From a scientific paradigmatic perspective, this is a strength of this literature, as RCTs are viewed as the gold standard research design for demonstrating causal effects (Flay et al., 2005). Qualitative research may be used in the development of eHealth applications (Skinner, Maley, & Norman, 2006). However, such research is still typically conceptualized within the context of a scientific (rather than interpretive or critical––cultural) paradigm. Thus, the exemplar studies described later in this chapter will all be scientific paradigm studies—and mostly RCTs.

---

eHEALTH APPLICATION ATTRIBUTES

Rather than thinking about eHealth as a set of different technologies, it may be more useful to think of it as a concept with a number of different applications, each of which has its own attributes (with some overlapping across applications and some unique to particular applications). Some of the major attributes are listed in Tables 15.1 and 15.2. Instead of arbitrarily picking an application type and then developing a particular eHealth application, it is more fruitful for a developer to think about what attributes he or she wants, select the application type with those attributes, and develop the particular eHealth application.

Another strength of this literature is that it is multidisciplinary, interdisciplinary, and even transdisciplinary in nature. That is, researchers developing and testing

Table 15.2 Overview of Several Types of eHealth Applications

Type	Description	Key Advantages	Applications	Effects	Cautions
Computer and Internet-based Interventions	Interactive programs designed to impact health; can make use of a great variety of features and thus can vary from one another in several ways	Interactivity and multimedia; individualized content; automated intervention	Numerous applications exist across most health domains	Several meta-analyses demonstrate significant effects of these programs on health behavior	Successful programs can be developed, but will people use them? How do we motivate people to maintain use of these programs over time?
Mobile Program (text messaging)	Programs and services designed to promote health using text-messaging as the sole or primary mode of communication	Reach individuals on the go with messages sent at opportune times; unique features such as location-based services; convenient for participants	Applications are rapidly growing, especially in areas such as smoking cessation, physical activity, and disease management	Evidence is building that text messaging may be an effective channel for behavior change and disease management, but more research is needed	Will people tolerate a variety of health texts on their phones? Will texting still be widely used with the proliferation of smartphones?
Mobile Program (apps)	Interactive programs designed for smartphones	Reach individuals on the go; use location-based services; convenient for participants; app stores provide easy dissemination of programs	While many health apps exist, most do not appear to be evidence based or to have been evaluated	Little is known about the effects of health apps; much more research is needed	How do consumers choose between apps with such varying quality and evidence behind them?

(Continued)

Table 15.2 Continued

Type	Description	Key Advantages	Applications	Effects	Cautions
Health Video Games	Games designed to improve health status	Fun to play; may be especially motivating for children and adolescents; exergames turn screen time into actual physical activity	A number of applications exist, with more being developed over time	Studies show that games can change behavior and help people manage disease, but more research is needed	Do these games simply encourage young people to engage in more screen time?
Social Media	Interventions and campaigns that use social media as a sole or primary communication channel	Youth increasingly spend time on social media sites; takes advantage of social networks; increases possibility of messages "going viral"; social media sites contain a wide variety of features	Applications are just beginning to appear	The first studies evaluating social media to promote healthy behaviors have now appeared; while promising, much more research is needed	Is social media a long lasting technology or a passing fad? Will people engage in social media for health?

eHealth applications have come from several disciplines, including communication, journalism, psychology, informatics, computer science, public health, and medicine, and at times researchers from several disciplines collaborate together on such applications. Moreover, as you will see, to date eHealth has been applied to numerous health and disease areas, including in major areas such as cancer, diabetes, obesity, and HIV/AIDS. I now discuss each of the major types of eHealth applications.

MAJOR TYPES OF eHEALTH APPLICATIONS

Computer and Internet-based Interventions

Health communicators have long been interested in using computers for health promotion, and there are many early examples of such applications (Conlon, 1997; Paperny, 1997). While early applications ran on CD-ROMs or locally on computers, today most programs are delivered over the Internet. **Internet-based interventions** can be described as "primarily self-guided, interactive Web-based programs, created with the goals of assisting users to make behavior changes that will prevent disease, monitor health status, and/or improve response to clinical treatment" (Buller & Floyd, 2012, p. 59). Such programs help people quit smoking, lose weight, increase physical activity, reduce alcohol use, and use condoms more often, among many other health areas.

One major strand of studies in this area is **computer-tailored interventions**, which are interventions that assess personal characteristics and provide tailored feedback and experiences to the user. For example, a program might assess a smoker's name, type of cigarettes they smoke, their readiness to quit smoking, and what motivates them to quit, and then provide tailored messages based on their answers. Tailored messages and programs are rated by users as more relevant to them than more generic messages/programs (Skinner, Campbell, Rimer, Curry, & Prochaska, 1999), which may account for their greater efficacy (Noar & Harrington, 2012a). Traditionally, these kinds of programs created tailored print materials (e.g., reports, newsletters) for the user, though increasingly such programs are delivered on the Internet.

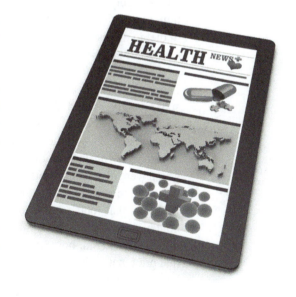

Given that computer and Internet-based interventions were one of the earliest areas of study in eHealth, there is a large literature on these interventions. Overall, the wealth of studies suggests that computer and Internet-based interventions can be effective in promoting a variety of health behaviors, including healthy diet, mammography screening, smoking cessation, safer sex, and alcohol reduction (Noar, Harrington, Van Stee, & Aldrich, 2011). This does not by any means suggest that all such programs work, nor do we currently have a "recipe" for what makes a perfect Internet-based intervention. Instead, the literature suggests that particular characteristics may improve the efficacy of such programs. These characteristics include using theory as a basis for an intervention, using messages tailored to the individual, engaging people with interactive features, and interacting with people for multiple sessions over time (Noar, Harrington, & Aldrich, 2009).

Tailoring exemplar. As computer-based interventions have been in existence for longer than most other eHealth programs, the exemplar that I discuss is one of the "classics." This particular study aimed to improve dietary behaviors in 558 adult patients recruited from primary care settings (Campbell et al., 1994). Participants were randomized to one of three conditions. The first group received a nutrition information newsletter tailored on stage of readiness to change dietary behaviors, dietary intake, and psychosocial variables based upon the health belief model (e.g., people's beliefs that their diet may or may not put them at risk for particular diseases; people's perceived barriers to changing their dietary behavior). Their tailored newsletter consisted of a profile of their current dietary behaviors and their level of interest in changing, tailored pages on both fat intake and fruit and vegetable intake, and tailored recipes and specific diet tips. The second group received a nontailored nutrition information newsletter consisting of standard risk information on the relationship of diet to disease. The third group was a no-treatment control group; they received no newsletter and simply completed the assessments.

Participants were assessed using a survey, and those in groups 1 and 2 were subsequently mailed the tailored (or nontailored) print materials. At four-month follow-up, 73% of the tailored group recalled receiving the nutritional information, whereas only 33% of the nontailored and 15% of the control group recalled receiving information (no information was sent to the control group). Those in the tailored group were also significantly more likely than the other groups to have read all of the information that was sent. Most important were the behavioral results: Findings indicated that total fat intake decreased by 23% in the tailored group, 11% in the nontailored group, and 3% in the control group. No differences on fruit and vegetable intake were found, however. Overall, this was one of the first studies to demonstrate that print materials that used messages tailored to an individual's unique beliefs could be effective in changing their dietary behaviors.

Mobile Programs

While representing a newer literature, studies using mobile devices for health promotion and disease management are rapidly appearing. **Text messaging** is particularly compelling given the huge saturation of mobile phones in society, as well as the fact that since we have our mobile phones with us most or all of the time, messages can be sent at opportune times (e.g., when it's time to go to the gym; when a smoker has a craving for a cigarette). According to Fjeldsoe, Miller, and Marshall (2012), text messaging is being applied to health in four ways: (a) to enhance the use of health services, (b) to mass distribute health messages, (c) for management of chronic disease, and (d) to deliver personalized health promotion messages. Texting can be used by itself or in conjunction with other intervention modalities such as Internet websites or provider advice.

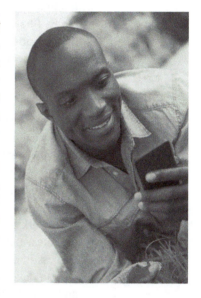

While evaluations of text-messaging programs have shown promise, recently two studies synthesized the effects of the first generation of text-messaging health programs (Free et al., 2013; Head, Noar, Iannarino, & Harrington, 2013). Both of these studies concluded that text messaging appears to be an effective communication channel for health behavior change. Those areas in which effects were strongest were smoking cessation, physical activity, and HIV/AIDS medication adherence. One of the studies also examined what features of text-messaging programs may make them most effective (Head et al., 2013). This study found that texting programs were most successful when they included tailoring of messages to the individual and when they *varied* the schedule of when participants received messages (instead of following a *fixed* message schedule). This same study found that programs that relied on text-messaging alone were just as successful as those that used text-messaging plus other components, such as an Internet website. While this literature is still relatively new and growing, the evidence to date shows much promise for text-messaging interventions for health.

Health apps, or software programs that are available on phones such as iPhone and Android, are also used for mobile health promotion. To date, however, health apps have rarely been rigorously evaluated (Abroms, Padmanabhan, & Evans, 2012). This is the case because while the population is rapidly adopting smartphones, these phones have not been in existence for that long. Some existing research has examined what health apps exist out there in the marketplace, such as in Apple's app store. Unfortunately, this research shows that existing apps—in areas such as smoking cessation and weight loss—typically do not adhere to best practices in these areas, and many if not most

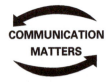

Steven M. Giles, Ph.D., Associate Professor, Department of Communication, Wake Forest University

As happens with many 40-something year old men, my waistline grew slowly but not imperceptibly through adulthood. I considered myself "healthy" so long as I remained active playing sports, or a little less portly than high school friends on Facebook. That changed when my wife asked me to partner with her in using MyFitnessPal, a free app that essentially assists users with counting calories and setting weight loss goals. I was initially resistant; I thought I could just "eat better" and lose weight. Upon using the app, however, I quickly realized how mindlessly I would eat foods with high caloric content and little nutritional value. Not only did my eating habits change as a result of using MyFitnessPal but I also took advantage of the app's ability to integrate with other health apps, like Striiv, which counts steps and adjusts calories. Seven months and 32 pounds *lighter*, I am now close to my college weight! More importantly, I have greater energy, less hunger, and fewer cravings as a result of eating better foods. Weight loss is not easy, but it is not complicated. I am definitely a fan of eHealth tools that simplify the dieting process and promote lifestyle change!

have *not* been evaluated for efficacy (Abroms et al., 2012). Thus, it is likely that many of the health apps available today are simply ineffective at helping people change their behavior—whether it be quitting smoking, losing weight, or some other health behavior.

In the coming years, there is little doubt that we will see many evidence-based health apps both developed and evaluated, and we will have a much better indication as to what works. It is also worth noting that apps share many similar features with Internet websites, and indeed some apps may run directly on mobile websites. Thus, given the success in developing effective Internet-based interventions, it stands to reason that we can develop efficacious health apps. Only time will tell what these will look like and how effective they will be, however.

Mobile exemplar. Perhaps the most rigorously evaluated mobile health program to date is the txt2stop text-messaging smoking cessation program (Free et al., 2011). While earlier studies suggested that text-messaging might be efficacious in helping people quit smoking, a rigorous long-term study had yet to be undertaken. Txt2stop is a smoking cessation program that encourages all participants to set a quit date within two weeks of beginning the program. In the study, five text messages were sent per day for the first five weeks and then three messages per day for the next 26 weeks. Messages were motivational in nature (e.g., This is it! You can do it!) and also focused on behavior change techniques that can be helpful to smokers trying to quit (e.g., using distractions for cravings, handling stressful situations). The messages also promoted a smoking cessation telephone helpline and nicotine replacement therapy. Tailoring was used in this intervention—messages used demographic and other information to tailor some messages sent to participants (e.g., smokers concerned about weight gain after quitting received special messages on this topic). Further, participants could text words like "crave" or "lapse" to get on-demand messages addressing what to do about cravings and quit lapses, respectively.

This study randomized smokers to either the txt2stop group ($n = 2,915$) or to a control group ($n = 2,885$) and followed all participants for a six-month period of time. Control group participants received generic text messages that thanked them for being in the study and encouraged them to stay in the study. The six-month follow-up timepoint included biochemical validation of quitting smoking, something that makes the study especially rigorous (most studies simply use self-reported quitting smoking). At six months, results indicated that the txt2stop group had double the smoking cessation rate of the control group—approximately 10% and 5% quit rates, respectively. These results clearly indicated that the program was successful in helping people quit smoking.

Health Video Games

A game is "a rule-based activity that involves challenge to reach a goal that provides feedback on progress made toward that goal" (Lieberman, 2012, p. 110). Health video games, or games designed with an explicit health focus, also are characterized by the three components in this definition—rules, goals, and feedback. Thus, such a **health game** will have goals that the person is trying to reach, rules about how he or she can reach those goals, and feedback along the way regarding how he or she is doing.

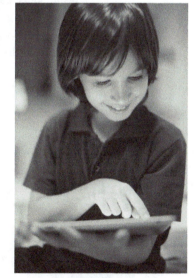

While many games are simply designed for the sole purpose of being fun, some games are designed with a specific purpose, such as for health, education, or training. Such games are sometimes referred to as *instructional* or *serious games* (Garris, Ahlers, & Driskell, 2002). In my view, this latter term (serious games) is not the best term to use because games with a purpose (e.g., health) are also supposed to be fun. Indeed, one of the most compelling attributes of games is that they *are* fun, and thus a person may be intrinsically motivated to play the game for that reason (Baranowski, Buday, Thompson, & Baranowski, 2008). Unlike Internet-based interventions, which research suggests people sometimes lose interest in over time, games may have better longevity and sustainability because of the ability to foster intrinsic motivation to play them.

Effective health games have been designed and evaluated in several different areas, including healthy diet, physical activity, asthma management, and cancer remission. In addition, game evaluations have demonstrated that in many cases, playing has led to improvements in health knowledge, attitudes, and even behaviors (Baranowski et al., 2011; Lieberman, 2012). While many games have been effective, additional research is needed to understand how generalizable these effects really are. The literature to date is promising, however, and the field is rich with new games being developed and evaluated all the time.

In addition to video games, another class of health games is exergames (also known as active games), or games in which people exert energy while playing (e.g., Wii fit, Xbox Kinect). This is a compelling area as it attempts to turn a typically sedentary activity—video games—into one that directly results in physical activity. Studies have shown that playing such games does indeed result in people expending energy in the form of light to moderate exercise (Peng, Lin, & Crouse, 2011), and playing these games can have mental health benefits, as well (Lieberman, 2012). While research on exergames to date is promising, more research is needed on game engagement and game effects.

Health video game exemplar. A recent study evaluated the impact of playing two health video games on the dietary and exercise behaviors of children (Baranowski et al., 2011). The games, called *Escape from Diab* and *Nanoswarm: Invasion from Inner Space*, were video games specifically designed to improve diet and exercise behaviors among children aged 10–12 years old. These games had appealing storylines that had

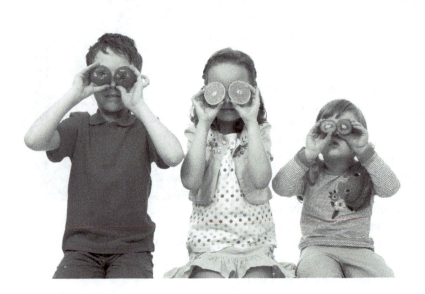

been tested with children, and they built in several theory-based strategies, such as goal-setting, problem solving, and mastery of material about nutrition and physical activity. The games also helped children to think about exactly how they would eat healthier and exercise more, with a video "menu" tailored to their particular eating and physical activity behaviors.

The study randomized 10–12-year-old children to either play nine sessions of each game ($n = 103$) or to a control group that played already existing web-based diet and physical activity games ($n = 50$). All children were assessed on fruit and vegetable intake, water intake, amount of moderate to vigorous physical activity, and body composition (e.g., weight) two months after the intervention ended. Results indicated that the intervention group significantly increased their fruit and vegetable intake, although no changes in water intake, physical activity, or body composition were observed. The study demonstrates that a carefully designed game can increase healthy eating behaviors among children.

EVIDENCE-BASED APPLICATIONS

Just because we develop an eHealth application does not mean that it will be successful in reaching its stated goal, whether that goal is weight loss, smoking cessation, or something else. This is why we rigorously test eHealth applications to understand precisely what the effects are. Those that are found to work are referred to as *evidence-based* programs. Once this evidence is demonstrated, efforts can be made to disseminate the program to as wide an audience as possible. A good example of this is the txt2stop program described in this chapter. In the absence of research showing that an application is effective, it cannot be considered an evidence-based program, and it should not be widely disseminated as it may not work, or even worse, it may do harm.

Social Media

While social media sites such as Facebook (founded in 2004) and Twitter (founded in 2006) have been in existence for only a decade or less, they are widely used today. They thus represent a very promising communication platform for health applications (Neiger et al., 2012; Taubenheim et al., 2012). Already, those interested in **social media for health** have written about the ways in which it could be used in this domain. According to Neiger et al. (2012), social media can be used in five ways: (a) to "listen" to consumers and learn about how they think about a particular health issue, (b) to establish and promote a brand, (c) to disseminate information to the public, (d) to expand the reach of a particular health communication initiative or campaign, and (e) to foster public engagement and partnerships. These functions can serve to impact several key outcomes of health communication efforts, such as increasing reach of a campaign, increasing frequency of exposure to health messages, and fostering engagement with a campaign's materials and messages.

Several studies have used social media as a part of multi-channel health communication campaigns, including high profile national campaigns such as the *Heart Truth* heart disease prevention campaign (Taubenheim et al., 2008) and the *VERB* physical activity (Huhman, 2008) campaign. Moreover, studies have now begun to test social media as a primary mode of delivering health behavior change interventions in areas such as safer sex (Bull, Levine, Black, Schmiege, & Santelli, 2012) and weight loss (Cavallo et al., 2012). All of these studies demonstrate the feasibility of using social media for health, and they show us *how* social media features can be applied to health. However, given the small amount of research in this area to date, we cannot yet make firm conclusions about the potential of social media to have a real impact on health behavior or health status.

Social media exemplar. One major study that has recently been completed in this area is the *Just/Us* study (Bull et al., 2012). The major goal of this study was to engage youth of color in sexual health education via Facebook. In particular, the study sought to evaluate whether an HIV prevention intervention delivered on Facebook can increase safer sexual behaviors relative to a news and current events control condition (also a Facebook page).

Participants were randomized to receive either HIV prevention education or the news and current events page. The intervention included HIV risk information, blogs where participants could post messages, videos to view online, and other topical information on safer sex and HIV. More than 1,500 (primarily African American and Latino) young adults were recruited into the study using various methods, including network methods where the participants themselves were asked to help recruit additional study participants. An original participant, referred to as the "seed," was randomized to a group, and all other participants referred by that "seed" were placed in the same study group (to avoid contamination across study conditions). All participants filled out a baseline assessment, as well as two follow-up assessments at two-month and six-month intervals. Results indicated that condom use significantly increased at the two-month assessment point in the intervention group (as compared to control). At the six-month assessment, however, the effect was not present, as both groups had approximately the same level of condom use. This is one of the very first studies to demonstrate that a Facebook-delivered intervention can be effective at changing sexual health behaviors.

DO RESEARCH RESULTS CONFLICT?

Given the fact that the eHealth field is in many ways fairly new, to date there are not an overwhelming number of conflicting findings. Rather, as illuminated above, what is needed is much more research in a variety of areas, particularly with newer technologies. The biggest conflicts in this field are perhaps over how to define and measure particular constructs. Indeed, even the term eHealth itself has been defined in a myriad ways, with one systematic review uncovering 51 unique definitions of the term (Oh, Rizo, Enkin, & Jadad, 2005).

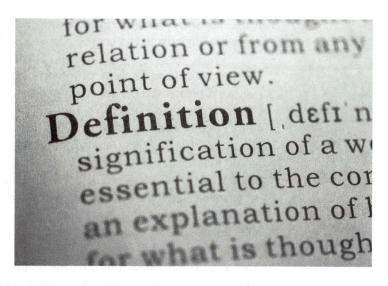

Researchers interested in concepts such as interactivity and presence (Hawkins et al., 2010), Internet-based interventions (Strecher, 2007), and other areas of eHealth must come to grips with the variety of terminology used in these areas. There is, in fact, a pressing need to standardize more of the terminology in eHealth. Some recent efforts have been undertaken thus far, such as efforts to standardize eHealth terminology (Hawkins, Kreuter, Resnicow, Fishbein, & Dijkstra, 2008; Kiousis, 2002) and reporting guidelines for published research (Baker et al., 2010; Harrington & Noar, 2012b). Still, we have a long way to go before we get to a place where folks are using terms such as interactivity, presence, customization, personalization, and many other terms in the same way. While this kind of definitional struggle is common to many fields (Abraham & Michie, 2008; Noar & Zimmerman, 2005), the fact that eHealth is so interdisciplinary makes the challenge even more daunting.

APPLICATION TO REAL WORLD SETTINGS

In some ways, there is a bit of a disconnect in the eHealth field. On the one hand, new technologies are here, and health organizations are using them in a myriad ways. On the other hand, we do not know if many of these technologies are effective, as the research to evaluate such technologies takes time. As one example of this, *LiveStrong* recently released a smoking cessation app for iPhone, called *MyQuit Coach*. While the app is based on evidence-based practices in smoking cessation (e.g., creating a personalized quit plan, gaining

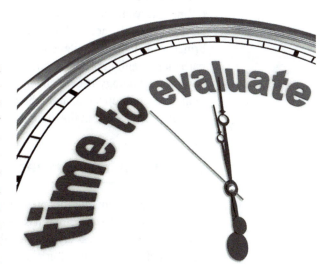

social support), it does not appear that any research yet exists evaluating whether this app is actually effective in helping people quit smoking.

This is simply one example of many where these technologies are being applied in the real world before we have data on whether they are effective or not. In another area, HIV/STD prevention, studies have broadly documented organizational use of websites (Noar, Clark, Cole, & Lustria, 2006), text-messaging programs (Lim, Hocking, Hellard, & Aitken, 2008), and social media (Gold et al., 2011) to promote sexual health. In many if not most cases, these programs have not been evaluated for their efficacy. Since so many people are online and using these technologies, however, organizations likely feel the need to pursue the use of such technologies. Current and future research can and should inform the most effective ways in which these technologies can be used for health promotion and disease prevention.

Another important area is dissemination and implementation research. In order for eHealth applications to have a real impact, they must be disseminated into the real world. Historically, researchers have been very good at developing efficacious interventions, but they have *not* done a very good job at ensuring that those interventions are disseminated into practice (Glasgow, Lichtenstein, & Marcus, 2003). An emerging field, **dissemination and implementation science**, focuses on how we can better translate interventions that work into practice (Rabin & Glasgow, 2012).

In eHealth, researchers are beginning to undertake studies to understand how eHealth applications can most easily be disseminated. In some ways, technology serves as a double-edged sword in this regard. On the one hand, the Internet is a delivery system that makes disseminating interventions into the real world easier than any type of offline intervention. For example, an iPhone app that is made available in the app store is instantly accessible to millions of people. On the other hand, technology brings with it new challenges, such as who will be responsible for maintaining a particular health application and providing updates and technical support for it. That is, since technology is ever changing, eHealth applications will constantly need to be maintained and updated, and who will do it and where the resources will come from are not entirely clear at this juncture.

DIRECTIONS FOR FUTURE RESEARCH

As is evident from this chapter, there are numerous fruitful directions for future research in eHealth (Harrington & Noar, 2012a). First, we need additional studies that test the efficacy of a variety of eHealth applications, especially in newer areas such as social media (Taubenheim et al., 2012) and smartphone apps (Abroms et al., 2012).

We need "proof of concept" studies in these areas to demonstrate that such technologies can effectively promote health. Second, we need studies that advance an understanding of *what it is* about particular eHealth applications that makes them effective (Buller & Floyd, 2012; Noar & Harrington, 2012a). For example, how do different types of interactivity and tailoring contribute to the efficacy of interventions? This latter area will likely require different research designs than the first area, as it will involve creating applications that vary on the particular components being tested (Strecher et al., 2008). Also, meta-analytic studies that combine the results of several eHealth trials and examine both overall effects and effects of particular components can contribute to both of these important areas of future research (Head et al., 2013; Noar, Benac, & Harris, 2007).

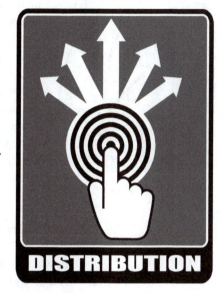

Moreover, as discussed above, current and future eHealth research should have a dissemination perspective built into it (Rabin & Glasgow, 2012). That is, we should not develop and test eHealth applications without a clear indication of how, if successful, such applications could ultimately be disseminated into a practice setting. If we do not do this, we run the risk of putting significant resources into testing interventions that will never see the light of day once the research has ended. This is not a theoretical concern, but a very practical one, as the track record for disseminating interventions into practice is not good. For example, one analysis found that it takes 17 years for 14% of research findings to be applied to practice (Green, Ottoson, Garcia, & Hiatt, 2009). Clearly, we should learn from the lessons of the past and do better in the eHealth arena.

Finally, since eHealth research uses technology, and technology is continually changing and advancing, research on new and emerging technologies in eHealth is needed. Already, studies on the use of virtual reality and avatars for health are beginning (Fox, 2012), but this research is in its infancy. Additional work is needed in this area, as well as other emerging areas. Indeed, one of the most compelling areas for research will involve electronic medical records (EMRs; see Chapter 12). We are only years away from when most patients in the United States will have an electronic medical record (Xierali et al., 2013). At that point, research to understand how various digital technologies can interface with those records to conduct effective health interventions may truly take off. For example, imagine a smoking cessation app that could interface with your EMR and tell you how your breathing function has improved since quitting smoking, or a physical activity app that could tell you how your blood pressure has improved since starting an exercise program. Given the fast pace at which technology is changing, and the extent to which healthcare is adopting technology, it will be nothing short of remarkable to see how the eHealth field changes in the coming decades. Research is the engine that will drive the effective use of these technologies in the years to come.

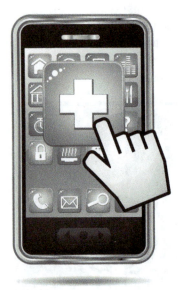

CONCLUSION

The eHealth field has developed rapidly, driven by the introduction of so many new technologies over a relatively short period of time. The use of the Internet to find health information is now as commonplace as a myriad other activities online, presumably because of accessibility and convenience. Much research has been completed, and much more is under way, to evaluate the effects of eHealth applications for health behavior change. To date, we have seen many eHealth applications achieve success in stimulating behavioral changes among targeted audiences. Significant challenges remain, however, including understanding what makes eHealth applications most effective, educating the public on fruitful ways to take advantage of eHealth tools, finding ways to quickly adapt to new technologies as they emerge, and learning the most effective and efficient ways to disseminate and promote eHealth applications that work.

DISCUSSION QUESTIONS

1. For what health behaviors might eHealth applications be most effective? Why?
2. Which populations are most likely to use eHealth tools? Which are least likely?
3. What do you think eHealth tools will look like 10 or 20 years from now?

IN-CLASS ACTIVITIES

1. Take a poll of the students in class: How many have used a computer or Internet-based intervention? How many have used a mobile health app? How many have played a health video game? How many have used social media for health? Divide the class into small groups based on their participation experience: Try to have one group for each major category. Have the groups discuss their experiences and then report back to the class. Are there similarities or differences across their experiences by category (e.g., mobile app versus game)?
2. Have students design their own eHealth application. Be sure to have them justify the health problem, population, technology, and features, as well as why they think eHealth can improve this particular health area.

RECOMMENDED READINGS

Baranowski, T., Baranowski, J., Thompson, D., Buday, R., Jago, R., Griffith, M. J., . . . Watson, K. B. (2011). Video game play, child diet, and physical activity behavior change: A randomized clinical trial. *American Journal of Preventive Medicine*, *40*, 33–38.

This study is a randomized controlled trial testing the ability of a health video game to increase the nutrition and physical activity behaviors of 10–12-year-old children.

Bull, S., Levine, D. K., Black, S. R., Schmiege, S. J., & Santelli, J. (2012). Social media-delivered sexual health intervention: a cluster randomized controlled trial. *American Journal of Preventive Medicine*, *43*, 467–474.

This study is a randomized controlled trial testing the ability of a Facebook-delivered intervention to increase safer sexual behaviors among diverse young adults.

Free, C., Knight, R., Robertson, S., Whittaker, R., Edwards, P., Zhou, W., . . . Roberts, I. (2011). Smoking cessation support delivered via mobile phone text messaging (txt2stop): a single-blind, randomised trial. *Lancet*, *378*, 49–55.

This study is a randomized controlled trial testing the ability of a text-messaging program to impact smoking cessation.

REFERENCES

Abraham, C., & Michie, S. (2008). A taxonomy of behavior change techniques used in interventions. *Health Psychology*, *27*, 379–387.

Abroms, L. C., Padmanabhan, N., & Evans, W. D. (2012). Mobile phones for health communication to promote behavior change. In S. M. Noar & N. G. Harrington (Eds.), *eHealth applications: Promising strategies for behavior change* (pp. 147–166). New York: Routledge.

Baker, T. B., Gustafson, D. H., Shaw, B., Hawkins, R., Pingree, S., Roberts, L., & Strecher, V. (2010). Relevance of CONSORT reporting criteria for research on eHealth interventions. *Patient Education and Counseling*, *81*, S77–S86.

Baranowski, T., Baranowski, J., Thompson, D., Buday, R., Jago, R., Griffith, M. J., . . . Watson, K. B. (2011). Video game play, child diet, and physical activity behavior change: A randomized clinical trial. *American Journal of Preventive Medicine*, *40*, 33–38.

Baranowski, T., Buday, R., Thompson, D. I., & Baranowski, J. (2008). Playing for real: Video games and stories for health-related behavior change. *American Journal of Preventive Medicine*, *34*, 74–82.

Bucy, E. P., & Tao, C.-C. (2007). The mediated moderation model of interactivity. *Media Psychology*, *9*, 647–672.

Bull, S., Levine, D. K., Black, S. R., Schmiege, S. J., & Santelli, J. (2012). Social media-delivered sexual health intervention: A cluster randomized controlled trial. *American Journal of Preventive Medicine*, *43*, 467–474.

Buller, D. B., & Floyd, A. H. L. (2012). Internet-based interventions for health behavior change. In S. M. Noar & N. G. Harrington (Eds.), *eHealth applications: Promising strategies for behavior change* (pp. 59–79). New York: Routledge.

Campbell, M. K., DeVellis, B. M., Strecher, V. J., Ammerman, A. S., DeVellis, R. F., & Sandler, R. S. (1994). Improving dietary behavior: The effectiveness of tailored messages in primary care settings. *American Journal of Public Health, 84*, 783–787.

Cassell, M. M., Jackson, C., & Cheuvront, B. (1998). Health communication on the Internet: An effective channel for health behavior change? *Journal of Health Communication, 3*, 71–79.

Cavallo, D. N., Tate, D. F., Ries, A. V., Brown, J. D., DeVellis, R. F., & Ammerman, A. S. (2012). A social media-based physical activity intervention: A randomized controlled trial. *American Journal of Preventive Medicine, 43*, 527–532.

Conlon, R. T. (1997). Introducing technology into the public STD clinic. *Health Education & Behavior, 24*, 12–19.

Cook, P. A., & Bellis, M. A. (2001). Knowing the risk: Relationships between risk behaviour and health knowledge. *Public Health, 115*, 54–61.

Eng, T. R. (2001). *The eHealth landscape: A terrain map of emerging information and communication technologies in health and health care*. Princeton, NJ: The Robert Wood Johnson Foundation.

Fjeldsoe, B. S., Miller, Y. D., & Marshall, A. L. (2012). Text messaging interventions for chronic disease management and health promotion. In S. M. Noar & N. G. Harrington (Eds.), *eHealth applications: Promising strategies for behavior change* (pp. 167–186). New York: Routledge.

Flay, B. R., Biglan, A., Boruch, R. F., Castro, F. G., Gottfredson, D., Kellam, S., . . . Ji, P. (2005). Standards of evidence: Criteria for efficacy, effectiveness and dissemination. *Prevention Science, 6*, 151–175.

Fox, J. (2012). Avatars for health behavior change. In S. M. Noar & N. G. Harrington (Eds.), *eHealth applications: Promising strategies for behavior change* (pp. 96–109). New York: Routledge.

Free, C., Knight, R., Robertson, S., Whittaker, R., Edwards, P., Zhou, W., . . . Roberts, I. (2011). Smoking cessation support delivered via mobile phone text messaging (txt2stop): a single-blind, randomised trial. *Lancet, 378*, 49–55.

Free, C., Phillips, G., Galli, L., Watson, L., Felix, L., Edwards, P., . . . Haines, A. (2013). The effectiveness of mobile-health technology-based health behaviour change or disease management interventions for health care consumers: A systematic review. *PLoS Med, 10*, e1001362.

Garris, R., Ahlers, R., & Driskell, J. E. (2002). Games, motivation, and learning: A research and practice model. *Simulation & Gaming, 33*, 441–467.

Glasgow, R. E., Lichtenstein, E., & Marcus, A. C. (2003). Why don't we see more translation of health promotion research to practice? Rethinking the efficacy-to-effectiveness transition. *American Journal of Public Health, 93*, 1261–1267.

Gold, J., Pedrana, A. E., Sacks-Davis, R., Hellard, M. E., Chang, S., Howard, S., . . . Stoove, M. A. (2011). A systematic examination of the use of online social networking sites for sexual health promotion. *BMC Public Health, 11*, 583.

Goldberg, L., Lide, B., Lowry, S., Massett, H. A., O'Connell, T., Preece, J., . . . Shneiderman, B. (2011). Usability and accessibility in consumer health informatics: Current trends and future challenges. *American Journal of Preventive Medicine, 40*, S187–S197.

Green, L. W., Ottoson, J. M., Garcia, C., & Hiatt, R. A. (2009). Diffusion theory and knowledge dissemination, utilization, and integration in public health. *Annual Review of Public Health, 30*, 151–174.

Harrington, N. G., & Noar, S. M. (2012a). Building an evidence base for eHealth applications: Research questions and practice implications. In S. M. Noar & N. G. Harrington (Eds.), *eHealth applications: Promising strategies for behavior change* (pp. 263–274). New York: Routledge.

Harrington, N. G., & Noar, S. M. (2012b). Reporting standards for studies of tailored interventions. *Health Education Research, 27*, 331–342.

Hawkins, R. P., Han, J.-Y., Pingree, S., Shaw, B. R., Baker, T. B., & Roberts, L. J. (2010). Interactivity and presence of three eHealth interventions. *Computers in Human Behavior, 26*, 1081–1088.

Hawkins, R. P., Kreuter, M., Resnicow, K., Fishbein, M., & Dijkstra, A. (2008). Understanding tailoring in communicating about health. *Health Education Research, 23*, 454–466.

Head, K. J., Noar, S. M., Iannarino, N., & Harrington, N. G. (2013). Efficacy of text messaging-based interventions for health promotion: A meta-analysis. *Social Science & Medicine, 97*, 41–48.

Hesse, B. W., Nelson, D. E., Kreps, G. L., Croyle, R. T., Arora, N. K., Rimer, B. K., & Viswanath, K. (2005). Trust and sources of health information: The impact of the internet and its implications for health care providers: Findings from the first health information national trends survey. *Archives of Internal Medicine, 165*, 2618–2624.

Huhman, M. E. (2008). New Media and the VERB Campaign: Tools to Motivate Tweens to be Physically Active. *Cases in Public Health Communication & Marketing, 2*, 126–139.

Kiousis, S. (2002). Interactivity: A concept explication. *New Media & Society, 4*, 355–383.

Lieberman, D. A. (2012). Digital games for health behavior change: Research, design, and future direction. In S. M. Noar & N. G. Harrington (Eds.), *eHealth applications: Promising strategies for behavior change* (pp. 110–127). New York: Routledge.

Lim, M. S. C., Hocking, J. S., Hellard, M. E., & Aitken, C. K. (2008). SMS STI: A review of the uses of mobile phone text messaging in sexual health. *International Journal of STD & AIDS, 19*, 287–290.

Neiger, B. L., Thackeray, R., A, Hanson, C. L., West, J. H., Barnes, M. D., & Fagen, M. C. (2012). Use of social media in health promotion: Purposes, key performance indicators, and evaluation metrics. *Health Promotion Practice, 13*, 159–164.

Noar, S. M., Benac, C. N., & Harris, M. S. (2007). Does tailoring matter? Meta-analytic review of tailored print health behavior change interventions. *Psychological Bulletin, 133*, 673–693.

Noar, S. M., Clark, A., Cole, C., & Lustria, M. L. A. (2006). Review of interactive safer sex web sites: Practice and potential. *Health Communication, 20*, 233–241.

Noar, S. M., & Harrington, N. G. (2012a). Computer-tailored interventions for improving health behaviors. In S. M. Noar & N. G. Harrington (Eds.), *eHealth applications: Promising strategies for behavior change* (pp. 128–146). New York: Routledge.

Noar, S. M., & Harrington, N. G. (2012b). eHealth applications: An introduction and overview. In S. M. Noar & N. G. Harrington (Eds.), *eHealth applications: Promising strategies for behavior change* (pp. 3–16). New York: Routledge.

Noar, S. M., & Harrington, N. G. (2012c). *eHealth applications: Promising strategies for behavior change*. New York, NY: Routledge.

Noar, S. M., Harrington, N. G., & Aldrich, R. S. (2009). The role of message tailoring in the development of persuasive health communication messages. *Communication Yearbook, 33,* 72–133.

Noar, S. M., Harrington, N. G., Van Stee, S. K., & Aldrich, R. S. (2011). Tailored health communication to change lifestyle behaviors. *American Journal of Lifestyle Medicine, 5,* 112–122.

Noar, S. M., & Zimmerman, R. S. (2005). Health behavior theory and cumulative knowledge regarding health behaviors: Are we moving in the right direction? *Health Education Research, 20,* 275–290.

Oh, H., Rizo, C., Enkin, M., & Jadad, A. (2005). What is eHealth (3): A systematic review of published definitions. *Journal Of Medical Internet Research, 7,* e1.

Paperny, D. M. N. (1997). Computerized health assessment and education for adolescent HIV and STD prevention in health care settings and schools. *Health Education & Behavior, 24,* 54–70.

Peng, W., Lin, J. H., & Crouse, J. (2011). Is playing exergames really exercising? A meta-analysis of energy expenditure in active video games. *Cyberpsychology, Behavor, & Social Networking, 14,* 681–688.

Pew Internet & American Life Project. (2010a). *Home broadband 2010.* Retrieved from http://pewinternet.org/Reports/2010/Home-Broadband-2010.aspx

Pew Internet & American Life Project. (2010b). *Social media & mobile internet use among teens and young adults.* Retrieved from http://www.pewinternet.org/~/media//Files/Reports/2010/PIP_Social_Media_and_Young_Adults_Report.pdf

Pew Internet & American Life Project. (2010c). *Teens and mobile phones.* Retrieved from http://pewinternet.org/Reports/2010/Teens-and-Mobile-Phones.aspx

Pew Internet & American Life Project. (2011a). *Health topics.* Retrieved from http://pewinternet.org/Reports/2011/HealthTopics.aspx

Pew Internet & American Life Project. (2011b). *Social networking sites and our lives.* Retrieved from http://pewinternet.org/Reports/2011/Technology-and-social-networks.aspx

Rabin, B. A., & Glasgow, R. E. (2012). Dissemination and implementation of eHealth interventions. In S. M. Noar & N. G. Harrington (Eds.), *eHealth applications: Promising strategies for behavior change* (pp. 221–245). New York: Routledge.

Rimal, R. N., & Adkins, A. D. (2003). Using computers to narrowcast health messages: The role of audience segmentation, targeting, and tailoring in health promotion. In T. L. Thompson, A. M. Dorsey, K. I. Miller & R. Parrott (Eds.), *Handbook of health communication* (pp. 497–515). Mahwah, N.J.: Lawrence Erlbaum Associates.

Skinner, C. S., Campbell, M. K., Rimer, B. K., Curry, S., & Prochaska, J. O. (1999). How effective is tailored print communication? *Annals of Behavioral Medicine, 21,* 290–298.

Skinner, H. A., Maley, O., & Norman, C. D. (2006). Developing Internet-based eHealth promotion programs: The Spiral Technology Action Research (STAR) model. *Health Promotion Practice, 7,* 406–417.

Strecher, V. J. (2007). Internet methods for delivering behavioral and health-related interventions (eHealth). *Annual Review of Clinical Psychology, 3*, 53–76.

Strecher, V. J., McClure, J. B., Alexander, G. L., Chakraborty, B., Nair, V. N., Konkel, J. M., . . . Pomerleau, O. F. (2008). Web-based smoking-cessation programs: Results of a randomized trial. *American Journal of Preventive Medicine, 34*, 373–381.

Tate, D. F., Jackvony, E. H., & Wing, R. R. (2006). A randomized trial comparing human e-Mail counseling, computer-automated tailored counseling, and no counseling in an Internet weight loss program. *Archives Of Internal Medicine, 166*, 1620–1625.

Taubenheim, A. M., Long, T., Smith, E. C., Jeffers, D., Wayman, J., & Temple, S. (2008). Using social media and internet marketing to reach women with the heart truth. *Social Marketing Quarterly, 14*, 58–67.

Taubenheim, A. M., Long, T., Wayman, J., Temple, S., McDonough, S., & Duncan, A. (2012). Using social media to enhance health communication campaigns. In S. M. Noar & N. G. Harrington (Eds.), *eHealth applications: Promising strategies for behavior change* (pp. 205–220). New York: Routledge.

Viswanath, K. (2005). Science and society: The communications revolution and cancer control. *Nature Reviews Cancer, 5*, 828–835.

Whiteley, L. B., Brown, L. K., Swenson, R. R., Romer, D., DiClemente, R. J., Salazar, L. E., . . . Valois, R. F. (2011). African American adolescents and new media: associations with HIV/STI risk behavior and psychosocial variables. *Ethnicity & Disease, 21*, 216–222.

Xierali, I. M., Hsiao, C. J., Puffer, J. C., Green, L. A., Rinaldo, J. C., Bazemore, A. W., . . . Phillips, R. L., Jr. (2013). The rise of electronic health record adoption among family physicians. *Annals of Family Medicine, 11*, 14–19.

16

Risk and Crisis Communication

Shari R. Veil and
Timothy L. Sellnow

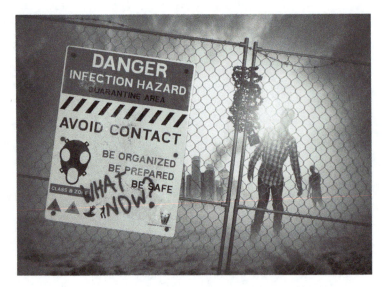

You made it! You finally reached the chapter that will be most useful in an actual zombie apocalypse. After all, if a rapidly spreading virus is causing people to eat each other's brains, you have definitely got a crisis on your hands. In fact, the **Centers for Disease Control and Prevention (CDC), Department of Homeland Security**, and **Federal Emergency Management Agency (FEMA)** have all used the zombie apocalypse as a tongue-in-cheek metaphor for a health crisis. This chapter will not only explain why we keep talking about zombies in a highly respected health communication textbook but also discuss how the field of risk and crisis communication has emerged from a melting pot of multidisciplinary, interdisciplinary, and transdisciplinary approaches where scientific, interpretive, and critical–cultural approaches are not only present but, in some cases, triangulated in the same study. When you're trying to save the world, arguments over whose research paradigm is superior seem to fade away—almost.

Barbara Reynolds, Ph.D., Senior Crisis Communication Advisor, Director, Public Affairs, Centers for Disease Control and Prevention

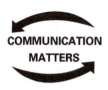

COMMUNICATION
MATTERS

What do you say when the unthinkable happens? The Centers for Disease Control and Prevention is the nation's health security agency—protecting people from health threats. When CDC responds to a national health emergency like a disease outbreak, a natural disaster or a deliberate attack, my job involves two important goals. I help people make the best possible choices to protect themselves, their loved ones and their community, and I help ensure CDC is viewed as a trusted source for that information. In national surveys, CDC consistently ranks as the most trusted federal agency, and we work every day to preserve that trust. We strive to ensure what we say is respectful and accurate. That means communicating from a set of values, not just using communication techniques. There are no communication gimmicks that will build you lasting trust, and without trust your message will fall flat. The communication stakes are never higher than when you are dealing with messages that can mean the difference between life and death. A job like mine gives me the opportunity to help save lives, and that's a job I hope more will aspire to do someday.

DEFINING RISK AND CRISIS COMMUNICATION

Broadly defined, **risk communication** is a process of informing people about risks and persuading them to modify their behavior to reduce risks (Seeger & Reynolds, 2007). Since much of the work in health communication focuses on reducing health risks, health communication is often similarly defined (Freimuth, Linnan, & Potter, 2000). Like all bourbon is whiskey but not all whiskey is bourbon, some would argue all health communication is risk communication but not all risk communication is health communication. Health communication messages are primarily based on an obvious or implied connection to a health risk. For example, health communication campaigns often focus on what you should or shouldn't do to be healthy (i.e., to not be at risk of illness, injury, or death). However, in addition to health and safety risks, risk communication scholars might study financial risk, environmental risk, political risk, economic risk, severe weather risk, cybersecurity risk, corporate reputation risk, or a variety of other risks. Thus, risk communication, like health communication, can be studied in silos.

That being said, some risk exigencies require a multidisciplinary approach, particularly when a risk manifests into a crisis. For example, British Petroleum's Deepwater Horizon explosion caused, at the very least, environmental, economic, political, corporate reputation, and health risks. In response to this amalgamation of risks, the **National Science Foundation (NSF)** sponsored a conference entitled *Collaborative*

Scientific Research Opportunities Relative to the Gulf Oil Spill and offered rapid response research grants to encourage interdisciplinary research. Interdisciplinary research centers such as the Department of Homeland Security's National Center for Food Protection and Defense (NCFPD) and Center for Risk and Economic Analysis of Terrorism Events were also tasked with considering implications of the BP spill on terrorism, an example of transdisciplinary research.

Despite the fact that risks almost always have a chance of becoming a crisis and the research on risk and crisis exigencies is rather fluid, in practice, crisis communication has only recently been applied to health concepts. Specific crisis events including 9/11, the subsequent anthrax attacks, the aftermath of Hurricane Katrina, and the threat posed by H5N1 illustrated that public health has an extensive role reaching far beyond informing the public about health risks. Crises create challenges for health communicators who must coordinate with other response agencies to address unexpected, fast-moving events in which there is often a great deal of uncertainty and threat (Reynolds & Seeger, 2005). Public health has, therefore, had to adjust to an expanded set of responsibilities.

These new responsibilities include a complex set of communication obligations that incorporate elements of both risk communication and crisis communication. As a function of public relations, the purpose of **crisis communication** is to prevent or lessen the negative outcomes of a crisis and primarily to protect the interests of the organization at the heart of the crisis (Coombs, 2012). Responses include instructional information for physical protection, adjusting information to help stakeholders cope psychologically with the crisis, and reputation management responses to protect the reputation of the organization both during and following the crisis (Sturges, 1994). While scholars agree the ethical imperative is to focus first on instructional messages that seek to explain the risks and what the public can do to protect themselves (Sellnow & Sellnow, 2010), failure to bolster the credibility of the communicating health organization can have a negative impact on public perception. Perceptions of the crisis response efforts are critical to maintaining confidence in the public health system (Ballard-Reisch et al., 2007; Ulmer, Alvey, & Kordsmeier, 2008).

The increasingly complex demands upon public health officials during emergency situations make the dynamic blending of risk and crisis communication both essential and practical (Veil, Reynolds, Sellnow, & Seeger, 2008). Both risk and crisis communication "share an essential purpose of seeking to limit, contain, mitigate, and reduce harm" (Reynolds & Seeger, 2005, p. 48). A significant difference between health risk communication messages and crisis communication responses is that, in addressing a risk that has not yet evolved into a crisis, communicators have the luxury of time to fully develop and test messages in an effort to maximize their effectiveness. When a

---

DEFINITIONS OF RISK AND CRISIS COMMUNICATION

Risk communication is a process of informing people about risks and persuading them to modify their behavior to reduce risks. As a function of public relations, crisis communication is meant to prevent or lessen the negative outcomes of a crisis and primarily protect the interests of the organization at the heart of the crisis; it includes instructional, adjusting, and reputation management messages. Both risk and crisis communication seek to "limit, contain, mitigate, and reduce harm"(Reynolds & Seeger, 2005, p. 48).

---

crisis causes additional risk, such as in the BP case, effective persuasive messages are needed to encourage action under the time constraints of an emergency. See Table 16.1 for a list of features that distinguish risk and crisis communication.

Public health emergencies create an intense and immediate need for information regarding what happened, who is in danger, what actions people should take, and how governments

Table 16.1 Distinguishing Features of Risk Communication and Crisis Communication

Risk communication	*Crisis communication*
Risk centered: projection about some harm occurring at some future date	Event-centered: specific incident that has occurred and produced harm
Messages regarding known probabilities of negative consequences and how they may be reduced	Messages regarding current conditions: magnitude, immediacy, duration, control/remediation, cause, blame, consequences
Based on what is currently known	Based on what is known and not known
Long term (precrisis stage)	Short term (crisis stage)
Message preparation (i.e., campaigns)	Less preparation (i.e., responsive)
Technical experts, scientists	Authority figures, emergency managers, technical experts
Personal scope	Community or regional scope
Mediated: commercials, ads, brochures, pamphlets	Mediated: press conferences, press releases, speeches, websites
Controlled and structured	Spontaneous and reactive

From Seeger, M. W., Sellnow, T. L., & Ulmer, R. R. (2003). *47 organizational crisis*. Westport, CT: Praeger.

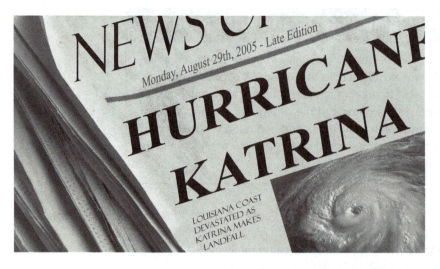

(local, state and federal) are responding (Sellnow & Seeger, 2001). Research by disaster sociologist Dennis Mileti and his colleagues (Mileti & Fitzpatrick, 1991; Mileti & Sorensen, 1990) identifies key elements to consider when crafting a message during a crisis. The recipients of the information must (a) receive the information, (b) understand that information, (c) understand that the message relates to them directly, (d) understand the risks they face if they do not follow the protective action provided, (e) decide that they should act on the information, (f) understand the actions they need to take, and (g) actually be able to take action. Ultimately, a response should include clear, concrete, and consistent messages with suggested actions to mitigate risk, presented by a trusted source (Windahl, Signitzer & Olson, 1992). All of these components must be considered in preparing a crisis response. Seeger and Reynolds (2007) note that many crisis scenarios pose a severe threat to psychological security and the associated socio-economic stability. Public health officials must, therefore, seek to understand the complex needs, background, and culture of audiences to determine the stressors impacting them and provide messages that reestablish a sense of personal control and thus reduce fears that may be unwarranted in the midst of a crisis (Veil et al., 2008).

CRISIS STAGE MODELS

While crises are unexpected events, they unfold in cyclical patterns. Crisis events follow a particular order with distinct communication strategies demanded at different points in the crisis cycle (Seeger, Sellnow, & Ulmer, 2003). Because, like health communication and risk communication, crisis communication can be studied in academic silos, the following models each emerged from a different perspective of crisis communication research. Interestingly, the approaches yield similar descriptions, albeit using different terms.

Fink (1986) was one of the first to develop a **crisis stage model**. While his research was primarily on for-profit corporations, Fink described crisis through the metaphor of a medical illness with four stages: (1) *prodromal*, when warning signals of a potential crisis emerge; (2) *acute*, when the trigger event and ensuing damage of the crisis occur; (3) *chronic*, when lasting effects of the crisis continue and clean up begins; and (4) *resolution*, when the crisis is no longer a concern to stakeholders. Fink describes crisis with a starting and ending point, yet he notes that warning signals emerge before the onset of a crisis.

Mitroff (1994) suggested there are opportunities to interrupt the **crisis lifecycle**. Also specific to organizational crises, his approach focused on strategic actions for crisis prevention through (1) *signal detection*, when warning signs can be identified and acted upon to prevent a crisis; (2) *probing and prevention*, when organization members should be searching for known crisis risk factors and working to reduce potential harm; (3) *damage containment*, the onset of crisis during which organization members try to limit the damage; (4) *recovery*, working to return to normal business operation as soon as possible; and (5) *learning*, which involves reviewing and critiquing the crisis management process. González-Herrero and Pratt (1995) extended Mitroff's work to include learning as a continuation of the recovery phase that will improve signal detection for organizations at the start of the cycle.

Drawing from emergency management and the work of Fink and Mitroff, Coombs (2007) described the crisis lifecycle through four interrelated factors: (1) *prevention*, detecting warning signals and taking action to mitigate the crisis; (2) *preparation*, diagnosing vulnerabilities and developing the crisis plan; (3) *response*, applying the preparation components and attempting to return to normal operations; and (4) *revision*, evaluating the crisis response to determine what was done right or wrong during the crisis management performance.

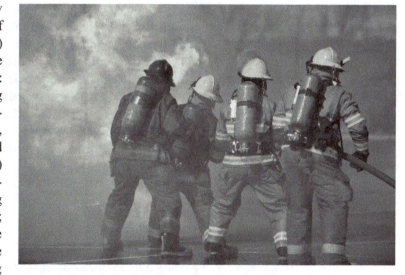

The three-stage approach is most commonly used to separate the events surrounding a crisis for further analysis (e.g., Seeger et al., 2003): (1) *precrisis* includes crisis preparation and planning; (2) *crisis* includes the trigger event and ensuing damage;

and (3) *post crisis* includes learning and resolution, which then informs the precrisis stage. This macro approach to crisis furthers the notion of a crisis cycle. If an organization survives the stages of precrisis, crisis, and post crisis, it will once again find itself in the stage of precrisis, only better equipped to prepare for another crisis (Coombs, 2007). While the cycle returns to precrisis, lessons learned from the crisis should inspire a different mindset in preparing for the next crisis (Veil, 2011).

CRISIS STAGE MODELS

There are a variety of different crisis stage models, each emerging from different perspectives of crisis communication research. Although they use different terms, the models have numerous similarities. The three-stage model, identifying precrisis, crisis, and post crisis, is the most common model used to separate the events surrounding a crisis for further analysis. Although scholars agree that effective communication is essential throughout all stages of a crisis, research has not been evenly distributed across these crisis stages.

One of the most widely adopted models for risk and crisis communication in a health context is **Crisis and Emergency Risk Communication (CERC)**. CERC was developed using a grounded theory approach based on communication practices tried and tested by CDC and public health officials. Grounded theory is inherently interpretive in nature, and applications of CERC seek to address both the urgency of crisis communication and the need to explain risks and benefits to stakeholders and the public. CERC follows a five-stage model of crisis and includes specific communication activities for each stage: (1) *precrisis*, risk messages, warnings, preparations; (2) *initial event*, uncertainty reduction, self efficacy, reassurance; (3) *maintenance*, ongoing uncertainty reduction, self-efficacy, reassurance; (4) *resolution*, updates regarding resolution, discussions about cause and new risks/understandings of risk; and (5) *evaluation*, discussions of adequacy of response, consensus about lessons, and new understandings of risks. Table 16.2 presents the CERC model.

Originally launched by the CDC in 2002, CERC was designed as a training program to educate and equip public health professionals for the expanding communication responsibilities of public health in emergency situations. CERC training covers definitions and descriptions of the crisis cycle, the psychology of a crisis, messages and audiences, crisis communication plans, spokespersons, working with the media, stakeholder and partner communication, communication channels, social and mobile media, terrorism, human resources, the role of varying levels of government agencies, and media and public health law. Throughout the CERC training manual, "reality

Table 16.2 A Working Model of CERC

I. Precrisis (Risk Messages, Warnings, Preparations)

Communication and education campaigns targeted to both the public and the response community to facilitate:

- Monitoring and recognition of emerging risks
- General public understanding of risk
- Public preparation for the possibility of an adverse event
- Changes in behavior to reduce the likelihood of harm (self-efficacy)
- Specific warning messages regarding some imminent threat
- Alliances and cooperation with agencies, organizations, and groups
- Development of consensual recommendations by experts and first responders
- Message development and testing for subsequent stages

II. Initial Event (Uncertainty Reduction, Self-efficacy, Reassurance)

Rapid communication to the general public and to affected groups seeking to establish:

- Empathy, reassurance, and reduction in emotional turmoil
- Designated crisis/agency spokespersons and formal channels and methods of communication
- General and broad-based understanding of the crisis circumstances, consequences, and anticipated outcomes based on available information
- Reduction of crisis-related uncertainty
- Specific understanding of emergency management and medical community responses
- Understanding of self-efficacy and personal response activities (how/where to get more information)

III. Maintenance (Ongoing Uncertainty Reduction, Self-efficacy, Reassurance)

Communication to the general public and to affected groups seeking to facilitate:

- More accurate public understandings of ongoing risks
- Understanding of background factors and issues
- Broad-based support and cooperation with response and recovery efforts
- Feedback from affected publics and correction of any misunderstandings/umors
- Ongoing explanation and reiteration of self-efficacy and personal response activities (how/where to get more information) begun in Stage II
- Informed decision making by the public based on understanding of risks/benefits

(Continued)

Table 16.2 Continued

IV. Resolution (Updates Regarding Resolution, Discussions about Cause and New Risks/ New Understandings of Risk)

Public communication and campaigns directed toward the general public and affected groups seeking to:
- Inform and persuade about ongoing clean-up, remediation, recovery, and rebuilding efforts
- Facilitate broad-based, honest, and open discussion and resolution of issues regarding cause, blame, responsibility, and adequacy of response
- Improve/create public understanding of new risks and new understandings of risk as well as new risk avoidance behaviors and response procedures
- Promote the activities and capabilities of agencies and organizations to reinforce positive corporate identity and image

V. Evaluation (Discussions of Adequacy of Response; Consensus About Lessons and New Understandings of Risks)

Communication directed toward agencies and the response community to:
- Evaluate and assess responses, including communication effectiveness
- Document, formalize, and communicate lessons learned
- Determine specific actions to improve crisis communication and crisis response capability
- Create linkages to precrisis activities (Stage I)

From Reynolds, B., & Seeger, M. W. (2005). Crisis and emergency risk communication as an integrative model. *Journal of Health Communication, 10,* 43–55.

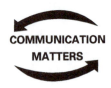

COMMUNICATION MATTERS

Shelley Roberts Bendall, MPA, Preparedness Coordinator, Division of Emergency Management/Division of Public Safety, Lexington-Fayette County Urban Government, Kentucky

As a preparedness coordinator for a local government, I know disaster preparedness can have tangible effects on my neighbors and my community. Whether it's listening to a tornado victim explain how she sleeps better at night with a NOAA weather radio by her bed, hearing a CERT volunteer recount using his skills to assist survivors of a car accident, or responding to requests for assistance in the EOC during a disaster, I see how being prepared for disasters not only saves lives, but can improve them, as well. The most rewarding aspect of my job is giving people the tools they need to better protect the health and safety of their families. Empowering people with the knowledge and tools they need to respond to a disaster better prepares our entire city, makes the jobs of our first responders easier, and allows us to recover more quickly from an emergency. Knowing I may have played a small role in increasing our community's resilience is extremely rewarding.

checks" are provided to debunk crisis myths and demonstrate how CERC concepts can be applied to different crisis scenarios. Specific communication activities for addressing different crisis types are described along with the expected relationships between the communication activities and outcomes.

In 2008, the journal *Health Promotion Practice* published a special issue on CERC and pandemic influenza, opening the practice-based applications of CERC to scholarly debate and discussion. What emerged was a more clearly defined theoretical framework for CERC and an alignment of the CERC model with community resilience and capacity building. The 2012 edition of the CERC program included contributions and reviews by dozens of crisis communication scholars to ensure the concepts aligned with the most recent research in risk and crisis communication. CERC advocates **six principles of effective risk and crisis communication**, which we present in Table 16.3. While CERC was developed using grounded theory in the interpretive paradigm, the translational research in the special issue of *Health Promotion Practice* helped CERC evolve from a stage model of crisis into a framework ripe for testing and analysis in the laboratory and field, both under the purview of the scientific paradigm.

CRISIS AND EMERGENCY RISK COMMUNICATION (CERC)

One of the most widely adopted models for risk and crisis communication in a health context is CERC. Originally launched by the CDC in 2002, CERC was designed as a training program to educate and equip public health professionals for the expanding communication responsibilities of public health in emergency situations. It follows a five-stage model of crisis: precrisis, initial event, maintenance, resolution, and evaluation.

THEORETICAL FRAMEWORKS AND APPLICATIONS

As noted, risk and crisis communication research incorporates a variety of approaches and paradigms. The theoretical foundation of crisis communication research in organizations continues to rely on **corporate apologia** (Hearit, 2006), **image restoration** (Benoit, 1997), and **situational crisis communication theory** (SCCT; Coombs, 2007), which all concentrate on determining the best strategy to protect the reputation of the accountable organization and not on the ethical imperative to protect the public first. Research on apologia and image restoration consider both the interpretive and critical–cultural paradigms by analyzing the meaning of corporate statements and, in some studies, how those statements prioritize the power of the corporation over the protection

Table 16.3 CERC Principles of Effective Crisis and Risk Communication

1. Be First: Crises are time-sensitive. Communicating information quickly is almost always important. For members of the public, the first source of information often becomes the preferred source.
2. Be Right: Accuracy establishes credibility. Information can include what is known, what is not known, and what is being done to fill in the gaps.
3. Be Credible: Honesty and truthfulness should not be compromised during crises.
4. Express Empathy: Crises create harm, and the suffering should be acknowledged in words. Addressing what people are feeling, and the challenges they face, builds trust and rapport.
5. Promote Action: Giving people meaningful things to do calms anxiety, helps restore order, and promotes a restored sense of control.
6. Show Respect: Respectful communication is particularly important when people feel vulnerable. Respectful communication promotes cooperation and rapport.

From Reynolds, B. J. (2010). Principles to enable leaders to navigate the harsh realities of crisis and risk communication. *Journal of Business Continuity & Emergency Planning, 3,* 262–273.

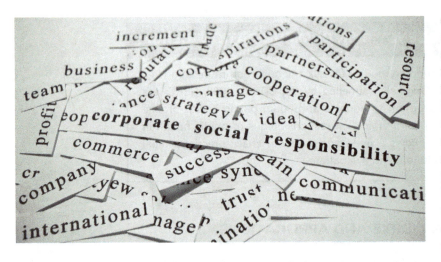

of the public. SCCT, on the other hand, follows the scientific paradigm by testing the strategies identified in interpretive and critical–cultural studies in experiments to determine the effects of corporate statements on public perceptions. While this borrowing of one paradigm from another would be an atrocity in some disciplines, in risk and crisis communication, this back and forth is commonplace.

Part of the challenge of theorizing crisis communication is that crises are largely event-specific. Therefore, the vast majority of crisis communication research has also been event-specific. **Case study research** is the primary method used to analyze and evaluate the communication strategies implemented by accountable organizations in a given crisis. While limited by the lack of generalizability, case studies "provide a method to investigate a contemporary event involving risk within a real life context, and they contribute to enhanced knowledge of complex social phenomena" (Sellnow, Ulmer, Seeger, & Littlefield, 2009, p. 54). A variety of data collection and analysis methods are used to develop the context of a crisis case, including qualitative methods such as interviews, focus groups, and narrative analysis and quantitative methods such as surveys and content analysis. In many case studies, extant data and media coverage of crises are used to determine power structures within a crisis exigency, clearly taking a critical–cultural approach to the case. While case studies are limited in scope, researchers are finding ways to test the effectiveness of crisis responses and media coverage using realistic message simulations in a laboratory setting, indicative of the scientific paradigm.

Next, we describe current applications of risk and crisis communication in research and practice according to the three-stage model of crisis. Although scholars may agree that effective communication is essential throughout all stages of a crisis (Ballard-Reisch et al., 2007), research has not been evenly distributed across crisis stages.

Precrisis

Pandemic influenza planning increased attention on operational healthcare prepared-ness; however, public preparedness in the precrisis stage has received very little research attention in risk and crisis communication research and practice. FEMA recommends that people have a plan and an emergency kit to sustain themselves for a minimum of three days after a disaster because it may take up to 72 hours for emer-gency personnel to reach a disaster site (FEMA, 2004). And yet, two-thirds of the general public still believes help will arrive within hours of a disaster (National Center for Disaster Preparedness, 2011). The immediate gratification of social media has exacerbated this assumption even further. In a 2010 American Red Cross survey, 74% of respondents who used social media expected help to come less than an hour after their tweet or Facebook post requesting help (American Red Cross, 2010). The National Center for Disaster Preparedness (2011) found that less than half the general public actually has an emergency plan and only one-third feel prepared for a disaster. FEMA Administrator Craig Fugate stated that "personal disaster preparedness is and must be a national priority," and in fact, "nothing will contribute more to saving and sustaining lives than a citizenry prepared and provisioned to live in a reduced-services environ-ment in the days immediately following a catastrophic disaster" (FEMA, 2009, p. 9).

Researchers have adapted the **transtheoretical model (TTM)** to better understand what factors influence individual preparedness (Paek, Hilyard, Freimuth, Barge, & Mindlin, 2010). The TTM posits that change occurs through a series of stages: (1) *precontempla-tion*, the stage where people have no intention to change behavior in the near future; (2) *contemplation*, where people are aware that a problem exists and are seriously thinking

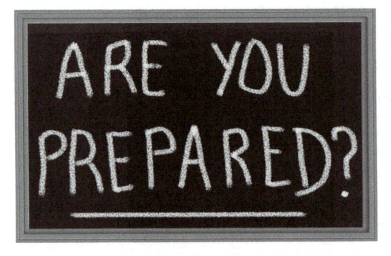

about overcoming it, but they have not yet made a commitment to take an action; (3) *preparation*, where people intend to take action and have started to make some changes; (4) *action*, where people modify their behavior or environment to overcome problems and reach certain goals; and (5) *maintenance*, in which people maintain behavior changes for at least six months or more (Prochaska & DiClemente, 1983). Paek and colleagues used the TTM to guide a research study to understand factors that influence the public's emergency preparedness. Let's take a closer look at their study.

Paek et al. (2010) used a professional research firm to conduct 15-minute telephone surveys with 1,302 adults in the state of Georgia in 2006. The survey sample was collected through a stratified, list-assisted, random digit-dialing method among the state's population. The survey included questions regarding the number of emergency items the participant had on hand through a series of yes or no questions. The stage of emergency preparedness was also determined through a series of yes or no questions such as, "Have you thought about planning for emergencies at all?" and "Have you updated your emergency plans or restocked your supplies for emergencies in the past 6 months?" Self-efficacy was determined with a four-point scale measuring responses to the question, "How confident are you about your own ability to manage an emergency?" Subjective norm was measured similarly with the question "How prepared do you think most people in the U.S. are for an emergency?" Finally, to measure media use, participants were asked about the amount of attention they paid to emergency preparedness news using a four-point scale ranging from "no attention at all" to "very close attention." Demographic and social status data related to education and income were also collected. Multiple regression models were computed to assess the predictive value of the variables. The researchers determined that self-efficacy (an individual's belief that he or she is capable of executing a particular behavior), subjective norm (belief about how one's significant others think she or he should engage in the behavior), and exposure to emergency news coverage were positively associated with possession of emergency kit items and advanced stages of emergency preparedness, including preparation, action, and maintenance. They advised researchers and practitioners to consider theory-based constructs such as a person's stage of change instead of superficial factors like demographics to help understand and influence emergency preparedness.

While studies measuring emergency preparedness are becoming more sophisticated, getting people to notice emergency preparedness messages when there is not an emergency is almost as difficult as convincing them to take action to prepare for something that may not happen. Before the start of hurricane season in 2011, the CDC tried a different approach by promoting preparedness for a zombie apocalypse. Finally, we're back to zombies! The social media campaign was created to target a younger, more media savvy demographic. While a typical CDC blog post might get between 1,000 and 3,000 hits, the CDC's blog had reached over 60,000 visits when the server was overwhelmed and went down (Reuters, 2011). Building on the attention, the CDC's Office of Public Health Preparedness and Response developed a zombie novella comic and webpage devoted to preparing for the zombie apocalypse, and both FEMA and the Department of Homeland Security joined the campaign (Caldwell, 2012; CDC, 2012).

Today, undergraduate courses are even being offered by the University of Kentucky to promote emergency preparedness in this captivating context.

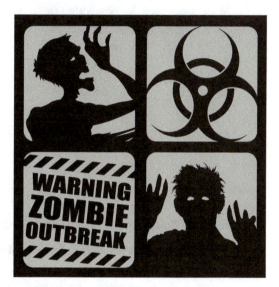

While the CDC, Department of Homeland Security, FEMA, and even the professor who teaches the zombie course at the University of Kentucky received criticism from humorless contrarians who clearly have not read the chapters in this book on audience analysis and message design, others have lauded the efforts to use a mainstay of popular culture to promote discussion of a truly life or death concept. Just think, if you had the option to take COM 316: Communicating Emergency Preparedness or COM 316: Communication and Humanity in a Zombie Apocalypse, which class would you register for next semester?

Crisis

Research on the crisis phase is very applied and has primarily focused on lessons learned from individual cases of pandemics (SARS, H5N1, H1N1), terrorist attacks (9/11, anthrax), and foodborne illnesses outbreaks (E. *coli, salmonella, hepatitis A*). In almost every crisis case, researchers find that communication could have been better. In 2006, the *Journal of Applied Communication Research* published a special issue on *Best Practices in Risk and Crisis Communication* to combine the various lessons learned into usable benchmarks.

Risk and crisis researchers worked together to propose a theoretical framework of best practices based on an extensive synthesis of literature and in-depth discussions of organizational crisis planning and response. Respected scholars contributed their perspectives to the theoretical conversation concerning the most effective strategies for risk and crisis communication. Seeger (2006) proposed the initial 10 practices list, while Heath (2006) and Sandman (2006) provided additions and critiques. In a later publication, Sellnow and Vidoloff (2009) expanded the list to 11 practices. Additional research studies have since applied, analyzed, and validated the best practices or used the best practices to assess the response strategies of accountable organizations (Sellnow et al., 2009; Ulmer et al., 2008; Veil & Husted, 2012; Veil & Sellnow, 2008).

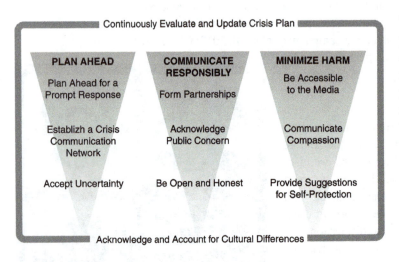

Figure 16.1 Best Practices in Risk and Crisis Communication.

Source: From The National Center for Food Protection and Defense (2009).

The best practices framework presented in Figure 16.1 most closely follows the three-stage model by serving as a guide to plan for a crisis, communicate responsibly in the acute phase of the crisis, and minimize harm in facilitating post-crisis response. While the best practices may seem intuitive to health risk communicators, in the heat of a crisis, many of these standard guidelines are forgotten or ignored and inevitably are included in the lessons learned in the next crisis response assessment. Consider for a moment the fear and embarrassment you feel when you have done something wrong. Next, consider how you would feel if the wrong you did caused significant pain and suffering to others. What if this wrong will cost you millions of dollars and potentially ruin your entire livelihood if anyone learns of it? Do you want to tell people what you did? It's not always easy to communicate with honesty, candor, and openness even when you know it's the right thing to do.

Here's another example. Your business is expanding but still has limited finances. There is only one property in the city you can afford that has the zoning regulations needed for the chemicals you use in your company. The surrounding neighborhood is upset and doesn't want you to move in even though you have every legal right to do so. You can't stay in your current location and grow your business. Do you go to the neighborhood association meeting to listen to public concerns? Or do you ignore the public and go about your business? The best practices provide a guide for how people *should* act in a risk or crisis situation, not how people always *want* to act. Following the best practices is much like following a moral business code in a crisis. The purpose is to always put the public's safety and well-being before profit—and ego.

Beyond best practices, there is a growing body of research specifically in food safety focused on the instructional dynamic of crisis communication. This research holds both crisis communicators and journalists accountable for delivering much needed health information (Sellnow & Sellnow, 2010). This line of research has examined instruction in crisis through two different methods: interpretive content analysis and scientific experimental study.

To draw attention to the lack of instructional messages for protection provided to the public in a food crisis, researchers content analyze official statements, press releases, website posts, and press conference transcripts of accountable organizations such as the FDA and CDC, as well as the resulting media coverage. Interpretive researchers have repeatedly found food safety crises are covered by the media as a horserace, with each news report focusing on how much bigger the recall is than the day before (Nucci, Cuite, & Hallman, 2009; Roberts & Veil, in press). The percentage of media coverage actually containing health information and instructional messages for self-protection was as low as 12% during the 2006 American spinach recall and 17% during the 2010 egg recall.

Researchers have also conducted experiments to determine the extent to which tailored instructional messages actually increase knowledge about food safety and self-efficacy (the belief that one can take action to protect oneself from foodborne illness; Frisby, Veil, & Sellnow, 2014). Not surprisingly, researchers have found that viewing a media clip with instructional messages for self-protection increases participants' level of knowledge and self-efficacy. However, when participants viewed a media clip that focused only on the size of the recall, they felt they were *less* knowledgeable about foodborne illness and *less* able to protect themselves than they did before watching the message (Frisby et al., 2014), suggesting an iatrogenic (harmful) effect of news coverage.

Indeed, the results of these studies imply that the vast majority of news coverage during a foodborne illness outbreak may actually be confusing the public rather than informing and protecting the public. A burgeoning model of instructional communication in crisis suggests tailoring messages so that individuals are provided (a) information detailing the scope of the risk, (b) concrete examples to internalize the risk and make it relevant, and (c) action-oriented instructions for self-protection (Sellnow & Sellnow, 2010). Whereas tailoring messages for health behavior change interventions requires collecting individual assessments along demographic, psychographic, and/or

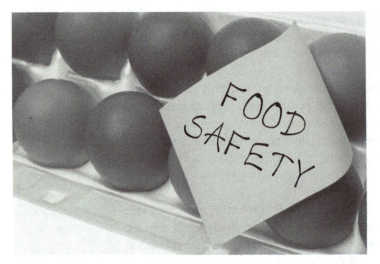

behavioral measures and then tailoring messages based on those assessments, the term tailoring is used here in the context of matching learning styles of the public to the crisis messages they receive. Specifically, by looking at how learning styles intersect in repeated studies over the years, Sellnow and Sellnow (2010) found that messages tailored using the instructional model match with the learning styles of most people, so individual assessment is not required.

Post Crisis

Chaos theory has been used as a metaphor to better understand the unexpected, dynamic, and complex events of natural disasters, terrorist attacks, and other public health crises (Seeger & Reynolds, 2007; Sellnow, Seeger, & Ulmer, 2002; Sellnow, Ulmer, Seeger, & Veil, 2008). Chaos theory argues that systems experience breakdowns or bifurcations as a result of complexity of a system or complex interactions with other systems. However, out of this complexity and chaos, a predictable pattern of organization occurs. Researchers have analyzed health crises to identify patterns of relationships, engagement of community groups, and organizational structures that emerge to mitigate harm and assist in crisis recovery (Seeger & Reynolds, 2007).

Research examining **renewal discourse** has demonstrated that a shared, prospective vision that honors the victims of a crisis while simultaneously focusing on learning and rebuilding from the crisis can assist organizations and communities in crisis recovery (Janssen, 2013; Seeger & Ulmer, 2001; Veil, Sellnow, & Heald, 2011). Ulmer et al. (2007) suggest renewal discourse is most successful when (a) crises are natural disasters rather than human caused, (b) responding organizations have strong precrisis relationships with stakeholders, (c) responding organizations can demonstrate a commitment to making changes and building a better organization and response system, and (d) the discourse allows the organization's publics and stakeholders to change the rhetorical frame of the crisis into a prospective vision for the future. Much like the best practices approach to crisis response, renewal discourse focuses on lessons learned. The key difference is that in post crisis, organizations can concentrate on preparing for the future and not just evaluating the past.

THEORY, METHOD, AND PRACTICE

Risk and crisis communication research draws on multiple paradigms. Similarly, risk and crisis researchers use multiple methods to inform their investigations, including interviews, surveys, and experiments. Case study research is the primary method used to analyze and evaluate the communication strategies implemented by organizations in a crisis. The best practices in risk and crisis communication provide a guide for how we *should* act in a risk or crisis situation, not how we always *want to* act.

THE EVOLVING ROLE OF MEDIA

The media play an essential role in disseminating necessary information during a crisis. Indeed, media are considered the "most important information path" during a crisis event (Larsson, 2010, p. 716). Television, specifically, is the most common medium used in times of risk and crisis in the United States due to its delivery of immediate information with visual aids (Heath & O'Hair, 2009). According to the **Pew Research Center** (2012), television remains the most popular news platform, with 55% of Americans getting their news from television. However, the Internet, both through online newspapers and social media sharing, has become the second most

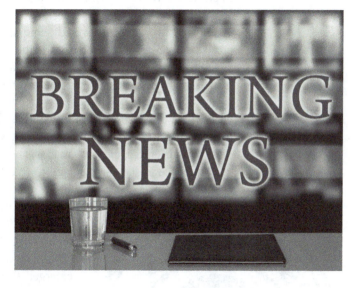

popular news platform, with 39% of Americans getting their news online or on a mobile device. In 2012, 38% of Americans got their news from a blend of offline and online news sources, up from 34% in 2010. While as early as 2003, 67% of organizations used their websites to communicate during a crisis (Perry, Taylor, & Doerfel, 2003), due to the growth of online usage, approaches to crisis communications have had to change (González-Herrero & Smith, 2008). Communicators must now carefully design messages effective in eliciting appropriate action and work closely with both traditional and online media to deliver those messages in crisis situations, especially crises that suddenly increase health risks.

Crisis communication scholars describe ideal media relationships as "equal communication relationships . . . established through honest and open dialogue" (Ulmer, Sellnow, & Seeger, 2007, p. 35). Researchers have found evidence of emergency manager–media partnerships in certain cases (Veil & Ojeda, 2010), but this is clearly not the norm. In general, Lowry et al. (2007) found problematic communication between journalists and public health public information officers (PIOs), resulting in PIOs providing hurried information beyond their comfort level and journalists exercising their watchdog duties by questioning government information. In the midst of a crisis, when information is most needed, researchers have observed trends in which health officials try to control the situation by limiting information (Lewis, 2008), and journalists withhold information already known in order to create a desired story angle (Veil, 2012). Veil identified stereotypical judgments, a lack of trust, paradoxical challenges, and unrealistic expectations between emergency managers and journalists as primary barriers to positive media relations in disaster response and recovery.

While we have already covered some applications of media research regarding the presence or absence of health information and instruction in the media in a foodborne crisis, researchers have also recognized a dearth of health risk information following natural disasters (Cohen, Vijaykumar, Wray, & Karamehic-Muratovic, 2008). And yet, as noted by social cognitive theory, researchers have found that without direct experience with a risk, people must rely on the vicarious information provided by the news media to make risk judgments (de Jonge, Van Trijp, Jan Renes, & Frewer, 2010). "In these circumstances, the news media is not only the messenger but also has an identifiable influence on the risk perception" (Kuttschreuter & Gutteling, 2004, p. 4).

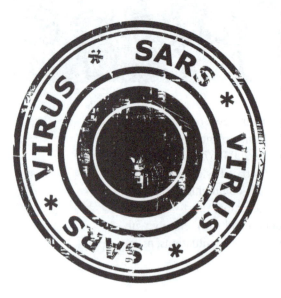

The narrative of a crisis, as depicted by the media, can greatly influence how society understands and responds to a crisis. According to Heath, Li, Bowen, and Lee (2008), during the SARS epidemic, competing narratives emerged that confused the public. Internationally, the media reported that SARS was out of control, and many reports pointed to China as the source of the virus. The **World Health Organization** warned people not to travel to China and for those in China to remain indoors. And yet, officials of the Ministry of Health in China insisted, "The SARS in part of China is under control; it is safe to work, to live and to tour in China" (Meng, 2003, n.p.). These confounding narratives created unnecessary uncertainty and fear and created the impression that the crisis was indeed out of control. Particularly in China, the competing narratives damaged the public's trust in the government's ability to bring the epidemic under control (Liu, McIntyre, & Sellnow, 2008). To move past the chronic phase of the crisis, crisis communicators employed by the Chinese government promoted a narrative of heroism in which medical heroes worked fearlessly on the frontline of the war against SARS by putting patients' safety over their own. In the SARS case, the Chinese government was eventually able to adjust the crisis narrative using state-run media to promote the desired narrative. However, in countries where there is a free market press, crisis communicators must work with journalists to frame the crisis narrative. The best practices of coordinating networks and remaining open and accessible to the media are essential in a health crisis.

Social Media

Today, crisis communicators have many new platforms and media choices available to facilitate the complex distribution and flow of information in a health crisis. In particular, technological advances have given rise to social media and networks that function very differently from more traditional media. The news of a crisis can be shared and re-shared across personal networks, reaching millions of people without the intervening presence of journalists or other command-and-control information centers. Such word-of-mouth news is tremendously influential and is often perceived as just as, or more trustworthy than mainstream media in some instances (Colley & Collier, 2009). In 2009, the CDC used widgets, games, graphic buttons, online video, podcasts, eCards, RSS feeds, microblogs (e.g., Twitter), image sharing, social networking, email, and book marking and sharing tools to raise awareness about the H1N1 virus (Aikin, 2009; Reynolds, 2010).

Research shows that onsite and online crisis response activities are becoming increasingly "simultaneous and intertwined" (Palen, Vieweg, Sutton, Liu, & Hughes, 2007, p. 2). While community members have always served as integral volunteers in crises (Scherp et al., 2009), social media makes the community part of the crisis communication response. For example, Twitter was used to share initial information and updates during the 2008 California wildfires, 2008 Mumbai massacre, 2009 crash of US Airways Flight 1549, 2010 Haiti earthquake, and 2011 Tunisian uprisings (Beaumont, 2008; New America Media, 2011; Smith, 2010). In even more recent examples, Google's crisis center and their *Person Finder* social media tool helped people find each other by providing updates on missing persons from the earthquake and tsunami disaster in Japan, the Christchurch earthquake, the Arab Spring protests, and Hurricane Sandy (Google, 2012).

The primary challenge for communicators is relinquishing control of the information shared on social media and trusting users. Online communities will self-correct misinformation, often before organizational representatives have the chance to

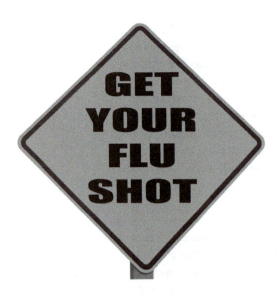

respond. During the H1N1 pandemic, the CDC wanted people to feel free to post their beliefs and concerns, even if they were counter to CDC's science and recommendations (Reynolds, 2010). The CDC did not censor or delete comments that were inaccurate or made claims that went against accepted science. While this openness allowed several posts on the CDC's Facebook page about flu vaccines causing the flu and vaccines causing autism, within a couple of posts the user community would counter the claims and even provide links to online articles debunking the myths from multiple sources, including the CDC.

In the midst of the pandemic, CDC's American Customer Satisfaction Index jumped from 74 to 82 (out of 100), and those who used social media gave the CDC higher satisfaction ratings than those who did not (Reynolds, 2010). Even more, "compared with a sampling of other federal agencies, the CDC scored highest for online participation, collaboration and trust" (Reynolds, 2010, p. 21). By understanding the audience's need to post opinions and allowing the online community to self-correct misinformation, rather than trying to control the conversation, the CDC demonstrated trust in the user community while establishing itself as a trusted resource.

Unfortunately, even social media cannot bridge the **digital divide**, signified by low-education and low-income groups having more restricted access to communication technologies (USDHHS, 2000). While the use of social media in most cases is free, the technology needed for access is not. Subscriptions are needed to read the newspaper, televisions are needed to view the news, and access to a computer or cell phone is needed to take part in the online interaction. Therefore, additional research and resources are needed to reach those without access who are often most vulnerable in health-related crises.

THE ROLE OF MEDIA IN CRISIS COMMUNICATION

The media play an essential role in disseminating necessary information during a crisis. Television is a particularly important channel. Today, however, social media outlets such as Facebook and Twitter are becoming important sources of information in crisis situations.

ETHICAL ISSUES AND STANDARDS

The best practices for risk and crisis communication promote communicating with honesty, candor, openness, compassion, concern, and empathy. Unfortunately, these recommendations are often ignored when the focus is on protecting organizational reputation and maintaining scientific credibility. Anthony and Sellnow (2011) describe this misalignment of values as a violation of first and second things. They apply C. S. Lewis' essay on first and second things to crisis communication by arguing, "organizations must be *first* concerned with clear communication and the well-being of all their stakeholders" (p. 442). Any emphasis on reputation or profit occurring at the expense of getting the best information available out to the public during a crisis is seen as unethical.

The ethical standard for identifying and communicating the best information available during crises is **significant choice**. The ethic of significant choice is founded on the principle that when a group has vital information the public needs in order to make important decisions, that information must be disseminated as completely and accurately as possible (Nilsen, 1974). Even if all the information is not yet known, communicators must accept the uncertainty of the 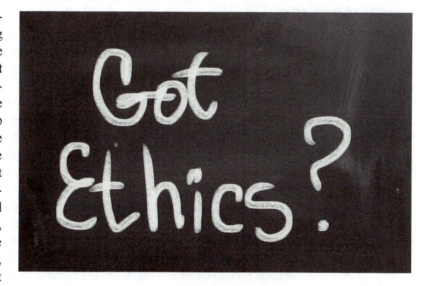 situation and communicate what precautionary measures could be taken for self-protection. In addition, technical communication provided without compassion is unlikely to reach audiences in a way that allows them to internalize the risk and make it relevant in order to take actions to minimize harm (Sellnow & Sellnow, 2010).

There is no point in a crisis where ethical considerations should diminish. Groom (2012) emphasizes that ongoing reflection by organizations is essential for maintaining ethical communication at all stages in a crisis. Groom explains that crisis narratives are formed via the interaction of many individuals in an organization. Thus, narratives emerge from the "interplay between these different kinds of advisors" (p. 94). Groom advocates the process of "questioning back" throughout the crisis in order to constantly reflect on the accuracy and impact of what was communicated (p. 95). This reflection establishes a "point of orientation whereby action can be procured amidst uncertainty" (p. 98). In short, remaining ethical in one's crisis response requires a continuous commitment to reflection and refining the crisis response.

CONCLUSION

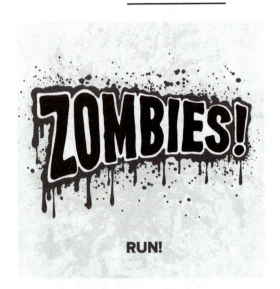

RUN!

This chapter discussed how the field of risk and crisis communication has emerged from a melting pot of multi-disciplinary, interdisciplinary, and transdisciplinary approaches. While much of the research in health communication focuses on the scientific paradigm, and to a lesser extent, the interpretive paradigm, risk and crisis communication is one area where the critical–cultural paradigm continues to hold ground. As we have shown in this chapter, many lines of research incorporate all three perspectives. While purists might see this as completely unacceptable, in risk and crisis communica-tion, the ethical questions are often simply too strong to ignore. If an organization, or country for that matter, can exert power over people that causes them to be in the dire straits of a crisis, that power must be exposed. Turf wars in academia will always exist. Henry Kissinger once said, "University politics are vicious because the stakes are so small." Perhaps the reason risk and crisis communication scholars have been able to collaborate across paradigms is because the stakes are high in a world-wide pandemic, culture-devastating hurricane, deadly terrorist attack, and even potential zombie apocalypse.

DISCUSSION QUESTIONS

1. The CDC, FEMA, and DHS have all used the zombie apocalypse to promote emergency preparedness. Do you think this attention-getting tactic minimizes the importance of emergency preparedness planning? Why or why not?
2. Keeping in mind the importance of journalistic freedom in the United States, should journalists be required to provide instructional messages for self-protection to the public in a crisis? What strategies can communication specialists use to work with journalists?

3. How can scholars advance theories of crisis communication without being able to predict crisis outcomes?

4. What other theories have you learned about in this class that could be applied to crisis contexts?

5. How long do you think you could survive in your current home if a mandatory shelter-in-place order was issued and there was no running water? What supplies would you need to survive for 72 hours? A full week?

IN-CLASS ACTIVITIES

1. Identify a crisis in the news that is likely to pose health risks. Compare three news stories from three different sources and analyze the stories for presence or absence of instructional messages for self-protection.

2. Choose one of the following health crisis scenarios and write a two-minute press conference statement following the best practices in risk and crisis communication (see Table 16.3) and present it to the class:

   a) 300,000 turkeys are being recalled due to Salmonella contamination. CDC says more than 500 people are confirmed ill and four are in the hospital, including a three-year-old girl who is now in a coma. You are the communications specialist for the CDC.

   b) A train carrying anhydrous ammonia has derailed just outside the city. The immediate area has been evacuated, and hospitals are crowded with people complaining of burning eyes and throats. You are the public information officer for the fire department.

   c) A devastating ice storm has hit your state. Power is out across town and likely will be for the next several days. Temperatures are forecasted below freezing tonight. You are the communications specialist for the city.

   d) Due to contamination at the largest vaccine supplier, there is a shortage of the flu vaccine this year, and the current strain is particularly dangerous, killing more people in the first month of flu season than all of last year. You are the communications specialist for local public health.

RECOMMENDED READINGS

Cohen, E. L., Vijaykumar, S., Wray, R., & Karamehic-Muratovic, A. (2008). The minimization of public health risks in newspapers after Hurricane Katrina. *Communication Research Reports*, 25(4), 266–281.

This article describes how media framing can reduce public concerns while increasing public risks.

Frisby, B. N., Veil, S. R., & Sellnow, T. L. (2014). Instructional messages during health-related crises: Essential content for self-protection. *Health Communication, 29*(4), 347–354.

This study compares standard media coverage of a food borne outbreak to the instructional messages recommended by research.

Reynolds, B., & Seeger, M. W. (2005). Crisis and emergency risk communication as an integrative model. *Journal of Health Communication, 10*, 43–55.

This essay provides the background of the CDC's CERC model.

Seeger, M.W. (2006). Best practices in crisis communication: An expert panel process. *Journal of Applied Communication Research, 34*(3), 232–244.

This article outlines the original best practices in risk and crisis communication.

REFERENCES

Aikin, A. (2009). Communicating during a novel emergency: How to make your messages viral by using social media. *Social Media for Crisis Communications in Government*, Washington, DC. Retrieved from http://www.aliconferences.com/conf/social_media_crisis1109/day1.htm

American Red Cross. (2010, August 9). *Web users increasingly rely on social media to seek help in a disaster. Retrieved from* http://newsroom.redcross.org/2010/08/09/press-release-web-users-increasingly-rely-on-social-media-to-seek-help-in-a-disaster

Anthony, K. E., & Sellnow, T. L. (2011). Beyond Narnia: The necessity of C.S. Lewis' *First and Second Things* in applied communication research. *Journal of Applied Communication Research, 39*, 441–443.

Ballard-Reisch, D., Clements-Nolle, K., Jenkins, T., Sacks, T., Pruitt, K., & Leathers, K. (2007). Applying the crisis and emergency risk communication (CERC) integrative model to bioterrorism preparedness: A case study. In M. W. Seeger, T. L. Sellnow, & R. R. Ulmer (Eds.), *Crisis communication and the public health* (pp. 203–219). Cresskill, NJ: Hampton.

Beaumont, C. (2008). *Mumbai attacks: Twitter and Flickr used to break news*. Retrieved from http://www.telegraph.co.uk/news/worldnews/asia/india/3530640/Mumbai-attacks-Twitter-and-Flickr-used-to-break-news-Bombay-India.html

Benoit, W. L. (1997). Image repair discourse and crisis communication. *Public Relations Review, 23*, 177–186.

Caldwell, A. A. (2012, September 6). Zombie apocalypse: 'The zombies are coming,' Homeland Security warns. *Huffington Post*. Retrieved from http://www.huffingtonpost.com/2012/09/06/homeland-security-warns-the-zombies-are-coming_n_1862768.html

Centers for Disease Control and Prevention. (2012). *Zombie preparedness*. Retrieved from http://www.cdc.gov/phpr/zombies.htm

Cohen, E. L., Vijaykumar, S., Wray, R., & Karamehic-Muratovic, A. (2008). The minimization of public health risks in newspapers after Hurricane Katrina. *Communication Research Reports, 25*(4), 266–281.

Colley, K. L., & Collier, A. (2009, Spring). An overlooked social media tool? Making a case for wikis. *Public Relations Strategist, 5(2)*, 34–35.

Coombs, W. T. (2007). Protecting organization reputations during a crisis: The development and application of situational crisis communication theory. *Corporate Reputation Review, 10*, 163–176.

Coombs, W. T. (2012). *Ongoing crisis communication: Planning, managing, and responding* (3rd ed.). Thousand Oaks, CA: SAGE Publications, Inc.

de Jonge, J., Van Trijp, H., Jan Renes, R., & Frewer, L. J. (2010). Consumer confidence in the safety of food and newspaper coverage of food safety issues: A longitudinal perspective. *Risk Analysis, 30*(1), 125–142.

Federal Emergency Management Agency. (2004). *Are you ready? An in-depth guide to citizen preparedness.* Retrieved from www.FEMA.gov

Federal Emergency Management Agency. (2009). Post-Katrina: What it takes to cut the bureaucracy and assure a more rapid response after a catastrophic disaster. *Statement of Craig Fugate Before the House Committee on Transportation and Infrastructure, Subcommittee of Economic Development, Public Buildings and Emergency Management U.S. House of Representatives Washington, DC.* Retrieved from http://www.fema.gov/pdf/about/testimony/072709_fugate.pdf

Fink, S. (1986). *Crisis management: Planning for the inevitable.* New York: AMACOM.

Freimuth, V., Linnan, H. W., & Potter, P. (2000). Communicating the threat of emerging infections to the public. *Emerging Infectious Diseases, 6*(4), 337–347.

Frisby, B. N., Veil, S. R., & Sellnow, T. L. (2014). Instructional messages during health-related crises: Essential content for self-protection. *Health Communication, 29*(4), 347–354.

González-Herrero, A., & Pratt, C. B. (1995). How to manage a crisis before—or whenever—it hits. *Public Relations Quarterly, 40*(1), 25–29.

González-Herrero, A., & Smith, S. (2008). Crisis communications management on the web: How internet-based technologies are changing the way public relations professionals handle business crises. *Journal of Contingencies and Crisis Management, 16*(3), 143–154.

Google. (2012, Oct. 28). *Google crisis response.* Retrieved from http://www.google.com/crisisresponse

Groom, S. A. (2012). Questioning back: Engaging in organization's narrative for ethical communicative responsiveness in crisis situations. In S. A. Groom & J. H. Fritz (Eds.), *Communication ethics and crisis* (pp. 87–100). Madison, NJ: Fairleigh Dickinson University Press.

Hearit, K. M. (2006). *Crisis management by apology: Corporate response to allegations of wrongdoing.* Mahwah, NJ: Lawrence Erlbaum Associates.

Heath, R. L. (2006). Best practices in crisis communication: Evolution of practice through research. *Journal of Applied Communication Research, 34*(3), 245–248.

Heath, R. L., Li, F., Bowen, S. A., & Lee, J. (2008). Narratives of crisis planning and infectious disease: A case study of SARS. In M. W. Seeger, T. L. Sellnow, & R. R. Ulmer (Eds.), *Crisis communication and the public health* (pp. 1301–156). Cresskill, NJ: Hampton.

Heath, R. L., & O'Hair, H. D. (Eds.). (2009). *Handbook of risk and crisis communication.* New York, NY: Routledge.

Janssen, C. I. (2013). Corporate historical responsibility (CHR). Addressing a past of forced labor at Volkswagen. *Journal of Applied Communication Research, 41*(1), 64–83.

Kuttschreuter, M., & Gutteling, J. M. (2004). Experience-based processing of risk information: The case of the millennium bug. *Journal of Risk Research, 7*(1), 3–16.

Larsson, L. (2010). Crisis and learning. In W. T. Coombs & S. J. Holladay (Eds.) *The handbook of crisis communication* (pp. 713–717). Malden, MA: Wiley.

Lewis, M. (2008). Breaking news and health crisis. In M. W. Seeger, T. L. Sellnow, & R. R. Ulmer (Eds.), *Crisis communication and the public health* (pp. 257–271). Cresskill, NJ: Hampton Press, Inc.

Liu, M., McIntyre, J. J., & Sellnow, T. L. (2008). Less ambiguity, more hope: The use of narrative in Chinese newspaper reports on the SARS crisis. In M. W. Seeger, T. L. Sellnow, & R. R. Ulmer (Eds.), *Crisis communication and the public health* (pp. 111–130). Cresskill, NJ: Hampton.

Lowry, W., Evans, W., Gower, K. K., Robinson, J.A., Ginter, P. M., McCormick, L. C., & Abdolrasulnia, M. (2007). Effective media communication of disasters: Pressing problems and recommendations, *BMC Public Health, 7*(97), 1–8.

Meng, X. (2003). *SARS crisis under globalization.* Retrieved from http://www.rieti.go.jp/jp/events/04011601/pdf/xiao.pdf

Mileti, D. S., & Fitzpatrick, C. (1991). Communication of public risk: Its theory and its application. *Sociological Practice Review, 2*(1), 20–18.

Mileti, D. S., & Sorensen, J. H. (1990). *Communication of emergency public warnings: A social science perspective and state-of-the-art assessment* (ORNL-6609). Oak Ridge, TN: Oak Ridge National Laboratory.

Mitroff, I. I. (1994). Crisis management and environmentalism: A natural fit. *California Management Review, 36*(2), 101–113.

National Center for Disaster Preparedness. (2011). *The American preparedness project.* Retrieved from http://www.ncdp.mailman.columbia.edu/files/Marist2011.pdf

New America Media. (2011). Social media made Tunisian uprising possible. *New America Media.* Retrieved from http://newamericamedia.org/2011/01/social-media-made-tunisian-uprising-possible.php

Nilsen, T. R. (1974). *Ethics of speech communication* (2nd ed.). Indianapolis, IN: Bobbs-Merrill.

Nucci, M. L., Cuite, C. L., & Hallman, W. K. (2009). When good food goes bad: Television network news and the spinach recall of 2006. *Science Communication, 31*(2), 238–265.

Paek, H.-J., Hilyard, K., Freimuth, V., Barge, J. K., & Mindlin, M. (2010). Theory-based approaches to understanding public emergency preparedness: Implications for effective health and risk communication. *Journal of Health Communication, 15*, 428–444.

Palen, L., Vieweg, S., Sutton, J., Liu, S. B., & Hughes, A. (2007, October). Crisis informatics: Studying crisis in a networked world. *Third International Conference on e-Social Science*, Ann Arbor, MI. Retrieved from http://ess.si.umich.edu/papers/paper172.pdf

Perry, D. C., Taylor, M., & Doerfel, M. L. (2003). Internet-based communication in crisis management. *Management Communication Quarterly, 17*(2), 206–232.

Pew Research Center (2012). In changing news landscape, even television is vulnerable: Trends in news consumption: 1991–2012. Retrieved from http://www.people-press. org/2012/09/27/in-changing-news-landscape-even-television-is-vulnerable

Prochaska, J. O., & DiClemente, C. C. (1983). Stages and processes of self-change of smoking: Toward an integrative model of change. *Journal of Consulting and Clinical Psychology*, *51*, 390–395.

Reuters. (2011, May 19). CDC "Zombie Apocalypse" disaster campaign crashes website. Retrieved from http://www.reuters.com/article/2011/05/19/us-zombies-idUSTRE74I7H420110519

Reynolds, B. J. (2010). Building trust through social media. *Marketing Health Services*, *30*(2), 18–21.

Reynolds, B., & Seeger, M. W. (2005). Crisis and emergency risk communication as an integrative model. *Journal of Health Communication*, *10*, 43–55.

Roberts, H. A., & Veil, S. R. (in press). Health literacy and organizational crisis: Communication in the 2010 egg recall. *Journal of Public Relations Research.*

Sandman, P. M. (2006). Crisis communication and best practices: Some quibbles and additions. *Journal of Applied Communication Research*, *34*, 257–262.

Scherp, A., Schwagereit, F., Ireson, N., Lanfranchi, V., Papadopoulos, S., Kritikos, A., . . . Smrs, P. (2009). Leveraging Web 2.0 communities in professional organizations. *W3C Workshop on the Future of Social Networking*. Barcelona, Spain. Retrieved from http://www.w3.org/2008/09/msnws/papers/ScherpEtAlLeveragingWeb2 Communities.pdf

Seeger, M. W. (2006). Best practices in crisis communication: An expert panel process. *Journal of Applied Communication Research*, *34*(3), 232–244.

Seeger, M. W., & Reynolds, B. (2007). Crisis communication and the public health: Integrated approaches and new imperatives. In M. W. Seeger, T. L. Sellnow, & R. R. Ulmer (Eds.), *Crisis communication and the public health* (pp. 3–20). Cresskill, NJ: Hampton.

Seeger, M. W., Sellnow, T. L., & Ulmer, R. R. (2003). *Communication and organizational crisis*. Westport, CT: Praeger.

Seeger, M. W., & Ulmer, R. R. (2001). Virtuous responses to organizational crisis: Aaron Feuerstein and Milt Cole. *Journal of Business Ethics*, *31*, 369–376.

Sellnow, T. L., & Seeger, M. (2001). Exploring the boundaries of crisis communication: The case of the 1997 Red River Valley flood. *Communication Studies*, *52*(2), 154.

Sellnow, T. L., Seeger, M. W., & Ulmer, R. R. (2002). Chaos theory, informational needs and the North Dakota floods. *Journal of Applied Communication Research*, *30*, 269–292.

Sellnow, T., & Sellnow, D. (2010). The instructional dynamic of risk and crisis communication: Distinguishing instructional messages from dialogue. *The Review of Communication*, *10*(2), 112–126.

Sellnow, T. L., Ulmer, R. R., Seeger, M. W., & Littlefield, R. (2009). *Effective risk communication: A message-centered approach*. New York: Springer.

Sellnow, T. L., Ulmer, R. R., Seeger, M. W., & Veil, S. R. (2008). Terrorism as chaos: A chaos model for managing random acts of terror. In D. O'Hair, R. Heath, K. Ayotte, & G. Ledlow (Eds.), *Terrorism: Communication and rhetorical perspectives* (pp. 411–424). Cresskill, NJ: Hampton Press.

Sellnow, T., & Vidoloff, K. (2009). Getting crisis communication right. *Food Technology*, *63*(9), 40–45.

Smith, B. G. (2010). Socially distributing public relations: Twitter, Haiti, and interactivity in social media, *Public Relations Review*, *36*(4), 329–335.

Sturges, D. L. (1994). Communicating through crisis: A strategy for organizational survival. *Management Communication Quarterly*, *7*(3), 297–316.

Ulmer, R. R., Alvey, R. J., & Kordsmeier, J. (2008). Best practices in public health communication: Managing West Nile virus in Arkansas from 2002–2003. In M. W. Seeger, T. L. Sellnow, & R. R. Ulmer (Eds.), *Crisis communication and the public health* (pp. 97–110). Cresskill, NJ: Hampton.

Ulmer, R. R., Sellnow, T. L., & Seeger, M. W. (2007). *Effective crisis communication: Moving from crisis to opportunity*. Thousand Oaks, CA: Sage.

U.S. Department of Health and Human Services. (2000). *Healthy people 2010*. U.S. Government Printing Office, Washington, DC. Retrieved from http://www.healthypeople.gov/Document/pdf/Volume1/11HealthCom.pdf

Veil, S. R. (2011). Mindful learning in crisis management. *Journal of Business Communication*, *48*(2), 116–147.

Veil, S. R. (2012). Clearing the air: Journalists and emergency managers discuss disaster response. *Journal of Applied Communication Research*, *40*(3), 289–306.

Veil, S. R., & Husted, R. A. (2012). Best practices as an assessment for crisis communication. *Journal of Communication Management*, *16*(2), 131–145.

Veil, S. R., & Ojeda, F. (2010). Establishing media partnerships in crisis response. *Communication Studies*, *60*(4), 412–429.

Veil, S. R., Reynolds, B., Sellnow, T. L., & Seeger, M. W. (2008). Crisis & Emergency Risk Communication as a theoretical framework for research and practice. *Health Promotion Practice*, *9*(4), 26S–34S.

Veil, S. R., & Sellnow, T. L. (2008). Organizational learning in a high-risk environment: Responding to an anthrax outbreak. *Journal of Applied Communications*, *92*(1), 75–93.

Veil, S. R., Sellnow, T. L., & Heald, M. (2011). Memorializing crisis: The Oklahoma National Memorial as renewal discourse. *Journal of Applied Communication Research*, *39*(2), 164–183.

Windahl, S., Signitzer, B., & Olson, J. T. (1992). *Using communication theory: An introduction to planned communication*. Newbury Park, CA: Sage

Epilogue

Nancy Grant Harrington

As a comedian, you have to start the show strong, and you have to end the show strong. Those are the two key elements. You can't be like pancakes . . . all exciting at first, but then by the end you're sick of 'em.

—Mitch Hedberg

I've had several people tell me over the years that no one ever reads the concluding chapter to a textbook. So I almost chose not to write one. However, having grown up watching a great deal of 1970s television, I let my compulsion to include an epilogue (thank you, Quinn Martin) override common sense, so here we are. I'll be brief so you don't get sick of me.

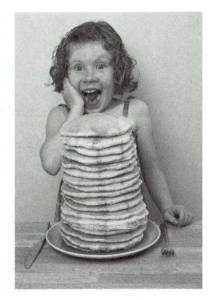

You've encountered a great deal of information in this book. You've learned about the experiences and perspectives of patients and healthcare providers. You've learned about some of the challenges and complexities in health communication at the individual, organizational, and societal levels. You've learned about health communication in the media and exciting developments related to technology. That's a lot to digest, but you made it through. Gold star!

Now that you've finished reading this book, I hope you have a more sophisticated understanding of health communication scholarship

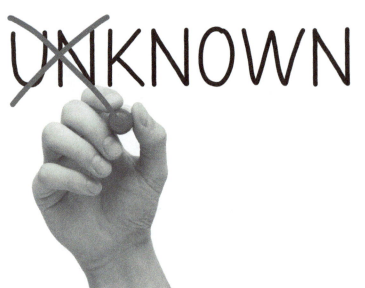

as informed both by theory and by multidisciplinary, interdisciplinary, and transdisciplinary research. I also hope you've developed an appreciation of the way that different metatheoretical perspectives approach health communication problems. I know metatheory can be a little cumbersome, but it highlights very important distinctions in the way we approach our research and what to make of the results. Still, whether it's a scientific approach that attempts to predict the effects of interventions and generalize results to populations, an interpretive approach that attempts to develop a rich understanding of unique and personal experiences, or a critical–cultural approach that attempts to explore and reveal issues of power inherent in the system and empower marginalized people to promote social change—it's all important to advance our knowledge of health communication.

Important, too, is our application of research. The translational research that you've

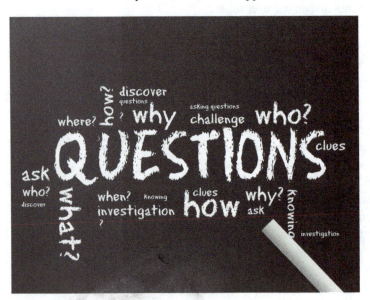

read about is having a real impact on the lives of others. It's helping patients to communicate more effectively with their physicians. It's helping healthcare providers to promote patient safety. It's helping people to improve their health literacy, to better navigate our healthcare system, to make healthier choices in life, and to avoid some of the unhealthier choices. As I said in the introductory chapter, health communication plays a *central role* in health promotion and disease prevention and treatment. It is a crucial role to play, and I hope you will be a part of it.

WHAT'S NEXT?

One of the things that researchers always do is to look for the next question. Although our studies give us answers, they also open up new directions for research. You saw how each chapter identified areas that should be explored or specific questions that should be asked next. Well, for this epilogue, I asked Teresa Thompson, Lewis Donohew, Barbara Sharf, and Mohan Dutta to answer the question, "What's next?" Specifically, I asked them, "What do you think is the most pressing unanswered question for health communication scholars today?" You can read what they had to say in their sidebars. Pay attention to what each scholar emphasizes, and you'll see the tremendous potential we have ahead of us. These are very challenging and exciting times!

Dr. Teresa Thompson, Professor at the University of Dayton and editor of our field's premier journal, *Health Communication*

COMMUNICATION
MATTERS

I think that this exciting opportunity to impact both actual health and health care delivery is also the aspect of health communication that is the most pressing, unanswered question for health communication scholars today, albeit a broad one: What are the pathways through which communication processes DO impact health? Although I mentioned in the first chapter the exciting findings that document fundamental impacts of communication on health, research with this focus has been disappointing to me in the 25+ years that I have been editing the journal *Health Communication*. Such scholars as Rick Street have been focusing on understanding these pathways, and I think that this line of research is fundamental to the contribution that we are able to make as we study health communication. Building on this concern, numerous scholars and practitioners of health communication have focused on training both providers and patients in communication skills to more adequately impact health care delivery. The work of Suzanne Kurtz and Don Cegala is exemplary in this regard. All of this work is an important start, but we need to more fully understand HOW communication impacts health and health care delivery in order to make the contributions that we are capable of making.

Dr. Lewis Donohew, Professor Emeritus at the University of Kentucky

In our everyday existence, humans select—or fail to select—messages out of the myriad of stimuli swirling around them. For those who design messages—and particularly persuasive messages about health, such as those employed in studies of prevention, or in doctor-patient communication—this can mean the difference between success and failure, both for the health of the person who failed to get preventive information and for the research project, as well.

Too often, communication researchers and those from other disciplines plunk messages in front of captive audiences and have them respond in some way. They may even run functional Magnetic Resonance Imaging (fMRI) studies on them, but the audiences are still captive. Then the researchers arrive at conclusions about what will work and what won't. But what if the messages never get attended in everyday life?

The biological process by which the human system selects messages to attend while allowing others to pass relatively unnoticed may have more to do with those parts of the brain, some of them primal, that pick up signals and transmit—or fail to transmit—them on to the more advanced brain centers for processing. We need to go beyond these studies to find out if it is the way the brain processes information that keeps some signals from being attended and how we can improve the chances of attracting and holding attention long enough for messages to be fully understood.

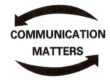

Dr. Barbara F. Sharf, Professor Emeritus at the Texas A&M University

In considering what might be the most pressing unanswered question for health communication scholars, I find myself both struggling and resisting the task. The scope of communicative phenomena that constitutes or relates to health is so vast and complex that any attempt to answer this query seems (to me) limiting and inadequate. There is important, urgent work to be done from the vantage points of a wide variety of contexts, problematics, and methodological approaches. What I believe I *can* respond to in a more concise, straightforward way are key questions that serve as *criteria* which health communication scholars should be applying to their own work, no matter what the specifics. We should be asking ourselves:

1. How does my work contribute to a more humane understanding of health-related beliefs, practices, and/or problems?

2. In what ways does my work enable and empower individuals to enact the rights and responsibilities of health citizenship?
3. (and/or) In what ways does my work inform social policies and public health practices?
4. Finally, what are concepts and findings emerging from my investigations in health contexts that enrich communication theory and disciplinary knowledge.

Dr. Mohan Dutta, Head of the Department of Communications and New Media at the National University of Singapore

COMMUNICATION MATTERS

In answering this question, let me begin by talking about what I believe we do know about communicating health. As health communication scholars, we know quite a bit about messages, under what circumstances do they work, what are the audience characteristics that drive message construction, etc. Similarly, we are starting to grow a body of work on narratives and meanings that explore the meanings of health and the ways in which these meanings are negotiated in health interactions at micro-, meso-, and macro-levels. Critical scholars have started to ask questions about power and inequality, documenting the ways in which unequal distributions of power in society contribute to the poor health of marginalized communities.

In this backdrop, one of the most pressing questions for health communication scholars relates to the role of communication in addressing the fast increasing global health inequalities. Even as unemployment and poverty continue to rise globally, a small percentage of the global elite continues to amass wealth and consolidate power. This vast inequality in the distribution of power plays out in the largely uneven burdens of health, large gaps in morbidity and mortality, and overall poorer health outcomes within highly unequal societies.

What are the dominant messages and meanings that circulate around these health inequalities, working together to normalize them, to make them acceptable and to consolidate power in the hands of the global elite? How then can these taken-for-granted assumptions, beliefs, and values be fundamentally transformed so as to work toward achieving a more just society? As health communication scholars develop sophisticated and complex understanding of the political and economic processes that fundamentally constitute health, what are the possible ways in which communication about health can work toward transforming these underlying inequalities? This calls for a fundamental shift in the orientation of health communication work, suggesting the need for productive collaborations among scholars with different frameworks to health communication working toward developing communication solutions that address the broader structural inequities that constitute health.

So at this point, I'll bring things to a close. I sincerely hope that you will be able to take what you've learned from this book and apply it in your life. Whether you have a career in the health communication field or find yourself in the role of patient, caregiver, or health media consumer, you should now be a more informed and enlightened participant.

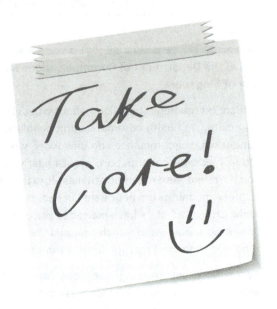

Subject Index

Author Index

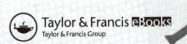